DATE DUE

Library Use Only			
SEP 4 '80			
SEP 23 '81			
GAYLORD			PRINTED IN U.S.A.

BASIC NEUROLOGY

BASIC NEUROLOGY

AN INTRODUCTION TO THE STRUCTURE AND FUNCTION OF THE NERVOUS SYSTEM

Second Revised Edition

J. P. SCHADÉ and DONALD H. FORD

76921   1973

ELSEVIER SCIENTIFIC PUBLISHING COMPANY

AMSTERDAM · LONDON · NEW YORK

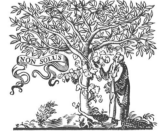

ELSEVIER SCIENTIFIC PUBLISHING COMPANY
335 JAN VAN GALENSTRAAT
P.O. BOX 1270, AMSTERDAM, THE NETHERLANDS

AMERICAN ELSEVIER PUBLISHING COMPANY, INC.
52 VANDERBILT AVENUE, NEW YORK, NEW YORK 10017

FIRST EDITION 1965
REPRINTED 1967
SECOND REVISED EDITION 1973

LIBRARY OF CONGRESS CARD NUMBER: 77-168914
ISBN: 0-444-40940-8
WITH 215 ILLUSTRATIONS AND 6 TABLES.

PRINTED IN THE NETHERLANDS

Preface to the second edition

The second edition of BASIC NEUROLOGY presents a cross section of knowledge of neuroanatomy and neurophysiology. An attempt has been made to present a synthesis of basic knowledge concerning the structure and function of the human nervous system. The very favourable reception of the first edition has prompted the authors to bring the text up to date. The scope, however, remains the same: a multidisciplinary approach to the study of the nervous system.

In order to enhance the value of the illustrated part of the book all figures have been redesigned. The use of an additional colour in the illustrations will, as is hoped, facilitate the "reading" of the figures.

We hope that this book will convey to the reader the fact that neurology is a living and changing science.

Acknowledgements

It is a pleasant obligation to express our indebtness to those who have been helpful in the preparation of this book. We are most grateful to the following colleagues for critically reading the chapters or putting illustrative material at our disposal: K. AKERT, J. W. BROWN, M. B. BUNGE, J. C. ECCLES, H. VAN DER LOOS, H. PAKKENBERG, J. D. ROBERTSON, H. DE F. WEBSTER, and many others.

The authors cannot express too strongly their obligation to the secretarial and graphic arts departments of the Institutes in Amsterdam and New York for their continuous cooperation in all matters.

This book is dedicated with affection and gratitude to all those who have assisted us in the preparation.

J. P. SCHADÉ
D. H. FORD

Preface to the first edition

While the subject matter of neuroanatomy, neurophysiology, neurochemistry and neuropsychology may still be considered as separate sciences, the recent trend is towards some unification of thought between these disciplines. Ultimately this trend may well become so established that the term neurobiology will be more descriptive than any other for this whole field of investigation. Other areas of study such as neuroendocrinology, neuroembryology and neurocybernetics would also logically fit into such a discipline. The synthesis of all these disciplines is paramount in the ultimate understanding of the function of the human brain.

The title *Basic Neurology* was chosen for this introductory textbook because an attempt was made to present the building stones of the neurological sciences in an interdisciplinary way. Thus the first section dealing with anatomy contains many references to the physiological state of brain areas as well as anatomical information necessary for comprehending the physiological processes. The section on physiology provides a framework for understanding how nerve cells work and how they interact with each other. The chapter on biochemistry then illustrates how the basic metabolic processes occur in the brain. Finally there is the section devoted to behavior. This is indeed a complex field and any interpretation of the results of behavioral experiments in laboratory animals and man is dependent on a thorough understanding of the structure and function and metabolic interaction of the individual components of the central and peripheral nervous system.

The book has been extensively illustrated so that a wide range of students from various disciplines may readily "see" what they are reading. Although this text may be considered introductory in relation to all the details known for each of the subsections represented, it should be useful to a wide audience, such as freshmen medical, dental-school and psychology students. The extensive use of illustrations should also make this a useful text in schools of nursing and physical therapy. The scope of the book is such that it may also be used for review of the basic sciences in post-doctoral training programs in neurology, psychiatry and neurosurgery. Physicists and chemists interested in the brain sciences may find some useful information.

References appropriate to each subject are given at the end of each section. For those students desiring additional details, an annotated bibliography is included which lists many of the standard, classical, or most recent volumes devoted to the special fields discussed.

Contents

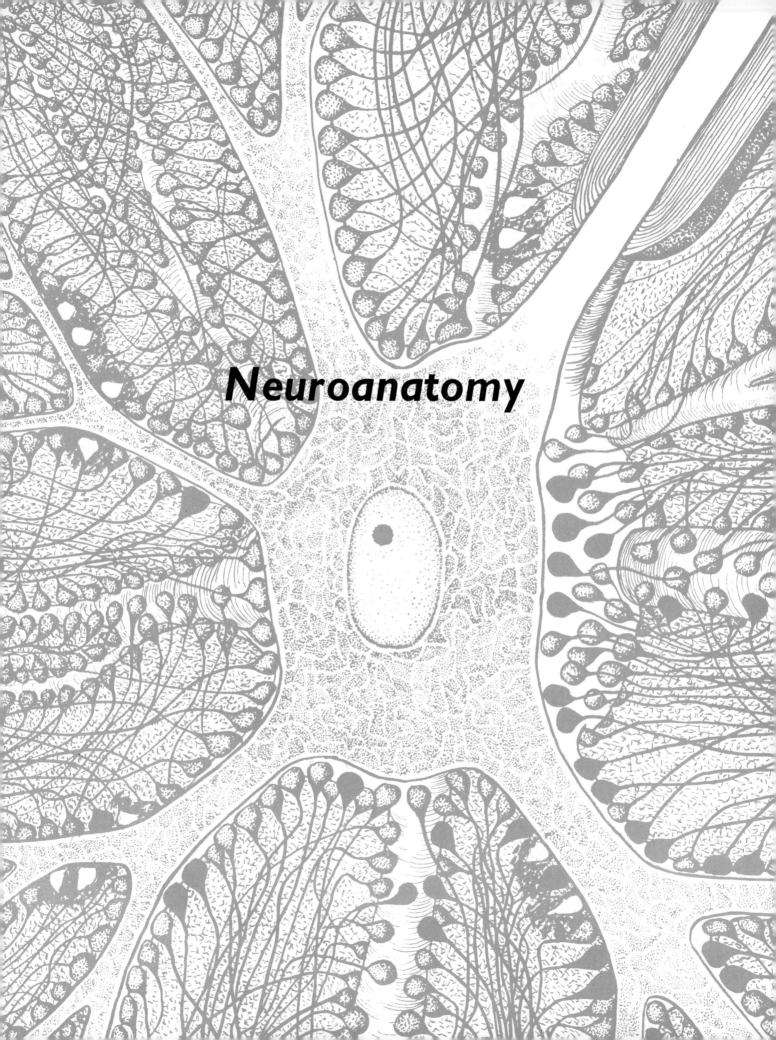

Neuroanatomy

Survey of Contents

1. Introduction

Neuroanatomy is the branch of the neurological sciences concerned with the study of the structure of the nervous system.

The nervous system can be said to comprise the nerves, the ganglia with which they are connected, and the mass of tissue from which they emerge. Expressed in cellular terms this would include all the nerve cell bodies, their processes (fibers, tracts, etc.) and supporting cells and membranes. Physiologically speaking the nervous system is that component of a living system which is specialized for carrying information and for integrating the reactions to the environment.

Fig. 1. The nervous system is usually divided, for convenience, into *central* and *peripheral* parts. The central nervous system (CNS) comprises the parts contained within the skull and vertebral column, while the latter term includes the ganglia and the fiber bundles which connect the central portion of the system with the sense organs and with the effectors of the body (muscles, glands, etc.). The central part may further be subdivided into the *brain* (*i.e.*, the enlarged anterior end, contained within the skull) and the *spinal cord* (contained within the vertebral column). The peripheral part is subdivided into *cranial* and *spinal nerves*.

The spinal nerves are connected to the CNS by two roots (ventral and dorsal), while cranial nerves are variable in their connection. These nerves are actually bundles of fibers, each connected to a single nerve cell body.

One can furthermore distinguish an *autonomic* nervous system, which also has a central and a peripheral part. It consists of an aggregation of nerves and ganglia through which the heart, blood vessels, viscera, glands, etc. receive their innervation. These organs which are regulated 'involuntarily' receive a double innervation, one component from the *sympathetic* and the other from the *parasympathetic* division of the autonomic nervous system. The actions of the two are generally opposite, so that the activity level of these organs is determined by the relative strengths of excitatory and inhibitory nerve actions upon it.

We presently regard the nervous system as the principle coordinator of all activity in the body but this concept has undergone quite an evolutionary series of convictions and ideas.

(1) Among the early Egyptians about 40 centuries

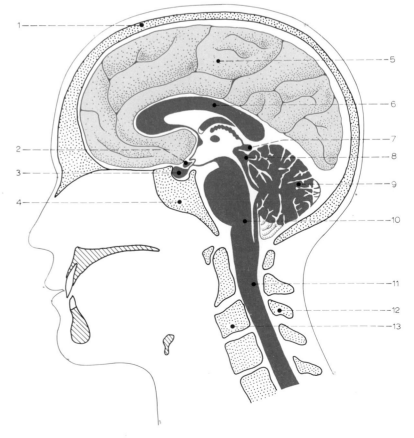

Fig. 1. Midsagittal section through the human head.
1, skull; **2**, optic chiasma (crossing point of the two optic nerves); **3**, pituitary body; **4**, base of the skull; **5**, cerebrum; **6**, corpus callosum; **7**, pineal gland (epiphysis cerebri); **8**, superior and inferior colliculi; **9**, cerebellum; **10**, brain stem; **11**, spinal cord; **12 + 13**, vertebra.

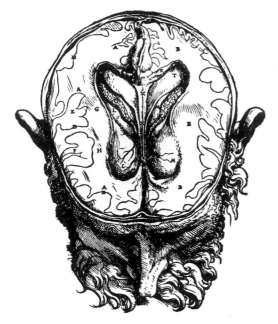

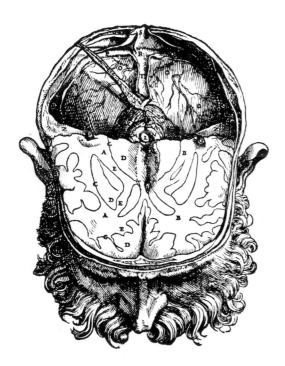

Fig. 2. Two drawings of the human brain, reproduced from *De Humani Corporis Fabrica*, by A. Vesalius (1514-1564).

B.C., the existence of at least certain parts of the nervous system was known, but no special significance was attached to it. They removed the brains of the deceased, who were embalmed in the following way (described by the Greek historian, HERODOTUS). First they would take a bent piece of metal and pull out the brain through the nostrils, in this way disposing of part of it. The other part would be removed by washing the skull with liquids. Considering the elaborate ritual ceremonies performed particularly over the abdominal cavity, we must assume that they attached very little significance to the brain. From HOMER we know that they considered the heart and the liver as the seat of emotions and paid hardly any attention to the brain and spinal cord.

(2) *By about 450 B.C.* there was some faint notion of the existence of the different parts of the nervous system, but only the shape was considered to be of any real importance. PLATO, dealing with the problem of localization of the essential attributes of the soul (desire, passion and reason) considered that reason could only be located in the brain and this because it possessed the most ideal shape, *viz.* that of a sphere. HIPPOCRATUS (about 420 B.C.) gave his views as follows: "*Man should be fully aware of the fact that it is from the brain and from the brain only that our feelings of joy, of pleasure, of laughing arise as well as our sorrow, our pain, our grief and our tears. We are thinking with the brain and we can see and hear and we are able to draw a distinction between ugliness and beauty, bad and good and what is pleasant and unpleasant*". He came to this conclusion mainly by his accurate study of epileptic patients.

(3) *The third era* was marked by a more or less detailed analysis of the gross anatomy. Some of the investigators attached specific significance to particular parts of the brain. HEROPHILUS (325–280 B.C.) analyzed the bodies of criminals and oxen. He described in detail among other things the four cerebral ventricles (the small chambers inside the brain). In these cerebral ventricles he thought all the powers responsible for the functions of the body to be present.

(4) *From then on* neuroanatomy slowly became a science. VESALIUS published his *De Humani Corporis Fabrica* in 1555[137]. This publication is the outstanding contribution of the sixteenth century to the anatomical study of the nervous system. The beautiful drawings (**Fig. 2**) are the first step towards careful analytical research.

In subsequent centuries neuroanatomy changed from extreme analysis into a synthetic approach. We may call this the multidisciplinary period, characterized by synthesis of separate approaches from various disciplines.

It is the purpose of this section to introduce the subject of the structure of the nervous system in very general terms. To accomplish this, it will be necessary to consider briefly embryology, histogenesis, histology and gross morphology. Some thoughts concerning function will also be introduced in an attempt to provide additional significance for the structure.

2. Embryology and Development

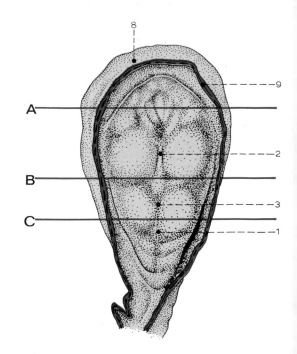

Fig. 3. The brain of man and other vertebrates is derived from the embryonic ectoderm. In the development of the human embryo, the nervous system forms from the ectoderm in relation to two structures, the *primitive streak* (**1**) and the *notochord* (**2**). At the end of the first three weeks, the embryo is a more or less oval disc about 1.5 cm long. Its long axis is established by the presence of the primitive streak in the posterior quadrant of the embryonic disc. This streak may be considered as a thickened longitudinal area. Just rostral to this primitive streak, there is another thickening of the ectoderm forming what is known as *Hensen's node* or the primitive node. The center of this node becomes invaginated by an inward movement of the surface cells, forming a pit, the *blastopore* (**3**). A cord of cells then migrates rostrally from Hensen's node between the ectoderm and entoderm, forming the *notochord* (**2**). This cord becomes attached to the *prochordal plate* (**4**) at the rostral end of the embryonic disc. As this is progressing, the blastopore invaginates further, extending into the notochord, forming an extension of the amniotic cavity called the *notochordal canal*.

Fig. 4. The ectoderm (**5**) overlying the notochord then becomes thickened, induced some believe by the notochord and the prochordal mesoderm to which the notochord attaches. This thickened ectoderm forms the *neural plate* (**6**), which will invaginate to form a *neural groove* (**7**) and eventually a long hollow tube just below the ectodermal surface from which it breaks away. The actual transformation of the neural plate into the hollow tube was said to be due to forces within the plate itself as long ago as 1895 (Foux). This folding takes place even when the plate itself is removed from the embryo. When the raised folds of the neural plate meet, they fuse forming the neural tube (**8**). The freed epidermal layers from which the neural tube has separated also come together fusing the neuro-ectodermal junctions over the top of the newly formed neural tube. The tube, as formed is enlarged at its rostral end in an area which will form the brain. The caudal smaller portion will develop into the spinal cord.

The first part of the neural tube to close forms the *rhombencephalon* or hindbrain. Closure of the tube then proceeds caudally, forming that part of the neural tube associated with the spinal cord. A rostrally directed closure of the neural groove occurs more or less simultaneously with that forming the cord segment. The rostral closure adds first the *mesencephalon* or midbrain and then the *prosencephalon* or forebrain as suprasegmental units above the rhombencephalon. The last part of the neural groove to

Fig. 3. Model of the dorsal aspect of an 18-days old embryo showing the medullary plate. Representative sections for planes at **A, B** and **C** are shown in the lower figures. Description in text. **5**, embryonic ectoderm; **6**, neural plate; **8**, yolk sac; **9**, amniotic ectoderm; **10**, embryonic mesoderm; **11**, entoderm.

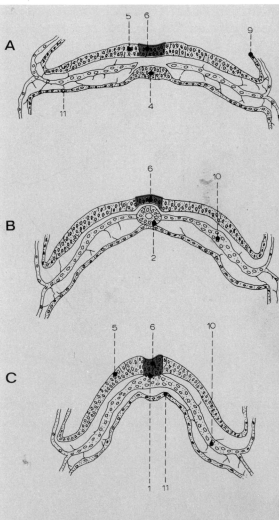

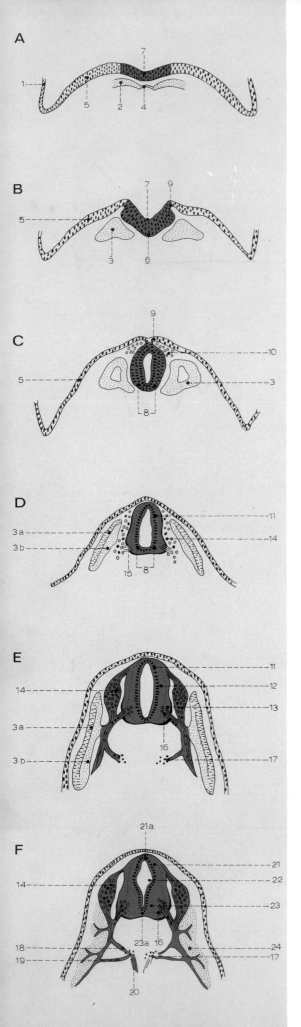

close rostrally is a small opening at the most cephalic end called the *anterior neuropore* (Fig. 14).

The slit-like shape of the normal neural tube cavity has been shown to depend on the presence of the underlying notochord (Fig. 4A, **4**). As the neural tube (**6**) is closing over, ectodermal cells at the lateral edge of the neural groove are extruded away, creating an elongated column of cells on either side of the tube, the *neural crest* (**10**). The process whereby this tube is formed has been termed *neurulation*. At the completion of neurulation, the embryo, which previously lacked an axis of symmetry, has acquired such an orientation. Cephalization is now apparent and there is a true head and tail end.

What are the underlying forces which induce the formation of the notochord, neural tube and its derivatives? While a conclusive answer is not yet available, it is believed that these morphologic changes in the embryo are preceded by the establishment of a metabolic gradient which is related to the subsequent cephalocaudal orientation. The metabolic variations are thought to be related to the existence of chemical gradients. Thus, in fish and amphibian embryos, there is a high concentration of glycogen in the presumptive ectoderm which will form the neural tube, while notochordal and endodermal levels of glycogen are very low. There is, furthermore, a cephalocaudal glycogen gradient. Furthermore, in areas in which morphogenesis is occurring, protein synthesis is understandably higher than in areas not undergoing differentiation. This high rate of protein synthesis has been associated with elevated nucleoprotein concentrations which undergo diminution as the differentiation in that particular region nears completion. This may then be succeeded by a new region of high nucleoprotein concentration which again appears to slightly precede morphogenesis. The neural plate region is one of the areas which has been characterized by a high concentration of ribonucleoproteins, again with a cephalocaudal gradient, which is presumably then indicative of increased protein synthesis in the region, as might be expected to occur during closure of the neural tube. The above gradients also coincide with gradients in respiratory enzyme metabolism. While conclusive proof of the relatedness of the above factors is still lacking, the concept of a relationship between cephalocaudal gradients during morphogenesis of the neural tube and RNA and protein formation seems quite logical.

Once the neural tube is formed (Fig. 4C, **8**), cells of the neural crest (**10**) migrate laterally, giving rise to the dorsal root ganglion (Fig. 4E, **14**), the peripheral postganglionic neurons of the visceral motor (sympathetic)

Fig. 4. Different stages in the development of the neural tube from the neural plate, and the subsequent formation of motor, sensory, and autonomic subdivisions. See text. **1**, amnion; **2**, mesoderm; **3**, somite, **3a**, dermatome; **3b**, myotome; **12**, mantle layer; **13**, marginal layer; **14**, dorsal root ganglion; **15**, anterior spinal root; **16**. anterior horn cells; **17**, sympathetic ganglion; **18**, preganglionic ramus; **19**, postganglionic ramus; **20**, visceral ramus; **21**, alar (sensory) plate; **21a**, roof plate; **22**, sulcus limitans; **23**, basal (motor) plate; **23a**, floor plate; **24**, muscle.

system, the Schwann cells which form the lipid (myelin) covering of peripheral nerves, supporting (satellite) cells of the dorsal root ganglion nerve cells, plus some of the cells which form the inner two of the outer membranous coverings (leptomeninges) of the central nervous system. The neural tube itself undergoes some changes as a result of proliferation of cells lining the central canal. This *ependymal layer* (**11**) is the proliferative zone which gives rise to the neuroblasts which become nerve cells and the spongioblasts which become the glial cells supporting the nervous system.

As a result of differential rates of cell division and accumulation, the central canal becomes constricted by two pairs of longitudinally oriented plates of cells (*cf*. Fig. 9). The more dorsal or *alar plates* (Fig. 4F, **21**) may be considered sensory in function in the spinal cord and lower brain stem, while the ventral or *basal plates* (**23**) have a motor function. The groove which separates these two plates is termed the *sulcus limitans* (**22**). The two alar plates are joined to each other dorsally by a *roof plate* (**21a**), while the two basal plates are joined together ventrally by a *floor plate* (**23a**). Rostral to the medulla there are many structures derived from the alar plate which are not sensory but motor, associative or relay in function (*i.e.*, cerebral hemisphere, diencephalon, cerebellum, and the pontine nuclei). It may be pointed out that all lower motoneuronal systems (ventral horn cells and cranial nerve nuclei) which innervate muscles, glands, etc. are derived from the basal plate. Since there are no alar and basal plates rostral to the mesencephalon (midbrain), one can not equate sensory or motor components to such structures.

Fig. 5. The long hollow neural tube undergoes rapid changes subsequent to its formation. At an early stage (Fig. 5A) there is a demarcation into a long caudal tube which becomes the spinal cord (**4**) and a broader, short rostral segment which will become the brain. The cephalic end soon becomes segmented into three dilations, the *primary vesicles* (**A**). The cavities of these vesicles will be present in a modified form in the adult brain, forming the *ventricular cavities* and *cerebral aqueduct*.

The most rostral division is the *prosencephalon* or forebrain (**1**). It is followed by the *mesencephalon* or midbrain (**2**) while the third most caudal segment forms the *rhombencephalon* or hindbrain (**3**). In subsequent development the prosencephalon becomes further subdivided into the *telencephalon* (cerebral hemispheres and certain basal nuclear masses, **5**) and the *diencephalon* or interbrain (**6**). An optic evagination will grow out from the diencephalon on each side, forming the neural component of

Fig. 5. The developing brain. **A,** formation of the primary vesicles, up to the 4th week; **B-F,** formation of the secondary vesicles. **B, C,** late 4th week; **D,** 6th week; **E,** 8-9th week, culminating in the formation of the major subdivisions (**F**) by the 14th week. **3a,** isthmus of rhombencephalon; **7,** lamina terminalis.

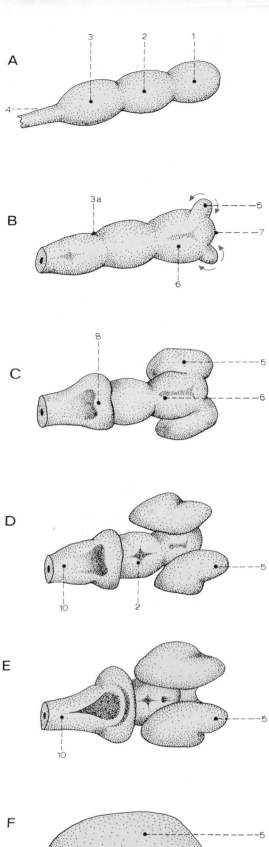

the eye. The *optic cup* formed by this outgrowth will induce changes in the surface ectoderm just overlying the optic cup (*cf.* Fig. 7) which will lead to the formation of the *lens*. The mesencephalon remains as one unit but undergoes considerable development into specialized reflex centers related to vision and hearing, as well as to primitive tactile sensations of pain, temperature, tickle, itch and erotic sensations. The rhombencephalon becomes subdivided into the *metencephalon* or afterbrain (*cerebellum* and *pons*, **8** and **9**) and *myelencephalon* or marrow brain (*medulla oblongata*, **10**).

2.1 Flexures

Accompanying these changes are certain bendings (flexures) in the neural tube resulting from differential growth rates of the various parts. At the conclusion of these changes, the telencephalon-diencephalon ends up being bent forward (anteriorly) at a right angle from the rest of the neural tube (*cf.* Fig. 7) at the mesencephalic (cephalic) flexure. Since much of the nomenclature of the brain has been based on animals in which this anterior flexure of the forebrain with the mesencephalon is not present, some difficulties in terminology have occurred. This may, however, be partially resolved if man is put into the position of a quadruped (Fig. 6) and the various terms for the parts of the brain now applied.

Figs. 7, 8. During the growth of the neural tube, various flexures occur as a result (partly) of more rapid growth in certain regions of the tube.

Fig. 6. A, sketch of the human primate in an anatomic position consistent with that of quadrupeds. This orients the brain and nerve roots in such a way that the anterior and posterior, rostral and caudal components may be compared with related structures of lower species. **B** and **C,** the common planes for sectioning the brain for anatomical or pathological study.
a, midsagittal; **b,** parasagittal; **c,** coronal; **d,** 15-20° from horizontal plane.

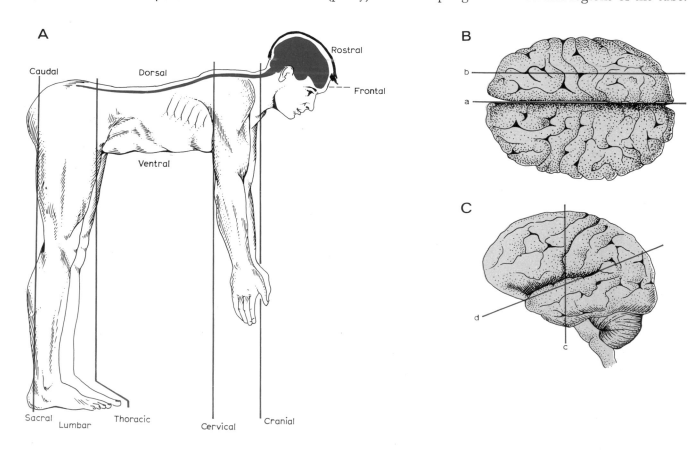

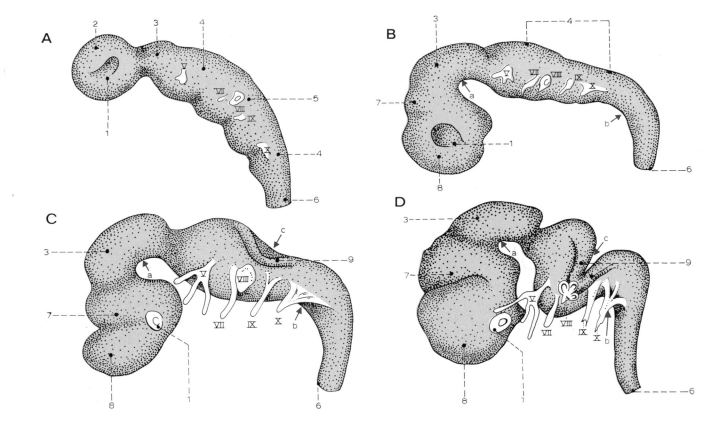

These flexures occur in such a way that the point where the forebrain is attached to the top of the buccopharyngeal membrane appears as a relatively fixed point in relation to the changes in position occurring with the rest of the neural tube. Thus, starting in the third week, very rapid growth rostrally and dorsally bends the neural tube anteriorly so that by the 4th week there is a flexure in the region which will form the mesencephalon (*cephalic* or *mesencephalic flexure*, **a**) and caudally at the junction of the myelencephalon with the spinal cord (*cervical flexure*, **b**). Somewhat later, during the fifth week, a third flexure starts to occur in the pontine region (*pontine flexure*, **c**) which is in the reverse direction of the two earlier flexures, and which is accompanied by an even increased bending in the region of the cephalic flexure (**a**). Eventually, all but the mesencephalic flexure disappear, leaving the CNS bent at almost a right angle at the mesencephalic-diencephalic junction.

Fig. 7. Lateral aspect of the developing brain from the 3rd through the 7th week illustrating the flexures occurring in the cephalic (**a**), cervical (**b**), and pontine (**c**) areas of the brain.
1, optic vesicle, eye; **2**, forebrain; **3**, midbrain; **4**, hindbrain; **5**, otic vesicle; **6**, spinal cord; **7**, diencephalon; **8**, telencephalon; **9**, rhombic lip.

Fig. 8. Diagram of the changes in position of the neural tube during the period in which the various flexures occur, due to firstly the rapid growth, and secondly that the tube is fixed at two points: the buccopharyngeal membrane (**1**) and in the region of the cervical somites (**2**); **3**, notochord. pink, stage 1; - - - - -, stage 2; ......, stage 3.

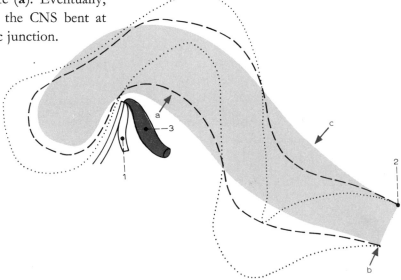

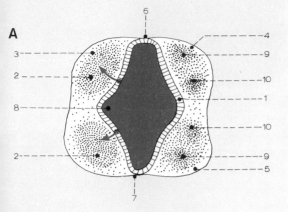

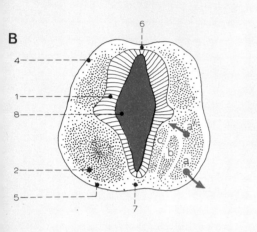

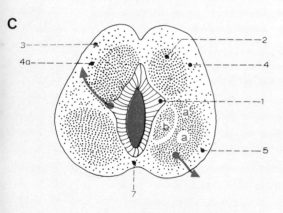

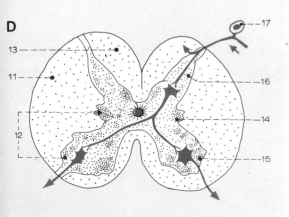

2.2 Regional development

2.2.1 Spinal cord

Fig. 9. During the early phases of development, the entire neural tube consists of three layers: the *ependymal* (**1**), *mantle* (**2**) and *marginal layers* (**3**). Neuroblasts migrate peripherally out from the ependymal or *germinal* layer into the mantle layer. Some of these neuroblasts are the precursor cells of neurons. Others are not truely neuroblasts, but spongioblasts which will form the glial elements. In that part of the neural tube which will give rise to the spinal cord, myelencephalon, metencephalon and mesencephalon, four parallel columns of neurons form in the mantle area (**2**). There are two *alar plates* (**4**) dorsolaterally and two *basal plates* (**5**) ventrolaterally. These columns are connected dorsally and ventrally by *roof* and *floor plates* (**6, 7**), while the longitudinally oriented *sulcus limitans* (**8**) separates the alar and basal plates. The basal plate, which contributes important elements to the motor units of the lower brain centers, does not extend rostrally past the mesencephalon. Thus, the telencephalon and diencephalon are derived entirely from the columns of cells in the alar plate.

During maturation of the spinal cord (Fig. 9**D**), the basal plate gives rise to the ventral horn cells (**15**) and cells of the intermediolateral cell column (**14**). As the mass of neuroblasts in the ventral basal plate enlarges, groups of indifferent nuclear masses are formed, so that the column of cells shows a series of regular enlargements, being thicker in the intersegmental intervals. This primitive segmental pattern of neuroblasts is evident as late as the 8- to 10-mm stage. In the stages of development which occur between the 8- and 15-mm embryos, these basal columns undergo a secondary longitudinal regrouping into 3 groups:

(i) A ventrolateral collection of cells (**a**), in which are 2 to 3 subsidiary peripheral columns. All give rise to neurons which enter the ventral root. The cells which will form the *intermediolateral cell column* (**a¹**) in the adult (*preganglionic sympathetic*) are derived from the dorsal part of this ventrolateral group.

(ii) A band of dorsomedially oriented cells (**b**), deep and medially placed to the cells in group **a**. The axonal processes from these cells pass through what will be the *ventral white commissure* to the other side.

(iii) A small group of neuroblasts (**c**) which appear to arise from the ependymal germinal cell area somewhat later and which lie between the ependymal layer and the cells of group **b** above. This group becomes important in the more rostral regions of the neural tube and appears to provide the cells for certain cranial nerve nuclei.

The alar plate (**4**) gives rise to the sensory, relay and internuncial

Fig. 9. Regional development of the spinal cord showing the growth from **A**, 8.0-mm, **B**, 15.0-mm, **C**, 35.0-mm stages to **D**, terminal, of alar and basal plates leading to the formation of the dorsal (**16**) and ventral (**15**) horns of the spinal cord grey matter (**12**). **9**, somatic and **10**, splanchnic functional areas.

neurons. The neuroblasts in the mantle zone of the alar plate grow and differentiate slowly, forming a massive condensation of cells dorsal to the basal plate by the middle of the second month. The derivation of neuroblasts from the part of the ependyma just dorsal to the sulcus limitans (8) appears to occur more quickly than in the more dorsal area near the roof plate (6). This results in a more lateral projection of the cells at the base of the alar plate (Fig. 9C). Some of these laterally migrating cells then proceed dorsolaterally around the more slower forming dorsal derivatives of the alar plate (4a).

Nerve fibrils from the alar plate cells can be seen projecting into the marginal zone as early as the 5th week (8.0 mm). These appear to be the short fibers which mature into the intersegmental connections found in the *fasciculi proprii* (a fiber system adjacent to the spinal cord gray matter (12) which interconnects segmental levels). These short fibers appear to be the first to be laid down and are just adjacent to the cells of the mantle zone. One might logically suppose that the longer projecting fibers in the *lateral funiculus* (11) might be laid down one upon the other, depending on length, such that there would be an orderly progression in development and position of ascending sensory fiber systems. There are, however, no data to support such a progression. The most lateral spinocerebellar fibers, however, do appear somewhat later than the preceeding medially placed fiber bundles. The fiber bundles of the *dorsal funiculus* (13) are for the most part provided by processes arising from the dorsal root ganglion cells (17). This bundle is very small in the 8-mm embryo and increases rapidly between the 15- and 35-mm stages, becoming displaced medially by 35-mm to form a true posterior (dorsal) column. There is some indication that the two bundles of fibers (*fasciculus gracilis* and *cuneatus*) which constitute the dorsal funiculus are formed separately. In the later stages of development, fibers from dorsal root ganglion cells may be observed to terminate among the neurons of the dorsal mantle layer mass and to form another tract dorsolateral to the cell mass, this tract becoming, in all probability, what is known as the *tract of Lissauer*.

The mitotic rate is apparently higher in the basal plate than the alar plate, since spontaneous movement occurs prior to the time when reflex responses may be elicited. Those motor units supplying the somatic musculature also mature more rapidly than do those of the higher centers (cerebellum and cerebral cortex). The overall rate at which nerve cells are formed is apparently the same throughout most of the cord, and is sufficient in magnitude to result in an overproduction of neurons for the musculature of the trunk. However, great numbers of cells in the thoracic cord disappear, leaving clusters of cells concerned with the innervation of specific muscle groups. Others become involved in the formation of the preganglionic cell group of the intermediolateral cell column (sympathetic division of the autonomic system).

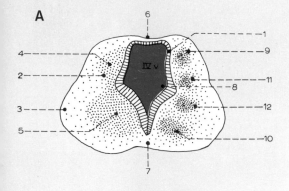

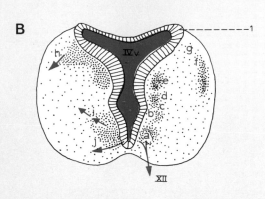

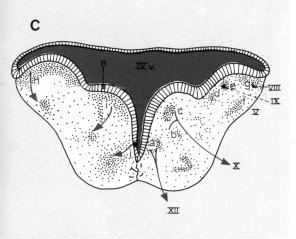

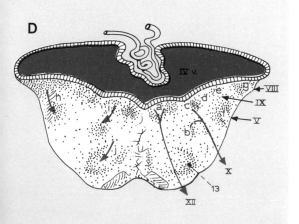

2.2.2 Myelencephalon

Fig. 10. The myelencephalon or medulla oblongata starts initially with a structure which is quite comparable to the spinal cord, having alar (**4**), basal (**5**), roof (**6**) and floor (**7**) plates. However, the alar-basal-plate area opens out like the covers of a book, the floor plate representing the back of the book. This occurs during the formation of the pontine flexure, and stretches out the roof plate (**6**), which becomes quite thin. The mesenchymal cells adjacent to the roof plate give rise to large numbers of hemocytoblasts and angioblasts to form a vascular plexus which invaginates the roof plate, eventually forming the choroid plexus of the fourth ventricle. The 'anlage' of a choroid plexus may be seen as early as six weeks (12 mm) in the human embryo when the formation of blood and vascular system cells is quite marked. By the 22-mm stage erythroblasts are present surrounded by strands of protoplasm from angioblasts which will provide for the endothelial cells for the vessels in the developing choroid plexus.

The alar and basal plates (**4**, **5**) undergo longitudinal cleavage so that four columns of cells are derived from the alar plate and three columns of cells from the basal plate (Fig. 10**B-D**). Certain of the cranial nerves will be derived from or associated with these columns. If one starts with the most medial column and passes laterally, the nerves derived from these columns are: (**a**) *hypoglossal* (gen. somatic efferent); (**b**) *ambiguous*–component of the *vagus* (spec. visceral efferent) – these cells will migrate ventrolaterally in later development; (**c**) *dorsal* nucl. of *vagus* (gen. visceral efferent); (**d**) *dorsal sensory* nucl. of *vagus* – nucl. of tract. solitarius (gen. visceral afferent); (**e**) *sensory* nucl. of *glossopharyngeal* – taste (spec. visceral afferent); (**f**) *descending sensory* component of *trigeminal* (gen. somatic afferent); (**g**) nucl. of *vestibulocochlear* nerve (spec. somatic afferent).

The sensory nuclei of trigeminal (gen. somatic afferent) and the motor nuclei of trigeminal and facial nerves (both spec. visceral efferents) are derived at the rostral end of the myelencephalic portion of the hindbrain and become located in the metencephalon secondarily. This occurs after the pontine flexure at which time the caudal metencephalic floor and rostral myelencephalic floor of the fourth ventricle (**IV v.**) become adjacent to each other (*cf.* Fig. 7). These two regions fuse together secondarily and provide for an impression that certain structures originating in the myelencephalon have originated in the metencephalon, whereas the metencephalic position of these structures in the adult brain is due

Fig. 10. Regional development of the medulla oblongata, **A**, 10.0-mm, **B**, 14.5-mm, **C**, 15.0-mm and **D**, 73.0-mm stage, illustrating the lateral movement of the alar and basal plates and thinning out of the roof plate which becomes invaginated by a vascular plexus to form the choroid plexus.

1, ependymal layer; **2**, mantle layer; **3**, marginal layer; **8**, sulcus limitans; **9**, somatic sensory nucl.; **10**, somatic motor nucl.; **11**, visceral sensory nucl.; **12**, visceral motor nucl.; **13**, inferior olive. **h**, cells from alar plate for **f**; **i**, cells from basal plate for **b**; **j**, cells from ependyma (**1**) for olivary complex (**13**).

primarily to the fusion of the two adjacent regions of the floor of the primitive fourth ventricle. The rostral components of the vestibular nuclei (VIII) are also in this category. The primitive abducens nucleus (VI) originates caudal to the VII nucleus and attains its more rostral medial position by a combination of the above mentioned fusion of myelencephalic and metencephalic areas and by a medial migration of the cells. It appears, therefore, that no cranial nerve nuclei are actually derived from cells formed primarily in the metencephalon (except perhaps for a small part of the main sensory and mesencephalic nuclei of V), and that their final position in the adult metencephalon may be ascribed to the processes of maturation and differentiation. Caudally, the gracilis and cuneatus (and external cuneate) nuclei form from the alar plate to provide a nuclear termination for fibers of the dorsal funiculus.

Fig. 11. The pons. In the seventh week (about 16 mm) the alar plate also gives rise to the cells which migrate ventrally and rostrally from the middle region of the myelencephalon to form the *pontobulbar body* and *arcuate nucleus* (Fig. 11**B, D**) on the ventral surface of the metencephalon. This pontobulbar body will form the pontine nuclei (**9**) when the cerebrospinal fibers reach them from above and pass among them. The formation of the *inferior olive* and *medial accessory olive* starts first at the 13-mm stage and has been classically described as being derived from the alar plate of the myelencephalon. Baxter[11], however, presents evidence demonstrating that these nuclei develop *in situ* by a condensation and proliferation of neuroblasts derived from the basal plate.

2.2.3 Metencephalon

The metencephalon may be considered in three parts; (i) a central axial nuclear part which is a direct rostral continuation of the medulla, (ii) the cerebellum, and (iii) the basal or fibrous pons.

Fig. 11C. (i) The axial part which is a continuation of the medulla oblongata contains the same alar-basal plate groups and has undergone the same spreading out, bookwise, which moves the alar plates quite far laterally. This has, of course, been accompanied by a thinning of the roof plate (**1**). However, there is no invagination or formation of a choroid plexus in the roof plate at this level. It will instead become overgrown with cells migrating from the alar plate, forming the cerebellar cortex (**5**) and deep cerebellar nuclei (**6**). The alar (**2**) and basal (**3**) plates of the metencephalon may also be associated with the formation (**b, c**) of various *reticular nuclei* (**7**) in this area.

Fig. 11. Regional development of the pons. **A**, 13.0-mm, **B**, 16.0-mm, and **C**, 100.0-mm stage, a diagrammatic representation of the migration of cells (a) which provide for the deep cerebellar nuclei (**6**) and cerebellar cortex (**5**) and **D**, the migration of cells from the dorsal surface of the medulla at **x** to **y**, to form the nuclei of the basal part of the pons. 1, ependymal layer of roof plate; 2, alar plate; 3, basal plate; 4, sulcus limitans; 7, reticular nuclei; 8, cortico spinal-cortico bulbar fibers; 9, pontine nucleus; 10, vesibulocochlear nerve; **IV, v,** fourth ventricle.

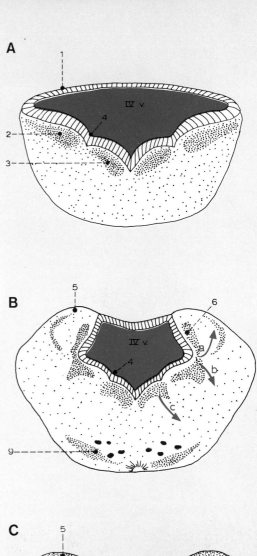

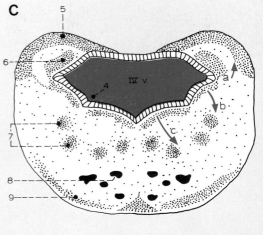

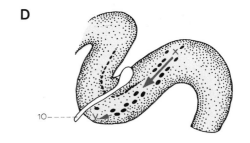

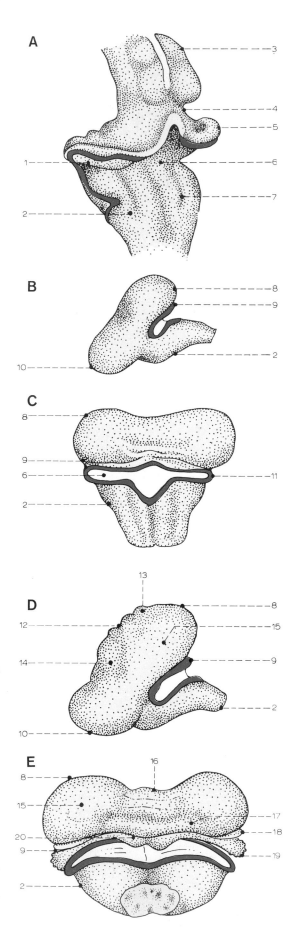

Fig. 12. (ii) The *cerebellum* develops in part from the *rhombic lip* (**5**) which is formed by the dorsal migration of alar plate cells just prior to the development of the pontine flexure. The cells in the rhombic lip come to lie at the junction of the roof and alar plate. During the pontine flexure, the rhombic lips are bulged out laterally (Fig. 12**B, C**), creating the site for the future *foramen of Luschka*. That part of the lip rostral to the future site of the foramina gives rise to the *flocculonodular lobe* of the cerebellum (**19, 20**) while the cells caudal to the aperture will contribute to the formation of the *vestibular nuclei*.

The *corpus cerebelli* (**8**), which is the largest part of the cerebellum in man, is developed from alar plate cells just rostral to the rhombic lips. These cells migrate dorsally and medially, finally fusing to form the *vermis* (**16**) in the midline. A rapid expansion then occurs on either side of the vermis, forming the *anterior and posterior lobes* (**14, 15**) of the cerebellar hemisphere. The first sulci which are formed in the cerebellum occur in the anterior part of the vermis (**16**), then in the remainder of the vermis after which sulcus formation slowly progresses laterally over the surface of the corpus cerebelli.

The alar plates of the metencephalon extend rostrally, roofing over the fourth ventricle (**6**) to meet in the 'roof' behind the *isthmus rhombencephali* (Fig. 12**A, 4**). These metencephalic projections actually proceed rostrally somewhat past the rostral limit of the metencephalon, meeting the midbrain tectum.

The inferior cerebellar peduncle *(restiform body)* develops about the same time as the spinal tract of the trigeminal nerve in the central part of the alar plate, and is lateral to the trigeminal fibers in the myelencephalon. It can first be recognized as a few fibers at the end of the 2nd month. These fibers extend rostrally into the alar plate of the metencephalon and thus reach the growing cerebellum. Their origin is in part from cells at the base of the dorsal horn (alar plate at this time) in the spinal cord. Other fibers from the myelencephalic olive and reticular nuclei will also enter into the formation of the restiform body. The superior cerebellar peduncle *(brachium conjunctivum)* appears at about the same time as small scattered fibers extending rostrally from the developing cerebellum into the mesencephalon. These fibers are the processes arising from the deep cerebellar nuclei.

Fig. 12. Regional development of the cerebellum. **A**, cerebellar and neighbouring region of the brain (oblique dorsal, 28.0-mm stage); **B, C** and **D, E**, lateral and dorsal views at 56.0-mm and 112.0-mm stages respectively. **A** illustrates the flaring out of the alar plates which occurs at the pontine flexure such that the most lateral aspect at the edges of the rhombic lip (**5**) becomes the site of the future *recessus lateralis ventriculi quarti* (foramen of Luschka).
1, primitive cerebellum; **2**, medulla; **3**, tectum of mesencephalon; **7**, sulcus limitans; **9**, posterolateral fissure; **10**, pons; **11**, lateral recess; **12**, primary fissure; **13**, postclival fissure; **14**, anterior lobe; **15**, posterior lobe; **17**, tonsilla; **18**, para flocculus.

2.2.4 Isthmus rhombencephali

Fig. 12A. The constriction (**4**) which this region represented in the more primitive brain undergoes many changes with the growth of the alar and basal plates. The *trochlear (IVth) nucleus* (gen. somatic efferent) develops at this junction from the basal plate. The nerve fibers run dorsally and at this stage decussate in the hindbrain caudal to the isthmus (12-mm stage). With further growth, the basal plate region containing the IVth nucleus moves rostrally so that the nucleus comes to lie in the midbrain by the 26-mm stage, and decussating fibers now emerge in the isthmus, as they do in the adult. The rostral displacement of the basal plate in this area at 12 to 16 mm is accompanied by similar displacement of the alar plate, bringing with it some of the rostral elements of the trigeminal nerve, placing them external to basal plate structures. Thus, the mesencephalic root of V and its cell bodies come to lie lateral to the tracts of the fourth nerve.

2.2.5 Mesencephalon

Fig. 13. This portion of the neural tube also has the same primitive alar and basal plate configuration as the spinal cord. The basal plate (**3**) gives rise to only one major nuclear mass (**5**), the *oculomotor nucleus* (III) (gen. somatic efferent) which is well defined by the end of the 3rd month. The alar plate provides for cells (**a**) which migrate dorsally to form the *nuclei of the inferior* (**7**) *and superior colliculi* (**13**) and possibly some cells which migrate ventrally to form the *red nuclei* (**c**) (3rd month) as well as some of the *reticular nuclei* (**b**). The details of formation of these 2 nuclei are not certain and many cells may be derived *in situ* by proliferation from the ependyma and basal lamina. The origin of the *substantia nigra* (**d**) is even more uncertain. It is not pigmented at birth, nor in fact for two or three years after birth. Somewhat later in development, two large fibrous masses *(basis pedunculi)* will be applied ventrally. These fibers arise from the cerebral cortex and are the motor units passing to lower centers.

The external growth of the alar and basal plates compress the ventricular cavity at this level until only a small canal, the *aqueductus cerebri*

Fig. 13. Regional development of the mesencephalon (**A**, 23.0-mm, **B**, 56.0-mm, **C**, 112.0-mm stage) showing migrations of cells from the ependyma (**1**) to form the oculomotor nucleus (**5**) and the other mesencephalic nuclei, whose precise origin is still uncertain. Note that the ascending and descending tract systems become associated with the ventral aspect of the mesencephalon. **2**, marginal region; **4**, floor plate; **6**, fibers from cerebellum; **7a**, developing collicular nucl.; **8**, sulcus limitans; **9**, cerebellar fibers around nucleus ruber; **11**, medial longitudinal fasciculus.

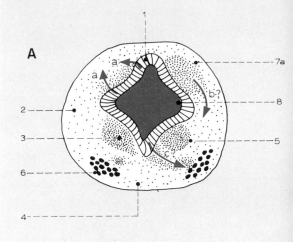

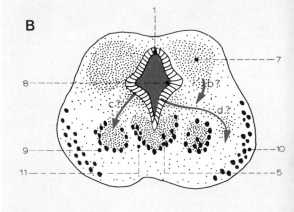

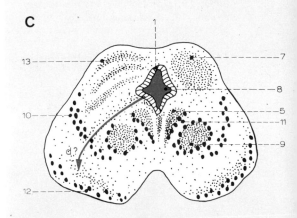

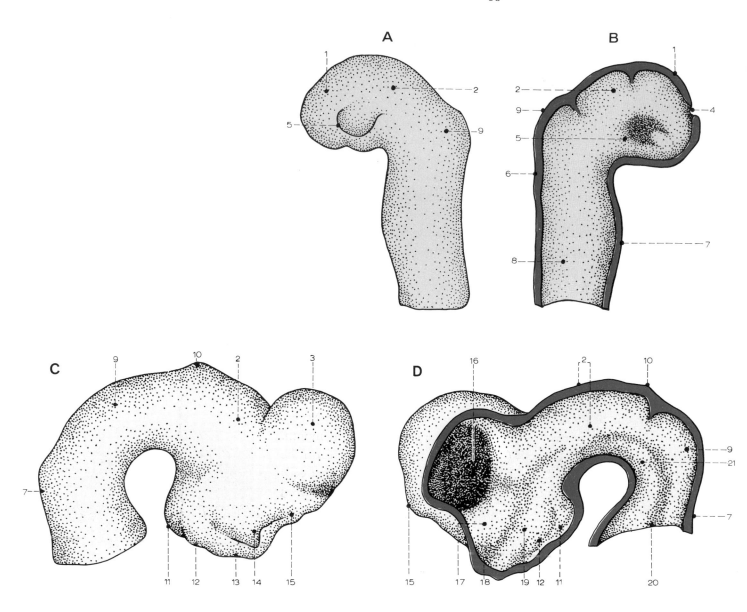

Fig. 14. Regional development of the forebrain showing the initial development of the telencephalon. **A, B,** 2.5-mm-, **C, D,** 10.2-mm stage; **B, D,** are mid sagittal sections. **6,** isthmus of rhombencephalon; **7,** pons; **8,** medulla; **9,** midbrain; **10,** pineal gland; **11,** mammillary region; **12,** tuber cinereum; **13,** hypophyseal pouch; **14,** optic stalk; **15,** olfactory lobe; **16,** foramen of Monro; **17,** striate body; **18,** optic recess; **19,** hypothalamus; **20,** sulcus limitans; **21,** basal plate.

remains. The fibers of the ascending *medial and lateral lemnisci* (**10**) enter among the alar plate derivatives and are spread over the lateral and ventral aspect of the midbrain during the third month. The descending corticospinal fibers (**12**) reach the midbrain somewhat later than the lemniscal fibers and are applied over them ventrally.

2.2.6 Prosencephalon

Figs. 14, 15. This, the most rostral part of the neural tube, the pallial region (**1**), is derived from the neural tube components rostral to the termination of the sulcus limitans and will become secondarily divided into the *diencephalon* (**2**) and *telencephalon* (**3**). The forebrain evolves as a secondary rostral projection from the anterior end of the neural groove, which is open at the *neuropore* (**4**) in this rostral area at this time. The open end of the groove is carried forward and the anterior neuropore finally closes over at the rostral end of these prominent forebrain structures just before the 3-mm stage is reached.

The forebrain, when first formed, appears as a short somewhat rounded terminal part of the neural tube, without any structures resembling a lateral hemisphere (**A** and **B**). From above it appears somewhat compressed rostrally, while caudally, the optic outgrowths project laterally from that part which will become the diencephalon (**2**). The curved postero-inferior portion of the diencephalon possesses a rounded prominence which is continuous laterally with the posterior inferior wall of the *optic outgrowth* (**5**). This prominence will be the site of the chiasmatic

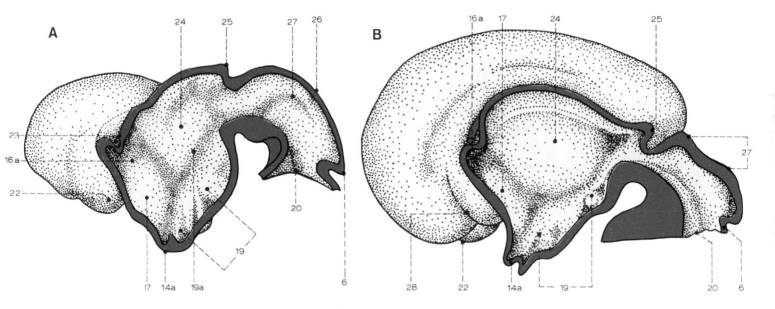

junction between the two eyes. At this time the telencephalon is only an indefinite area of thin wall at the rostral end of the forebrain. The telencephalic wall of the primary vesicle then evaginates dorsolaterally into two cerebral vesicles which will grow and mature to become hemispheres (Fig. 14**C** and **D**; see also Fig. 15). The cavities of these hemispheric vesicles will form the lateral ventricles. The connecting parenchymal portion between the two vesicles is at the rostral end of the neural tube and third ventricle and will be called the *lamina terminalis*. The roof plate of the hemisphere is very thin and is carried out into the telencephalon for a short distance rostrodorsally and almost reaches the midbrain tectum caudally. The remainder of the prosencephalon caudal to the telencephalic outgrowths (which are due to increased cell division in the telencephalic area) will become the diencephalon.

Fig. 15. Regional development of the forebrain (prosencephalon) showing the formation of some of the components of the diencephalon (**2**), corpus striatum (**17**) and rhinencephalon (**15**) from Fig. 14. **A**, 13.6-mm and **B**, 60.0-mm stage; **6**, isthmus rhombencephali; **14a**, optic chiasm; **16a**, interventricular foramen; **19**, hypothalamus; **19a**, hypothalamic sulcus; **20**, sulcus limitans; **22**, rhinencephalon; **23**, choroid fissure; **24**, thalamus; **25**, pineal gland; **26**, mesencephalon; **27**, quadrigeminal bodies; **28**, hippocampal fissure.

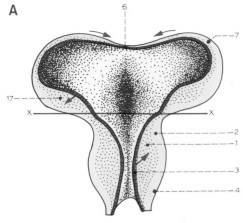

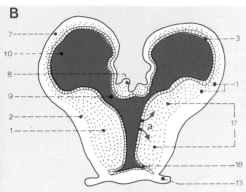

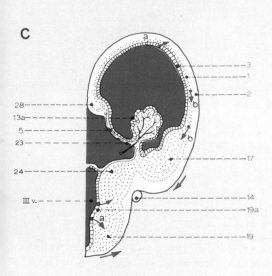

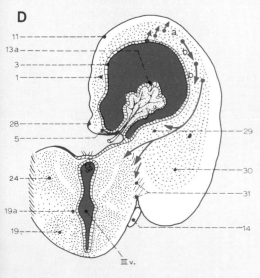

Fig. 16. The diencephalic part develops primarily through a massive thickening of the mantle layer (**1**), which becomes so extensive that there is virtually no marginal layer left (**2**). Some differentiation in cell division rates occurs between those areas which will form the *dorsal thalamus* (**24**) and a *ventral hypothalamus* (**19**). This results in the formation of a shallow groove along the ependymal wall recognized in the adults as the *hypo-thalamic sulcus* (**19a**). The optic cup also evaginates from the diencephalon at its ventral rostral aspect. The roof plate of the diencephalon becomes the roof of the 3rd ventricle, which becomes invaginated with a choroid plexus.

The telencephalic evagination continues to grow rostrally, dorsally and caudally, overhanging and covering over the diencephalon (Figs. 15 and 16). In its earliest stages, it is very thin walled and thus contains a large ventricular extension of the central canal of the primitive neural tube. The roof plate becomes even more stretched out during this growth and then becomes folded on itself as the hemisphere, grows up and folds over dorsomedially. This fold forms the *choroid fissure* (Fig. 15, **23**). An external capillary plexus which forms adjacent to the roof plate will invaginate the plate along the plane where it becomes folded on itself, forming the choroid plexus (**13a**) of the lateral ventricle.

The ventrolateral floor of the telencephalic 'bag' becomes thickened quite early as a result of a large area of very rapid localized cell division (10 to 20 mm). This thickened area forms the *corpus striatum* (**17**) which will become subdivided in the adult into the *caudate nucleus* (**29**), *putamen*, *globus pallidus* (lenticular nucleus) and *amygdala*. As the hemisphere of the telencephalon expands, the floor region (corpus striatum) moves medially and comes to lie against the diencephalon to which it fuses at about ten weeks (40 mm). The thin dorsal wall of the telencephalon is a virtually undeveloped saccular wall at the sixth week (12 mm), which is continuous with the thick striate mass everywhere along its base (Fig. 16). Since growth of the telencephalon is rather slow during the 3rd and 4th months, the cortical wall of the hemispheric vesicle increases in thickness and area slowly. Axonal sprouts start leaving the cortex after about 8 weeks (23 mm), many being directed caudally toward the diencephalon and lower centers (corticofugal fibers). As they pass away from the cortex, large groups of fibers will intersect the prominent nuclear mass of the corpus striatum and divide it into the isolated nuclear groups seen at birth and in the adult (Fig. 16**D**). Those fibers which do not terminate

Fig. 16. Regional development of the telencephalon, diencephalic part. **A**, horizontal, **B, C, D**, coronal sections. **B**, 12.0-mm stage, cut along line x in **A**; **C**, 17.0-mm stage; **D**, 40.0-mm stage, showing development of the cerebral cortical tissue, corpus striatum (**17**) and diencephalon (**4**) at 6, 7 and 10 weeks respectively. Note the growth of the inferior aspect of the telencephalon toward the diencephalon and the passage of nerve fibers along the plane of junction of the two units (**31**). This bundle of fibers will eventually form the capsula interna. **3**, ependyma; **5**, fimbria fornicis; **6**, lamina terminalis; **7**, cerebral vesicle; **8**, rostral thalamus; **9**, interventricular foramen; **10**, lateral ventricle; **11**, cerebral hemisphere; **13**, optic nerve; **14**, optic tract; **18**, optic recess; **19**, hypothalamus; **19a**, sulcus hypothalamicus; **28**, hippocampus; **30**, lenticular nucleus. **III v.**, third ventricle; **a**, migrating cells from ependyma; **b**, axon growth.

19

in the diencephalon or striatum follow a path along the plane of fusion of the base of the telencephalon with the diencephalon (**31**), forming the *internal capsule*. The fibers continue running caudally anterior (inferior) to the mesencephalon, forming the *crus cerebri*. This fiber mass penetrates the basal cell and fiber mass of the pons and finally emerges ventral to the medulla as the structure termed the *pyramid*. These fibers in the pyramids finally undergo a partial decussation and enter the spinal cord. Since these axons terminate on motor cells, some fibers will naturally be terminating at levels higher than the motor cells of the ventral horns of the spinal cord. Other fibers do not leave the hemisphere, but form associational bundles, which begin to be apparent at the end of the 2nd month.

Fig. 17. From the 11th to 12th week on, the cerebral hemispheres are recognizable for what they are although their form is perhaps more comparable to those of lower species than man. However, the development of fissures (sulci) very quickly begins to subdivide the hemisphere into the recognizable adult components. As the outer cortical part of the hemisphere expands, an area near the middle of its base fails to grow as rapidly and as consequence is overgrown by the rest of the cortex. This is the *insula* (**6**). The convolutions which finally result from this growth are relatively constant and have afforded a certain degree of localization based on anatomical variations in the lamination of cells in the cortex which has to some degree corresponded with the physiological concepts of localization. The parcelling out of such functional areas was of great interest to earlier investigators. While to some extent such localizations may be valid, there appears to be great individual variation as well as considerable disagreement as to the degree to which such concepts apply, particularly when dealing with abstract entities. Thus, the concept that the frontal lobe is solely responsible for the 'original thought' is inadequate. Surely the parietal lobe, considered by some to serve as a storehouse of information, must contribute to thought, since thought is undoubtedly concerned with past experience or memory. In addition, the area on the medial surface concerned with emotional behavior also affects thought. That 'original thought' may be associated with any one area is also contradicted by experience with patients. Reports based on studies where masses of cortical tissue have been removed suggest that a loss of cortex from any region may in some manner affect the thought or reasoning processes. Furthermore, the function of all these cortical regions will be influenced by available energy levels (glucose) and the levels of circulating hormones (thyroid and adrenal) which may influence intracellular electrolytes. The male and female hormones have also been shown to affect excitability of neurons.

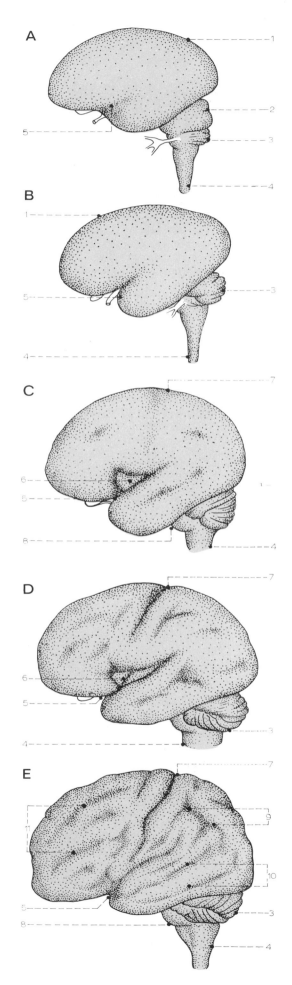

Fig. 17. A to E. Lateral aspects of developing cerebral hemispheres (at 11, 16-17, 24-26, 32-34 weeks, and newborn respectively) illustrating the formation of the fissura lateralis (**5**), sulcus centralis (**7**) and other sulci and gyri during maturation. (Adapted from Patten's Embryology, 1953.)
1, telencephalon; **2**, mesencephalon; **3**, cerebellum; **4**, medulla; **7**, sulcus centralis; **8**, pons; **9**, parietal sulci; **10**, temporal sulci; **11**, frontal sulci.

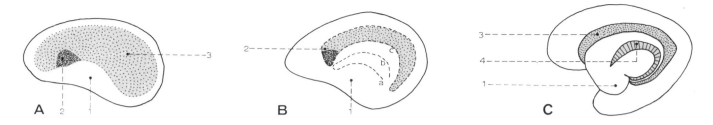

20

Fig. 18. A, B, C, illustrate the upward growth of the corpus striatum (1) from the lateral aspect of the floor of the telencephalic vesicle in stages a, b, c, which coincides with the downward and anterior growth from the occipital end of the brain to provide for the formation of a C shaped lateral ventricle (3).
2, foramen of Monroe (interventricular foramen); 4, capsula interna.
D, E, F, illustrate the development of the corpus callosum (6) and the manner in which it 'pushes' the hippocampus (10) and related structures caudally, leaving a thin stria of fibers as a hippocampal rudiment (7) passing over the dorsum of the corpus callosum.
7, supracallosal gyrus (rudiment of 10); 11, stria terminalis; 12, thalamus; 13, septum pellucidum.

Thus, while one may indicate some localization of function in regard to vision, hearing and sensory–motor activities, such abstract concepts as thought, memory and emotional response are much harder to define or to associate with any specific region.

Fig. 18. The *corpus callosum* (6) is one of the several commissural bundles which link right and left structures within the CNS. The corpus callosum, which is found at the beginning of the fourth month, represents a commissural band linking cortical structures. It starts in the lamina terminalis as a small group of transverse fibers lying immediately above the *hippocampal commissure* (5). It grows rapidly by acquisition of additional interhemispheric fibers and extends dorsally and caudally fairly rapidly. There is also an addition of fibers to the rostrodorsal portion of the callosum. During its caudal progression, the *hippocampal commissure* (5) and *fornix* (9) are shifted caudally. The position of the primitive *hippocampus* (10) is also altered in a caudal direction by this acquisition of fibers forming the corpus callosum. As the hemisphere grows and axons start to leave the primitive cortex, more and more fibers are directed into this bundle, which, as a consequence becomes quite large and is eventually believed to link every right and left cortical area to each other except the cortex of the primary visual cortex (area 17).

The *anterior commissure* (8) also runs through the lamina terminalis and serves to link the cortex of the *olfactory bulbs* to each other, as well as linking the *amygdaloid nuclei* and the cortex of the temporal lobes which just overlies the nuclei (pyriform cortex).

The *hippocampal commissure* (5) is a small bundle which links the two hippocampi. In the three month old fetus, this fiber bundle is just caudal and inferior to the corpus callosum (6). As the corpus callosum expands and grows caudally, the hippocampal commissure is carried back with it until finally it is found only near the splenium of the adult corpus callosum. One might regard it as that subdivision of the corpus callosum which is commissural for the hippocampal structures. The fornix (9) is

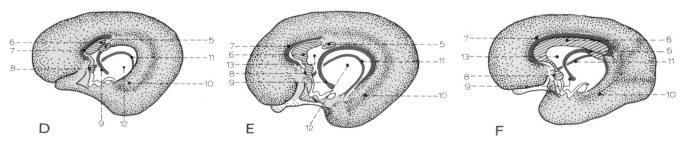

another prominent fiber bundle of the telencephalon. It arises from the hippocampus during the latter part of the third month and extends into the diencephalon and mesencephalon. As its fibers arch into the substance of the diencephalon, they form the anterior margin of the *interventricular foramen* (2) which links the lateral and third ventricles.

2.2.7 Pineal gland and Neurohypophysis

This structure, which is derived from neural ectoderm, arises as an evagination from the roof plate at the caudal end of the diencephalon as two processes which fuse to form a single parenchymal structure. The posterior pituitary lobe forms as an evagination from the diencephalic forebrain just above and caudal to Rathke's pouch ('anlage' for anterior pituitary lobe).

Changes in appearance of the cerebral hemisphere

Age in weeks	Crown–rump length (mm)	Brain development*
2.5	1.5	Neural groove indicated.
3.5	2.5	Neural groove prominent, closing rapidly, neural crest a continuous band.
4.0	5.0	Neural tube closed, three primary vesicles of brain represented, nerves and ganglia forming, ependymal, mantle and marginal layers present.
5.0	8.0	Five brain vesicles, cerebral hemispheres bulging, nerves and ganglia better represented (suprarenal cortex accumulating).
6.0	12.0	Three primary flexures of brain represented, diencephalon large, nerve plexuses present, epiphysis recognizable, sympathetic ganglia forming segmental masses, meninges indicated.
7.0	17.0	Cerebral hemispheres becoming large, corpus striatum and thalamus prominent, infundibulum and Rathke's pouch in contact, choroid plexuses appearing, suprarenal medulla begins invading cortex.
8.0	23.0	Cerebral cortex begins to acquire typical cells, olfactory lobes visible, dura and pia-arachnoid distinct, chromaffin bodies appearing.
10.0	40.0	Spinal cord attains definitive internal structure.
12.0	56.0	Brain attains its general structural features, cord shows cervical and lumbar enlargement, cauda equina and filum terminale appearing, neuroglial types beginning to differentiate.
16.0	112.0	Hemispheres conceal much of brain stem, cerebral lobes delimited, corpora quadrigemina appear, cerebellum assumes some prominence.
20–40	160–350	Commissures completed (20 weeks), myelinization in cord begins (20 weeks), cerebral cortex typically layered (25 weeks) cerebral fissures and convolutions appearing rapidly (28-30 weeks), myelinization of brain begins (36-40 weeks).

* From Arey-Embryology

The cerebral hemisphere, which starts as a bleb-like out pocketing on the dorsolateral surface of the prosencephalon grows quickly until it expands over the diencephalon and mesencephalon. During this process, its surface area becomes greatly increased by folding. The earlier phases in the gross morphological appearance are apparent in Figs. 14 to 16. The sulci and fissures so prominent in the adult do not begin to develop until about the 11th to 12th week when the lateral fissure starts to form laterally and the hippocampus and gyri cinguli begin to become discernable medially (Fig. 18). From this time on sulcus and gyrus formation is rapid (Fig. 17). While all the major gyri are present at birth, the degree of convolutional complexity is still rather simple, resembling the diagrammatic pictures portrayed in textbooks. This relative degree of 'textbook' order soon disappears so that by the first year of age the organization of gyri and sulci in different brains shows several variations in the minor unnamed sulci which tend to alter the overall appearance of the major gyri and sulci slightly. Variations in the rates of growth and maturation also lead to individual differences in the degree of gyral complexity at specific ages, which make it difficult to 'date' a fetal brain too precisely, such estimates being only to within half a month of the correct age.

3. Histogenesis

Initially, the neural tube consists of a single layer of columnar cells forming a neural epithelium. This becomes pseudostratified as the epithelium proliferates, and the wall of the tube thickens. At the outer margins of this epithelium individual cells lose their clear cut outlines and a syncytium is formed which becomes bounded externally by an external limiting membrane formed by processes of spongioblastic elements. There is also an internal limiting membrane which lines the central canal of the tube. The proliferative layer (germinal layer) provides for all the cell types of the central nervous system except the microglial cell and finally remains in the adult as the ependyma. In the spinal cord, the nerve cell elements tend to remain around the primitive central canal.

Fig. 19. The primitive neural tube in this region soon becomes differentiated into 3 layers. There is the inner *ependymal region* (3) containing the germinal cells (6), an intermediate zone (mantle layer, 2) into which the proliferated cells will migrate and an outer marginal layer (1) which in the adult spinal cord will contain the fibers arising from the cluster of nerve cells in the more central grey matter as well as long fiber systems which descend from higher centers.

The germinal or ependymal layer will provide the nerve cells and internal supporting (glial) cells of the central nervous system. Initially, the germinal cells divide into two daughter cells. One migrates into the mantle layer (2) and one remains in the germinal layer (3). The cell which migrates into the mantle layer may become an *apolar neuroblast*. This cell is thought to develop a process at each extremity becoming a *bipolar neuroblast* (14). One process will regress, leaving a unipolar neuroblast (15). This is followed by a sprouting of cytoplasmic processes

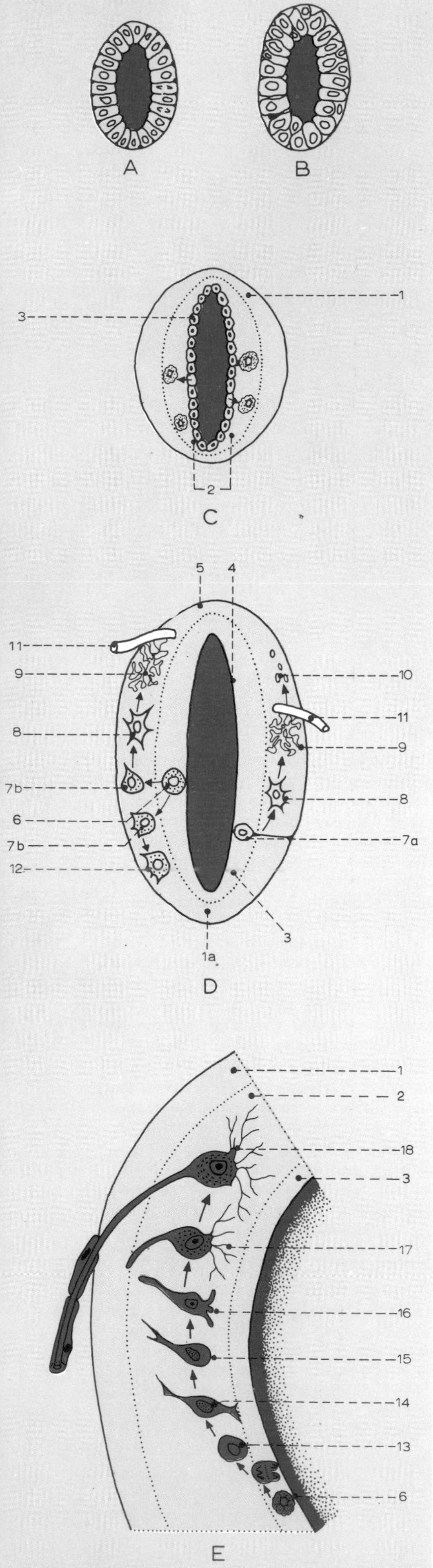

Fig. 19. Changes in the development of the neural tube. **A,** single columnar epithelium; **B,** pseudostratified neuroepithelium; **C,** formation of three primitive layers; **D,** formation of supporting glial elements; **E,** section of neural tube showing stages in the development of a multipolar neuron.
1a, combined mantle and marginal layer; **3,** ependyma; **6,** germinal cell; **18,** multipolar neuron with myelinated axon.

in the region of the previously regressed process (**16**). The new sprouts will form the dendrites of the adult cell. The cell is now a *multipolar neuroblast* (**17**), which by growth and further differentiation, becomes a mature neuron (**18**). All the changes following the apolar neuroblast stage occur in the mantle region.

Other developing cells (**7**, Fig. 19**D**) remain attached to the internal limiting membrane (**4**) deep to the ependymal layer (**3**) and send out peripheral processes which contribute to an 'external limiting membrane' (**5**). These are the *spongioblasts* (**7a**), which will become *astrocytoblasts* (**8**) upon loosening their attachment to the internal and external limiting membranes. Cells which maintain their attachment to the internal limiting membrane will mature as the ependymal cells which line the central canal and ventricular cavities of the adult nervous system. Many of these cells have cilia which have been observed to be capable of producing currents of flow in cerebrospinal fluid[148]. Other cells similar to the spongioblasts lose their attachment to the internal limiting membrane and become separated from the ependymal layer while still undifferentiated; these are the *medulloblasts* (**7b**). In the adult these cells will form the *oligodendrocytes* (**12**). Those cells derived from *spongioblasts* (**7a**) and the *medulloblasts* (**7b**) which become the adult *astrocytes* (**9**) and *oligodendrocytes* (**12**) form the internal supporting framework of the adult nervous system.

A third type of glial cells (*cf.* p. 22), is the *microglia* (**10**), accompanying a vessel (**11**).

Mesenchymal cells are found surrounding the external limiting membrane of the neural tube. From their location it seems likely that they contribute to the formation of the meninges.

3.1 Types of neurons

Neurons may be divided into 3 main categories depending on the number of processes arising from the cell body.

3.1.1 Unipolar cells

These cells have a characteristic distribution, in that with one exception they are all located in sensory ganglia (*i.e.*, dorsal root, trigeminal, petrosal, etc.). They are all more or less concerned with sensory perceptions which are not as specialized as vision or hearing. This includes pain, temperature, light touch, pressure, proprioception, vibratory sense and awareness of distance between two simultaneously applied pointed objects to the skin. Stereognosis, or texture sense which is more or less the summation of many of these sensations is also appreciated. These cells, while called unipolar, are actually bipolar units whose afferent and

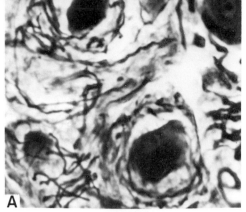

A

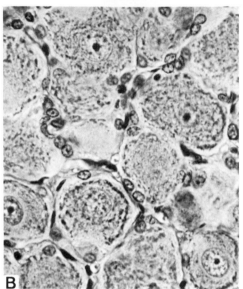

B

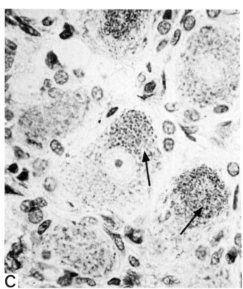

C

efferent limbs have become fused together when they approach the cell body. The cells are characteristically encapsulated with a glial type of element (satellite cell) which forms a very close investment into which project cytoplasmic processes from the ganglion cells (Fig. 20**A, D**). Connective tissue elements form a second outer capsule round these satellite cells (Fig. 20**A, B, C**). The unipolar cell is found in only one part of the central nervous system. This is in the nucleus mesencephalicus of the Vth nerve which is located in the ventral lateral margin of the *substantia intermedia centralis* of the midbrain. Its function is believed to be concerned with proprioception from the muscles of mastication.

3.1.2 Bipolar cells

Fig. 21, 1, 2. These are cells which have an axon and one dendrite. They are characteristically found in the visual, auditory and olfactory systems. The retina of the eye has, in a sense, two types of bipolar cells. One is the actual receptive cell which has an afferent light-sensitive process (rod or cone) followed by the cell body from which arises an axonal process which passes deeper into the retina to synapse with a second type of bipolar cell which has more the characteristics of a neuron. This in turn synapses with a cell which projects the light impulse further within the central nervous system to regions concerned with interpretation of the signal. The construction of the receptor element in the auditory system is somewhat analogous. It starts with a neuro-epithelial hair cell which is stimulated in some way by an auditory impulse. The next cell in the auditory pathway is a true bipolar (**1**) neuron. This cell has a dendritic (afferent) ending around the base of the hair cell. The cell bodies are accumulated in a spiral ganglion within the bony modiolus of the inner ear. Their axons project into the central nervous system.

The bipolar cell is also observed in the olfactory system. In this instance (at least in rabbit) there is a coarse rod-shaped process which terminates at the surface of the olfactory epithelium where its terminal end may show some specialization in structure. The centrally directed process which terminates on more typical neurons in the olfactory bulb is much finer. One might note that the bipolar cells which have been described are all located in the rather specialized sensory systems.

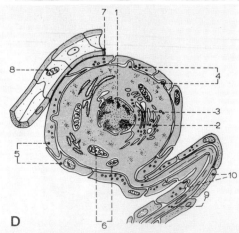

D

Fig. 20. A, silver preparation showing the complicated glomerular tangle of the single process of a dorsal root ganglion as it passes through the capsular elements; **B,** light cells in the dorsal root ganglion of young adult; **C,** dorsal root ganglion cells from an elderly person with accumulations of lipofuchsin in the cell (arrows); **D,** cell of the dorsal root ganglion with surrounding layer of satellite cells.
1, nucleus, **2,** nucleolus; **3,** Golgi apparatus; **4,** parafiti; **5,** satellites; **6,** mitochondria; **7,** basement membrane; **8,** capillary; **9,** neuronal process with **10,** periaxonic satellites.

3.1.3 Multipolar cells

Fig. 21, 4-13. The remaining neurons may all be classed as multipolar. They have a single axon but more than one dendrite. The further classification of these cells then depends on the morphology of the cell bodies, *i.e.*, fusiform, basket, stellate, and pyramidal. While the principal cell types of the cerebral cortex are pyramidal, stellate and fusiform, variations within these categories provide up to 60 different forms. This may be illustrated by referring to the pyramidal cells of the cortex. They may differ in size, ranging from very small cells found near the surface of the cortex to giant pyramidal 'Betz' cells of the primary motor cortex. Pyramidal cells (**4**) may also vary somewhat in shape. The latter differences may be observed in the hippocampus in which its three layered cortex has been divided into four areas by Lorente de Nó[88]: CA_1, CA_2, CA_3, CA_4. As noted by Cajal[19], the pyramidal cells in what Lorente de Nó called CA_1, do not have a morphology identical to those in CA_3. Certain multipolar cells in the cerebral cortex have been described and noted to differ from other cortical cells in that (a) their axons go to the surface of the cortex instead of being corticofugal or (b) have axons which pass parallel to the surface of the cortex (cells of Cajal). The total number of cortical cells in both hemispheres has been estimated to be from 5 to 10 billion[1, 118].

The above cells have been described as having processes of two types, dendrites and axons. Functionally, dendrites transmit an impulse toward (afferent to) the cell body and form the receptive pole of the cell. The cell body including the axon hillock may in general also be considered as a part of the receptive pole of a neuron since axonal synapses from other cells are made on these structures as well as on dendrites. The axon transmits impulses away (efferent) from the cell body and dendritic zone. While the axon and dendrite are described in a way which suggests that an impulse may travel in only one direction, such is only partially true. Only the synapse is unidirectional, while impulses may be propagated in both directions in the nerve fibers. The cell body or perikaryon plays a trophic role providing for synthetic functions through its RNA-protein components and may have nothing to do with the conducting polarization of a neuron[12] (see also p. 100).

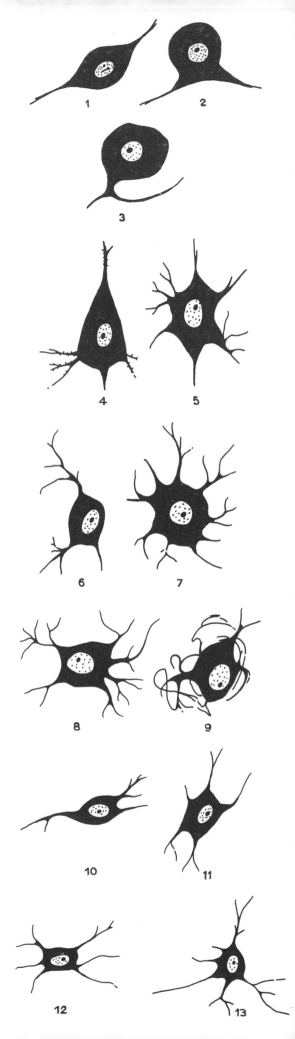

Fig. 21. Various neuronal cell types **Sensory neurons** — **1**, bipolar; **2**, pseudobipolar; **3**, pseudounipolar; **Motoneurons** — **4**, pyramidal cell; **5**, spinal cord; **6**, nucl. ambiguous; **7**, nucl. n. hypoglossi; **Sympathetic neurons** — **8**, stellate ganglion; **9**, sup. cervical ganglion; **10**, intermediolateral column; **Parasympathetic neurons** — **11**, myenteric ganglion; **12**, dorsal vagal nucl.; **13**, ciliary ganglion.

3.1.4 Glial cells

Figs. 22, 23. These are the inner supporting cells of the CNS. As previously indicated, there are three main types, the *astroglia* (**1**), *oligodendroglia* (**2**), and *microglia* (**4**). The term glia which is applied to these cells is most appropriate. The word glia ($\gamma\lambda\iota\alpha$) means glue and while these cells have other functions, they do literally glue the CNS together.

(i) *Astrocytes* (astroglia, also macroglia) are described as being of two types, fibrous and protoplasmic, depending on their morphological configuration with certain stains. They have irregularly oval nuclei with only a small amount of chromatin and although present in Fig. 23, nucleoli are not normally observed. The cytoplasm as seen in light-microscopic preparations is scanty. With the electron microscope, the cell emerges as a rather large unit, with many much convoluted processes interwoven around the fibers of the nerve cells. Many of these projections form foot like attachments around the capillaries, enclosing them so thoroughly that there is very little capillary surface not associated with an astrocyte[117]. Such capillary surface that does not contact astrocyte feet may be in contact with an oligodendroglial cell or be completely bare. The cytoplasm of these large cells is similar to that of neurons and mitochondria (*cf.* p. 106) and other normal cell constituents are to be found scattered in the greatly convoluted extensions of the astrocyte cell body. While cells with protoplasmic (fuzzy) much branched processes and fibrous astrocytes have been described by light microscopy as being somewhat different types of cells, the picture seen by electron microscopy suggests that these differences are partly due to a molding of the external morphology to conform with the nature of its environment. Thus, in the cellular areas, it would tend to have a more branched appearance than it would in the fibrous white matter. In either case, it is a cell which is uniquely placed between the capillaries and the nerve cell body and is believed to be actually concerned with the transport of materials from the blood to the neuron and possibly of wastes back to the blood. It also forms a cellular bridge between capillaries and the ependyma lining the ventricular cavities and thus may be involved in the transport of materials between these two fluid containing compartments as well as being in a position to relate both the vascular and cerebrospinal fluid compartment to at least some nerve cells (Fig. 68). Astrocytes also contain very fine fibrils – which can only be seen by electron microscopy – which further distinguishes them from oligodendroglia. These are most abundant in fibrous astrocytes.

(ii) *Oligodendroglia* are smaller than astrocytes and have more basophilic, smaller nuclei. They, like the astrocyte (Fig. 23, **2**) do not normally have a readily visible nucleolus (**3**). There are fewer cytoplasmic processes than in the astrocyte and they have a more granular cytoplasm. Despite

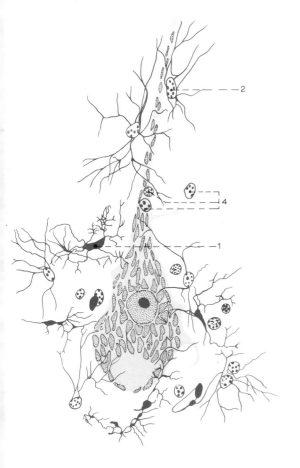

Fig. 22. A neuron surrounded by various glial elements.

these differences, the two may not always be easily distinguished by light microscopy although the more highly basophilic nuclens of the oligodendroglia cell is usually a dependable criterion. By electron microscopy the oligodendroglial cytoplasm is much denser than that of astrocytes, being filled with many more ribosomes. The presence of many transitional forms undoubtedly contributes to the problem, as does the presence of reactive forms.

Oligodendroglia are most numerous in the white matter and are responsible for the formation of myelin in the CNS. Those located in the nerve-cell rich areas are frequently found around the soma of neurons, hence the term satellite cell is frequently given to them in these locations. An increase in such satellites around a cell body has been observed in certain pathologic states. The complete understanding of the function of the glial cells as yet awaits resolution. It is apparent that oligodendroglia adjacent to nerve cells are not solely concerned with myelin formation or neuronophagia. Studies by Hamberger[58] suggest that oligodendroglia may have some trophic function in maintaining nerve cells while the astrocytes may be more specialized for transport activities. The problem is somewhat complicated by a lack of complete agreement as to the precise anatomical characteristics of astrocytes (**2**) and oligodendrocytes (**1**).

(iii) *Microglia* (**4**) are much smaller and more basophilic than the other types of glia. They spread by active migration through the CNS and have a phagocytic function. The nuclei are polymorphic and may be twisted into S or C shapes. A nucleolus is present. The cytoplasm is scanty under normal conditions and quite basophilic. Many long thin spiky processes arising from the cell body may be demonstrated with special techniques.

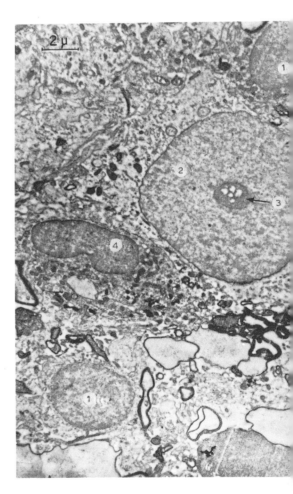

Fig. 23. White matter of an adult rabbit near a stab wound, containing various cell types (× 8000).
1, nucleus of oligodendrocyte; **2,** nucleus of astrocyte; **3,** nucleolus; **4,** nucleus of microglial cell.

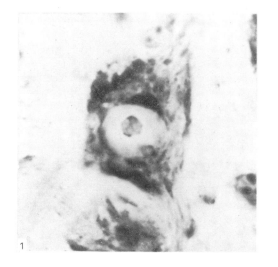

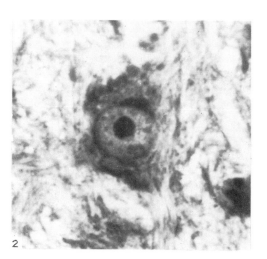

4. Maturation in the nervous system

4.1 Prenatal changes

The study of maturation and aging in the nervous system may be subdivided into two major areas. There are first developmental and morphological changes which are usually covered in embryology. Associated with these structural changes are increases in the protein and nucleoprotein content of the tissue as the cells become more differentiated. There are then those changes occurring after birth (in man and in many other mammals) which are initially concerned with maturation (growth, protein synthesis and myelinization). These are then succeeded by degenerative changes in older persons.

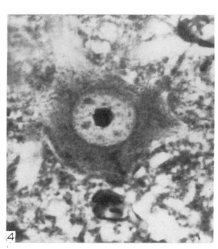

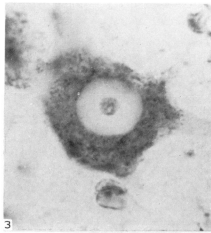

Fig. 24. 1 and 3 are chromatolytic cells of a 19- and 24-day-old hamster resp., after axon severance 4 days earlier (at 15 days and at 20 days). Buffered thionin stain for nucleic acid components.
2 and 4 are the same cells which were 'de-stained' and then restained for protein with mercuric bromphenol blue. In both cells, the distribution pattern of Nissl material is equivalent to that seen with thionin.
Diffuse chromatolysis and swelling occur only in the 20-day operative; 'focal' chromatolysis without swelling occurs in the 15-day operative.

Toward the end of gestation, gross examination indicates that myelinization has become evident, particularly in the more primitive systems and that the surface morphology resembles that of the adult. Various chemical changes have also occurred. Perhaps one of the most dramatic is the change in certain enzyme systems which enable the brain to convert its metabolic pathways from those which are anaerobic to those which are aerobic. Thus, as reported by Flexner et al.[45-49], the capacity of guinea pig cerebral cortex for aerobic glycolysis increases two-fold just prior to birth to reach adult levels of performance. The enzymes which Flexner demonstrated to be increased in activity in the last trimester of pregnancy or just before birth in the guinea pig are succinic dehydrogenase, succinoxidase, adenyl pyrophosphatase, and aldolase, while alkaline phosphatase levels decrease after birth[46, 49]. Whether or not identical changes occur in man can only be inferred. It may be noted, however, that the newborn human, like other mammalian species, can survive anoxia considerably longer than the adult. Acid phosphatase has been reported to change its location in the human Purkinje cell, being cytoplasmic at birth and extracellular in the adult[96]. How much of this may be related to postmortem artifact is difficult to ascertain, since the autopsies were performed 12–24 hours after death and it is well known that phosphatase diffuses readily.

Fig. 24. Some rather interesting changes in the nucleic acids precede the various changes in enzyme concentration in experimental animals. Cells of guinea pig cerebral and cerebellar cortex, the motor nuclei of the facial, trigeminal and 5th cervical nerves, the sensory ganglion cells of the trigeminal and 5th cervical nerves, and the mesencephalic nucleus of the trigeminal nerve were studied using techniques which demonstrated DNA and RNA[83]. During early development, the nerve cell nucleolus appears as a DNA rich structure, the chromocenter or fetal nucleolus. The DNA of the structure then appears to move peripherally until only a rim of DNA (Feulgen-positive material) is left. The remaining structure is Feulgen-negative and thionin-positive and is largely RNA plus protein.

The size and degree of thionin basophilia of the RNA 'adult type' of nucleolus vary from cell type to cell type. Regenerating neurons frequently show a reversion to the less mature nucleolar pattern in that the DNA Feulgen-positive material appears to become more dispersed through the nucleolus which then resembles that seen in less mature nucleoli. Lavelle[83] notes that the first sign of nucleolar maturation was always closely accompanied by a noticeable increase in Nissl substance in the cytoplasm. When nucleolar development was about intermediate in maturation, most of the 'DNA' chromocenter material was at the periphery, and Nissl substance was becoming more coarse and spicular. In mature cells, the less the quantity of Nissl substance, the less well advanced is the structure of the nucleolar apparatus. This is perhaps most clearly demonstrated by the granule cells of the cerebellar cortex which have a relatively Feulgen-positive, less mature nucleolus and relatively little Nissl substance in the cytoplasm. The changes which Lavelle reports for the nucleolar apparatus and Nissl substance are well under way by the 25th day of pregnancy in the guinea pig (68-day gestation period) and coincide with the first movements observed in fetal guinea pigs following stimulation of the forelimbs[13]. By 36 days, more fetuses per litter exhibit typical movements to stimulation (winking of an unopened eye, movements of the pinna and jaw)[20]. The correlation between the various studies suggests a definite relationship between the degree of behavioral response which may be elicited and the extent of development of the nucleolar-Nissl picture. Olszewski has called at-

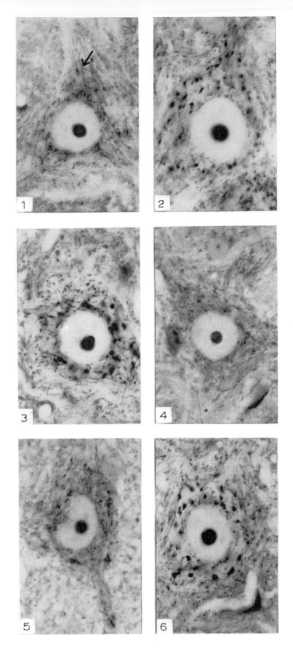

Fig. 25. Facial motor nerve cells of the postnatal hamster. Basic fuchsin-aniline blue stain for mitochondria. All magnifications are the same, taken with a 97 × objective and a 10 × eyepiece. **1,** is from the non-operated nuclear group at 24 days postnatal age. **2,** showing swollen mitochondria, is from the operated side of the same animal after axon severance 4 days earlier at 20 days of age. **3,** showing swollen mitochondria, is from a 50-day-old hamster after axon severance at 20 days. **4** and **5** are control and injured cells, respectively, from a 19-day-old hamster after facial nerve was severed 4 days earlier at 15 days postnatal age. **6** is a cell in a 46-day-old animal after axon severance at 15 days of age with mitochondrial swelling. **7** and **8** are control and injured cells, respectively, from an 11-day-old hamster operated 4 days earlier at 7 days of age. **9** is an injured cell from a 39-day-old hamster, after nerve severance at 7 days of age. Mitochondrial swelling is evident only in the older animal.

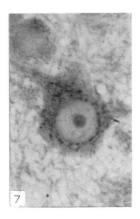
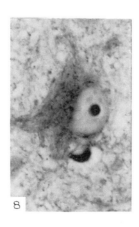
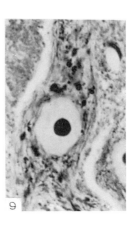

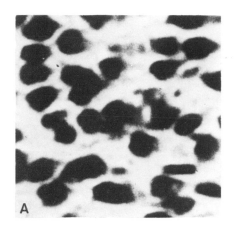

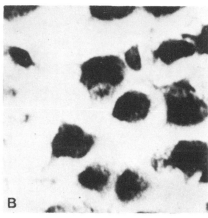

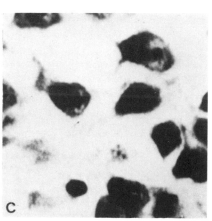

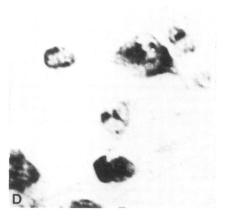

tention to similar nucleolar-Nissl relationships in the hippocampus of the human[97].

A considerable literature exists dealing with the appearance of behavioral responses to stimuli in the human fetus[16, 62–64, 145]. If one may summarize briefly, it would appear that different reflexes appear at different times, those associated with the 'avoidance' type reactions as might be related to the more primitive pain and temperature systems being extremely early. Those associated with oral function also occur quite early, and may reflect the phylogenetically primitive oral relationship of an animal toward its environment. The ability to demonstrate the reflex depends on the establishment of neuronal connections between physiologically active receptors and effectors. Some degree of dependence on the formation of Nissl substance in the nerve cell appears important in the functioning of the cells involved in the reflex reactions during these early periods. As the reflexes become more complex, some reliance on increased collateralization also seems apparent.

4.2 Postnatal changes

4.2.1 Maturational changes

Fig. 26. Study of the cerebral cortex of subprimates may provide much information useful in understanding what occurs in man[101]. The rat, guinea pig and rabbit have been extensively used, even though the extent of development at birth is not entirely the same as in man. At birth, the cerebral cortex of the rat shows an extremely dense neuronal pattern with the individual cortical laminae very hard to observe[36]. By the 6th day, there is an increase in cell size (increase in synthesis of protein) and layers III and IV are distinguishable. By the 18th day, all the cortical layers are visible. Few axons are present at birth. Those occurring first run tangential to the cortical surface. Bundles of radially oriented fibers, presumably thalamic afferents do not appear until between the 12th and 18th days. Very few dendrites appear before the 6th day, but exhibit rapid growth and multiplication after the 12th day. Thus, at birth the cortex of the rat consists largely of cells, both neuronal and glial. The neurons are small, containing little Nissl substance and do not yet possess their characteristic (pyramidal, stellate, etc.) shapes. Dendrites and axons are very sparse. Extremely rapid growth and protein synthesis ensues accompanied by enlargement in cell size, growth of axons and dendrites with the establishment of neuronal connections[113]. Structures such as

Fig. 26. Micrographs of Nissl-stained preparations to show changes in packing density of cortical neurons and in the appearance of the Nissl substance. **A,** layer II/III of the cerebral cortex of a 2-day-old rabbit; **B,** 10-day-old animal; **C,** 20-day-old animal; **D,** adult rabbit.

the corpus callosum, which contains commissural fibers, are not well developed. These cortical growth patterns seem to occur later than those noted previously for the Vth and VIIth nerves for man and other animals. Thus, lower brain stem and cord maturation, to the point of there being well developed neurons with an established neuropil (nerve cell processes, glial and vascular structures) in which synaptic connections and established reflexes are found, appears to occur earlier than in the higher cortical centers.

TABLE 1

SOME NEURONAL PARAMETERS DURING POSTNATAL MATURATION OF THE HUMAN CEREBRAL CORTEX

(Layer III, middle frontal gyrus)

	Newborn	6 Months	24 Months	Adult
Packing density ($\times 10^3$/mm^3)	99.0	30.5	20.1	12.5
Volume cell body (μ^3)	240	610	990	1040
Number of branching points of dendrites	3.1	15.6	16.7	40.8
Total length of dendrites (μ)	203	2367	3259	6836

Similar studies have been done with man[115]. It was found that the nucleus of cortical cells in the human newborn, like those of the neonatal rat, is very large in proportion to the volume of cytoplasm. However, the stratification of the human cortex at birth is almost identical to the adult, indicating a considerable advance over the rat. Cell size increases considerably with age, the rate being greatest in the first 3 months for the pyramidal cells of layers II and layer VI. The increase in cell size appeared more gradual for the granule and small pyramidal cells of layer IV. An increase in neuropil was also noted since the nerve cell density decreased from 60.5 ± 5.7 in the newborn to 6.0 ± 0.7 in the adult in cortical layer V (mid frontal gyrus).

This was accompanied by a change in the grey cell coefficient (GCC) which changed from 36 to 66 for the same layer. The GCC is a measure of the ratio of the volume of grey matter to the volume of nerve cells in it. Thus the only two-fold increase in the GCC, while the neuron density decreased 10-fold, raises the question as to how the neuron density can change so greatly. It must be remembered that layers V and III contain the larger pyramidal cells which will have a greater increase in volume/cell ratio than will occur for cells in layer IV. Thus, while the cell number/unit area may decrease markedly in layers III and V (as pointed out by Brody[14]) the volume of cortex occupied by the nerve cells in the pyramidal cell layers does not change as drastically. Brody[14] performed cell counts on human cerebral cortex and noted a marked decrease in number with age, there being from 2,500 to 3,800 cells/unit area at birth and only from 864 to 1,382/unit area in the adult. The decrease in cell number/unit area was noted to be more apparent than real, however, since the extreme expansion of the components of the neuropil greatly thickens the cortex, while dispersing the cells further from each other. Many cells may also be dying from varying causes. In the human brain no Nissl substance was present in any cell of the middle frontal gyrus (region reported in detail[115]) of the newborn. Dustlike particles were seen in some of the larger cells of layer V. The scarcity of Nissl substance in cortical cells is in contrast with the marked development of Nissl substance in neurons of the brain stem and spinal cord at birth and earlier. At 3 to 6 months of age the Nissl substance is more advanced and by two years of age, the Nissl material is almost comparable to that of the adult. The changes observed in regard to DNA and RNA in the nucleolus of the guinea pig[82] were also observed in the cells of the human middle frontal gyrus cortex in the 3, 6 and 15 month old infant.

Fig. 27. At birth, the dendritic pattern of the human newborn cerebral cortex is hardly better than the rat and doesn't begin to approach the adult state until 24 months, when the complexity is still somewhat less than that of the adult. At birth, only the pyramidal cells of layer V show any degree of basal dendrite formation, while the dendrites of stellate cells of layer V and VI are rather well developed (the unbranched stalks of the apical dendrites are well developed). However, the closer one approaches to the surface of the cortex, the less well developed is the dendrite pattern of even these cells. The number of branches per dendrite

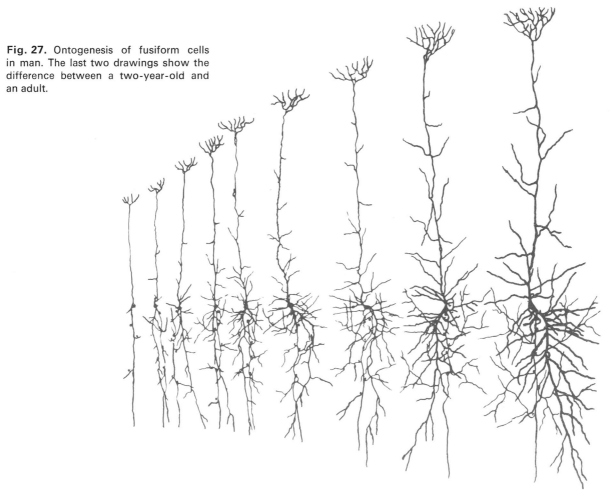

Fig. 27. Ontogenesis of fusiform cells in man. The last two drawings show the difference between a two-year-old and an adult.

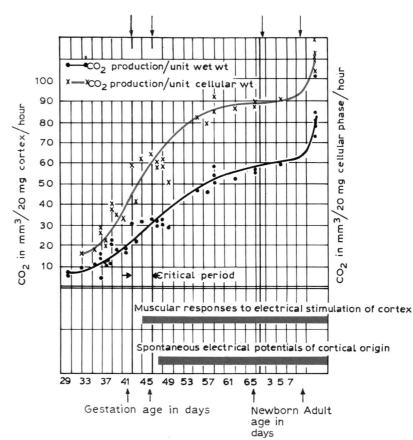

Fig. 28. Example of interdisciplinary developmental study of the cerebral cortex of the Guinea pig. Acetylcholinesterase activity of the motor cortex of the fetal and adult Guinea pig per unit total wet weight and per unit of cellular wet weight.

and the length of the dendrite was observed to increase from birth to adulthood. Thus, man, like the rodent, has relatively incompletely developed cortical neurons at birth. This refers not only to the branching processes but to the Nissl substance associated with cellular synthetic processes[101]. One must presume that the extent to which development occurs, with the formation of synaptic connections, plays some role in the subsequent performance of the individual. One might note from studies by Eayrs[35-37] on the effect of protein starvation and hypothyroidism that the dietary state and hormonal situation are both very important in the development of neurons, both starvation and hypothyroidism serving to depress maturation markedly.

Electron microscopy of the developing cortex of the cat after birth (Pappas[101]) reveals the greatly changing picture in relation to dendrites most clearly. At birth they are not only very poorly developed, but possess few axonal synaptic junctions. By six days, numerous synaptic terminations have occurred and the dendrites have developed a rather extensive degree of branching. By 12 days, the cat cortex is essentially comparable to that of the adult as far as the development of fine dendrite processes and the establishment of synapses goes.

The rat, cat and other mammals, have been utilized in studying the maturation of the cerebellar cortex[106]. It, like the cerebral cortex, undergoes considerable maturation after birth, which can be readily visualized with ordinary staining procedures. At birth, the rat cerebellum is grossly very poorly developed, with only a few folia. Twenty-four hours after birth is a period in which cell types are not easily recognized. Purkinje cells are not greatly larger than granule cells and Nissl substance is not

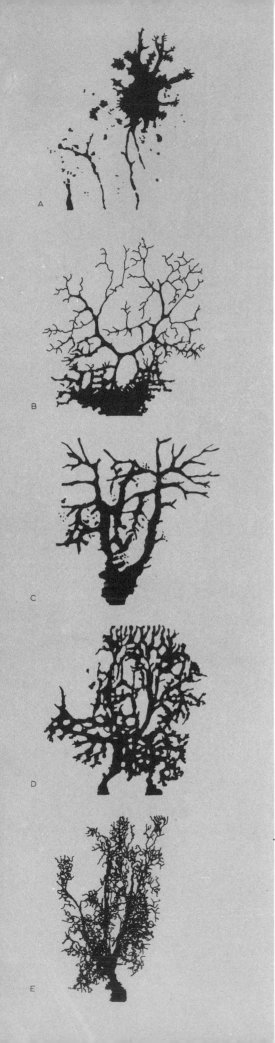

clearly evident since the nucleus takes up so much of the cell volume. The most outstanding observation is the presence of two well developed granule layers. There is an external layer which blends with the pial-glial membrane. The granule cells of this external layer appear to migrate slowly toward the deeper layer, as determined by radioautographic studies. The migration also seems apparent with ordinary preparations. The external granule layer is still present 17 days after birth, though reduced to being only about 4 cells deep. The slow reduction of the external granule layer is accompanied by a thickening of the deep granule layer until finally the external granule layer has completed its migration, being virtually absent in the adult. It has been postulated that this migration permits the establishment of synaptic connections. Since the details of the development of dendritic processes in these cells at this age remain uncertain, this claim may be premature. The external granule cell layer gives rise to both basket and stellate cells of the molecular layer.

Fig. 29. Purkinje cells are just discernable 4 days after birth in rat. Though Nissl substance is not well established, the cytoplasm is highly basophilic, indicating a high concentration of ribosomal material not associated with the endoplasmic reticulum. These cells are still larger at 17 days of age when their size appears comparable to that seen in adults. Nissl granules at 17 days of age in adults are still not clearly defined, though cytoplasmic basophilia was intense. It would appear that the Purkinje cells of different species can not be too closely compared, since clearly defined Nissl material was seen in the Guinea pig by the third trimester of pregnancy as well as after birth. In man, too, Nissl substance is clearly defined. The studies with the rat have, however, been useful in that it has enabled us to study the migration of the cells of the external granule layer into the deeper layer. This has answered a long standing question concerning the nature of the cells of the external layer. The same sequence of events has also been observed in the cat cerebellum[95]. Fig. 29 shows a series of Golgi studies on the postnatal maturation of Purkinje cells.

An external granule layer is also seen in man at birth and similar migrations occur. Of particular interest is the observation that some of the Purkinje cells of man are derived mitotically from the external granule layer. Toward the end of the third month of gestation cells migrate centripetally toward the internal granule layer, assuming an intermediate position. This lamina of cells will later become the Purkinje cell layer. Recognizable Purkinje cells have been reported in the anterior lobe of the vermis as early as the fourth month. Their differentiation in other parts of the cerebellar cortex occurs in later intra-uterine life. The matu-

Fig. 29. Microphotographs of Purkinje cells revealed in 200 μ thick Golgi–Cox sections of cerebellum in kittens of various ages. A, 2-day-old kitten. Main stem dendrites are short, occasionally branched and have several protuberances. Dendrite-like ramifications are seen emerging from the cell body. B and C, 2 different stages of Purkinje cell development seen in the same section but from different parts of the cerebellum in an 8-day-old kitten. D, 20-day-old kitten; E, 42-day-old kitten.

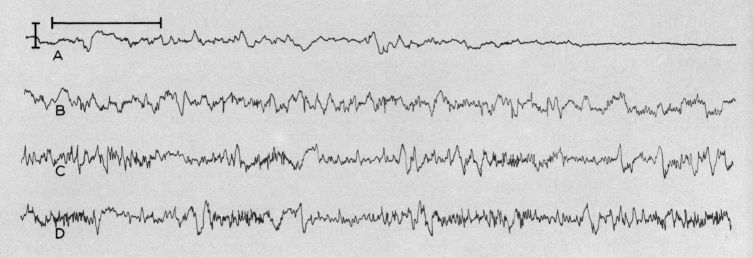

Fig. 30. EEG records during development, **A,** EEG of 8-day-old rabbit. Recording from frontal cortex, light urethane narcosis. **B,** EEG of 12-day-old rabbit. Recording from parietal cortex, light urethane narcosis. **C,** EEG of adult rabbit. Recording from parietal cortex, unanesthetized curarized preparation. **D,** EEG of same animal, lightly anesthetized with urethane. Calibration: horizontal line indicates 10 sec, vertical line indicates 1 mV.

ration of these cells spreads first over the rest of the vermis and later to the inferior and then superior surface of the hemispheres. Sulci formation in the human cerebellum parallels or follows closely the maturation of Purkinje cells. Thus, sulci appear, first in the vermis and then extend laterally, paralleling the march of histological differentiation across the cortex[32].

Studies on electrolytes of maturing rat brain tissue have revealed additional interesting facts[135]. Potassium increased while sodium and chloride levels decreased. Water also decreased from about 89 to 81%. The spinal cord showed similar changes but reached a lower level being only 70-71% in the adult. It has also been shown that there is less water in myelinated areas than in grey matter. With the decrease in total sodium and chloride, there was a decrease in the sodium and chloride space from about 45 to between 20 and 30%. This figure, long considered to represent the extracellular water space may actually be largely intraglial since there is only a small extracellular space in the brain.

Total nitrogen of the rat brain increased rapidly after birth, paralleling the increase in nerve cell size. Acid soluble nitrogen (free amino acid) remained constant from birth till adulthood. Bound protein, however, increased from 1.0 g/100 g of wet weight to about 1.5 g/100 g. Glutamic acid, γ-aminobutyric, aspartic acid and glutamine increased during maturation. The four amino acids which increased (of the four glutamic acid increases the most) are the four predominant free amino acids in the brain. Thus, protein increased with increase in cell size and number of processes and the protein increase is inversely proportional to the decrease in total water. In man, total CNS protein increases through fetal life (3.77 to 3.98% of fresh tissue) to 8.99% of fresh tissue at 35 years. By the 67th year a slight drop has occurred with the protein being 7.54%. This may be associated with an actual decrease in nerve cell population.

While the total amount of protein present/unit weight of brain in-

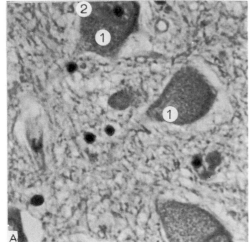

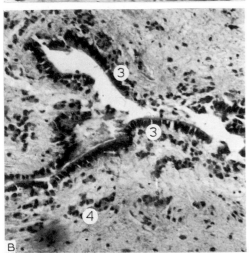

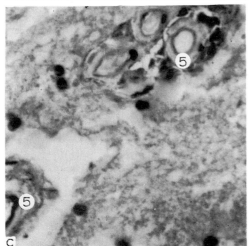

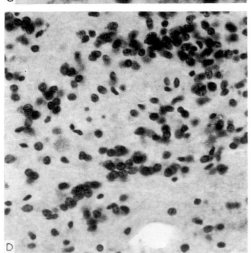

creases with age, certain other features of protein metabolism regress, at least in experimental animals. Winzler[147] noted that the ability of the adult mouse brain to synthesize amino acids from ¹⁴C-glucose was limited to glutamate, aspartic acid and glycine, while the newborn mouse showed a significant incorporation of the ¹⁴C label into essential amino acids as well. This infers a considerable change in enzyme activity which may be associated with the large increase in the glial components interposed between the nerve cells and capillaries which occurs with aging. At least the increase in these glial units has been used to explain the decrease in incorporation of labeled amino acids which occurs as the animals grow older. However, the greater rates and amounts of incorporation of amino acids into the brain protein in young animals may be closely related to the high rates of growth of neurons and myelinization rather than to any restrictive role played by the increased number of glial cells or to a blood–brain barrier.

The changes in brain protein are accompanied by a considerable increase in the brain lipids associated with the myelinization of axons[15, 50]. Those indicated in the following table for white matter (Table 2) demonstrate a marked increase in the total lipids as well as some of the components of cerebral lipids.

TABLE 2

SUMMARY OF THE RESULTS OF BRONTE[15] ON LIPID COMPOSITION OF BRAIN WHITE MATTER AT DIFFERENT AGES

(Expressed as percent weight of fresh tissue)

	Fetus 4-9 months	Child 2-5 months	Child 2-5 years	Child 10-19 years
Total lipid	2.88	7.60	14.10	18.60
Phosphatides	1.68	3.84	6.25	8.10
Cholesterol	0.45	1.38	3.06	4.23
Cerebrosides	0.31	1.58	3.34	4.20

Fig. 31. Various non specific changes which may occur in the brain with advancing age.
A, 1, cluster of lipofuscin loaded cells from the hypoglossal nucleus of a 102-year-old female (× 440). **B,** variation in the appearance of the adult central canal (of a man in his sixth decade) (× 275). During life, the ependymal cells (**3**) of the central canal are gradually encroached upon by an ingrowth of glial cells and fibers. This may start in early childhood. **4,** considerable increase in the number of surrounding glial cells. **C, 5,** adventitial fibrosis in the small arteries of the same spinal cord as in **B** (× 275). **D,** complete obliteration of the central canal in a man of about the same age (× 275).

4.2.2 Maturational myelinization

A further aspect of the maturation of the nervous system is concerned with the formation of myelin sheaths around the axonal processes. This aspect of structural differentiation does not proceed in a disorganized manner, but follows a predictable pattern in relation to anatomical locus or system of fibers. There is a primordial group in which myelinization started before birth (pre- and postcentral gyri, the calcarine cortex and adjacent areas, the gyrus uncinatus, the hippocampus and subiculum, the middle third of the gyrus fornicatus and the transverse temporal gyri). A second group consists of areas in which myelin formation starts at about the time of birth. This involves a fairly large area of cortex and consists of all those areas not listed in group one and three.

In the third group, myelinization occurs after birth and involves the middle and inferior frontal gyri, the inferior parietal lobule, the middle and inferior temporal gyri and part of the gyrus fornicatus. Those areas in which myelin first appears tend to be associated with those sulci and their adjacent gyri which first appear and which have an association with the reception of sensory information (sensory–motor, calcarine and auditory cortices), or have subcortical associations. These are also the phylogenetically older areas. Those areas in which myelinization occurs latest tend to be phylogenetically newer and tend to be concerned with intracortical connections.

4.2.3 Postnatal growth of the brain

At birth, the brain of the newborn child is exceptionally large in relation to the total body weight and may exceed 10% of the total weight. By adulthood, the weight of the brain is about 2% of the total body weight, despite having increased in size from about 350 g at birth to 1250 g in girls and 1375 g in boys. Most of this growth occurs during the first year when the weight increases from 350 to about 1000 g.

Since the only nerve cells of the mammalian brain known to exhibit cell division after birth are the granular cells of the hippocampus and cerebellum (primarily in rodents; Altman and Das[2, 3]) the considerable growth which occurs after birth must deal with growth of the nerve cell bodies and their processes and with an increase in the glial supporting elements, rather than with a further increase in the nerve cell population. The fact that neurons start to die after birth accentuates even further the fact that the postnatal growth of the brain is due to the growth of the approximately 20,000,000,000 neurons which are present at birth and with the myelinization of their fibers. Some additional weight increment may also be attributed to the proliferation of vascular units within the brain parenchyma. A large part of this weight increase must also be ascribed to the formation of myelin by the oligodendroglia.

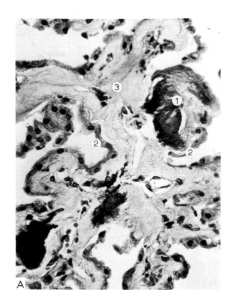

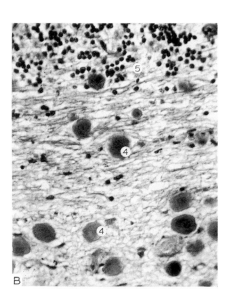

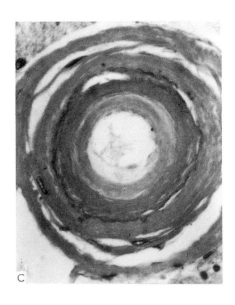

4.2.4 Vascular and metabolic changes

Fig. 31, 32. Vascular changes occur commonly with increasing age. Atherosclerosis of cerebral vessels, frequently quite advanced, is often seen at autopsy. The elastic lamina of cerebral vessels undergoes reduplication with advancing age and frequently loses its normal staining properties. The media undergoes fibrosis and may appear hyalinized. The vessel walls are in general thicker and less pliable in older individuals. The thickening of the arterial walls, frequently with atherosclerosis, decreases the blood supply to the brain, thus producing an ischemic state. There seems little room to doubt but that the changes in the vascular tree to the brain contribute considerably to the marked reduction of the nerve cells in extreme old age. It is questionable as to how effectively the remaining cells function with this reduced blood supply. Some intimation of the effect of these vascular changes has been reported[4, 22, 71].

For the general population of elderly people, there was a decrease in oxygen (18% for normal adult) and glucose utilization, in cerebral blood flow (ml/100 g tissue/min) and an increase in cerebrovascular resistance with increasing age. In contrast, a highly selected group of normal elderly men who functioned effectively in their communities and were free of disease (including vascular), had cerebral blood flow and oxygen utilization rates comparable to normal young men. A similar group of elderly men afflicted with mild asymptomatic or subclinical disease, chiefly vascular, all showed a significant decrease in cerebral blood flow. Oxygen consumption was lower, but not significantly depressed. All of the reduction in cerebral blood flow and oxygen consumption could be accounted for by the atherosclerotic subjects. Therefore, it would appear that when vascular disease is present, it may be an underlying factor in the 'age changes' which occur, since it would be associated with a relative cerebral circulatory insufficiency and hypoxia. This does not of course preclude other factors. Glucose utilization was significantly reduced in both normal and atherosclerotic subjects. In the normal group, this apparently had no serious sequelae, while in the atherosclerotic group it may have aggravated an already serious situation. In any event, alterations in carbohydrate metabolism occur in the aged which need not be paralleled by change in blood flow or oxygen consumption. The significance of decrease in glucose utilization remains to be resolved.

Fig. 32. A, section through the choroid plexus; **B,** section through the substantia alba of the cerebellum. Both represent certain non specific changes which occur with advancing age (102-year-old woman; × 275). There are commonly regions of calcification (**1**) seen in the choroid plexus of older individuals. The ependymal lining cells (**2**) become flattened and there is an increase in collagen fibers (**3**) in the stroma. Corpora amylacea (**4**) are frequently observed in the white matter near the ventricular cavities of older individuals, as in **B** where they may be observed in the cerebellar white matter. The adjacent granule layer (**5**) is also indicated. **C,** This is a large cerebellar artery within the pia which has undergone mineralization, which is typically concentric (102-year-old woman; × 440). Such changes are more commonly seen in the arteries of the globus pallidus, at the inner angle of the hippocampus and in the substantia alba of the cerebellum. The degree to which mineralization occurs is usually greater in the veins.

4.3 Gross and histologic changes with advanced age

Fig. 33. The changes in the brain vascular system which occur with age may be associated with certain gross changes in the CNS of elderly people. The word 'may' is used intentionally, since not all vascular systems show the same degree of 'aging'. Yet, the gross changes in the brain occur, even when the vessels are strikingly normal. A marked cortical atrophy, restricted frequently to the frontal lobe and superior parietal lobe is often seen. The sulci appear quite broad. This is accompanied by an increase in the size of the ventricular system and a decrease in white matter. This decrease in total brain parenchyma undoubtedly is the cause for reports of decrease in brain weight with age. The leptomeninges of such older brains are also thicker than in younger persons. Hypertrophy of the Pacchionian granulations is also said to occur, and there may be patches of calcification in the meninges. Cortical atrophy of the cerebellum is also apparent in that the anterior and posterior lobes may be seen to be retracted somewhat from the brachium pontis.

Certain histologic changes in neurons may also be observed. Thus, there may be an obvious decrease in the number of cells per volume of cortex, which exceeds that observed during the maturation of the cortex wherein the great expansion of the neuropil tends to disperse cells further from each other[76]. Purkinje cells appear particularly susceptible to varying 'environmental' conditions and are greatly reduced in number. The larger pyramidal cells of cortical layer V also seem to decrease relatively more rapidly than others, with the result that the primary motor cortex of a man in his 60's may be hard to identify on the basis of its cell population. Cells change in size, being smaller than in young adults, and there is a decrease in Nissl substance. The nucleus may be crenated or angular in outline and more basophilic (due to shrinkage). The nucleolus in many cells reverts to that seen in more primitive or regenerating cells in that the peripheral rim of DNA becomes less clumped and therefore becomes more obvious. Extra nucleoli and bilobed or double nuclear structures have also been reported in Purkinje cells, cells of the supraoptic and paraventricular nuclei and cells of the substantia nigra. Such multiple nuclear configuration is not necessarily restricted to older persons in that a teenage boy killed accidentally was observed to have many autonomic ganglion cells with double or even triple nuclei.

Changes in the neurofibrils have also been seen to occur with advancing age. They become thicker and more clumped together, with varicosities and thickened fused strands adjacent to the cell surface. The complex whorls of neurofibrillar material reported in Alzheimer's senile psychosis also apparently occur in more 'normal' aging individuals. Since the role of the neurofibril remains to be ascertained, the significance of these observations is uncertain.

The number of *amyloid bodies* (corpora amylacea) also increases with age (Fig. 32 **B, 4**). The precise origin of these round bodies of various size

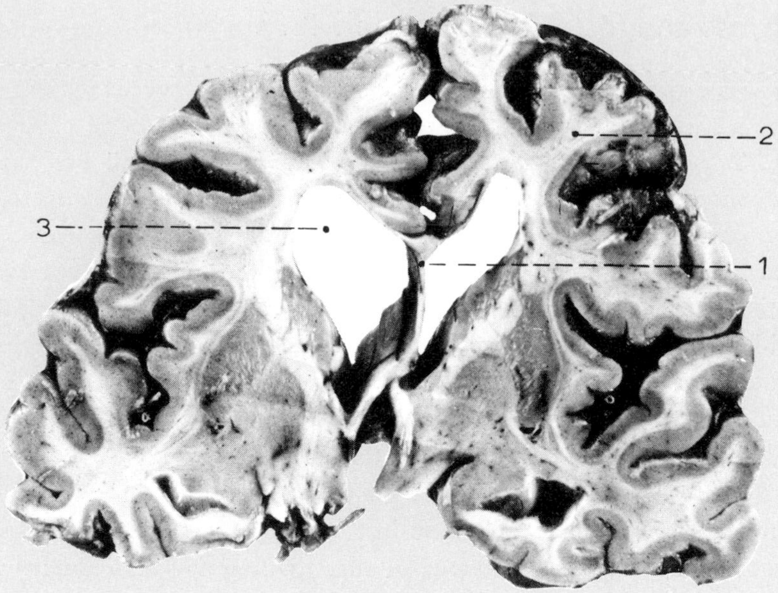

Fig. 33. Two sections in the coronal plane through the septum pellucidum (1). A, from an old man and shows marked shrinkage of the white matter (2), enlargement of cornu anterius of ventriculus lateralis (3), and extensive sulcal widening. B, from a male adult of 45 to 50 years of age.

A

is uncertain, although Liss[87] claims that they are the end products of degeneration of almost all of the cellular elements of the brain. The greatest accumulation occurs near ventricular surfaces.

Satellitosis is also said to increase with age, again with uncertain significance. In some instances, there is undoubtedly increased neuronophagia. Since the relationship between glial and nerve cells appears extremely complex, involving the vital trophic function of the nerve cells, an explanation for increased satellitosis based solely on neuronophagia appears an oversimplification with little proof to support it. Brownson[17] also notes an interesting change in the type of glial cell associated with the neuron, reporting a slight increase in the number of satellites which are oligodendroglia and a decrease which are astrocytes.

Very soon after birth, refractive granules appear in human neurons. They are stainable with osmium tetroxide and are faintly yellowish green when unstained, becoming darker with age. This material is what is termed 'lipofuscin' and is generally conceived as representing a 'wear and tear substance' (Fig. 31, A, 1). The pigment molecule seems to be a lipoprotein plus a complex chromophore which according to Hydén and Lindström[68] contains pterine. It is just detectable in anterior horn cells during the first decade of life. It may accumulate to such large amounts in subsequent years as to deform the cell. This is quite marked in the cells of the inferior olive. It is also present in sensory cells, but is never more than scantily present in Purkinje cells. It varies in amount in different areas of the CNS and is found in other primates, old cattle and guinea pigs. It has frequently been stated that this pigment does not interfere with the function of a nerve cell. However, since the cell content of RNA-P decreases at a rate roughly commensurate to the increase in pigment in anterior horn cells, one wonders if this is completely true. If RNA-P is essential for the synthesis of nerve cell protein and enzymes,

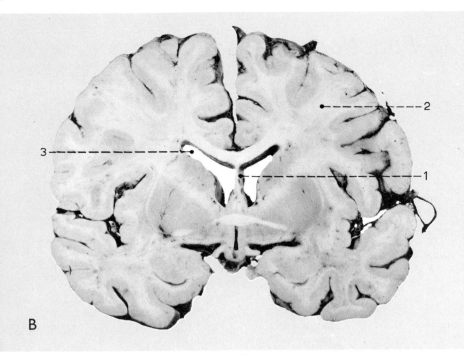

B

it would seem that a deficiency in the trophic functions of a nerve cell, which need not necessarily be accompanied by a deficiency in impulse propagation, might occur. Such neurons might be considered as fatiguing more readily.

4.4 Glial changes

Changes in astrocytes occur which are comparable to those in neurons. Some protoplasm often appears to contain a yellow rather granular pigment. In view of current ideas concerning the function of astrocytes as pathways between capillaries and nerve cells, such accumulations may eventually be shown to be deleterious to the function of the nerve cell. Glial fibers increase in the subpial zone, spreading deeper into the cortex, particularly along perforating vessels. There is also a general increase in glial fibers in the striatum with advancing years.

The accentuation of glial fibers around the vessels of the globus pallidus more or less parallels changes in the vessels which are prone to have a degeneration of the elastic layer with a deposit of calcium and iron. Oligodendroglia and microglia appear to undergo very little change with age though it has been said, with little proof, that microglia respond less rapidly as phagocytes in older brains.

The foregoing comments represent but a brief introduction to a subject which increases in importance each year. The longer life expectancy of man is introducing many new problems related to gerontology which are only recently being investigated. It is to be anticipated that our understanding will improve rapidly, however, as various investigators pool their interests in joint efforts directed toward extending our knowledge of the function of the normal and abnormal brain.

5. Functional subdivisions

5.1 Telencephalon

Figs. 34, 35. In the adult, the telencephalon becomes divided into frontal
(**1**), parietal (**2**), occipital (**3**) and temporal (**4**) lobes. Each of these
divisions becomes further subdivided by grooves (sulci) into smaller
elevations (gyri). A fifth 'lobe' may be described which includes parts
of the frontal, parietal and temporal lobes. This is the *limbic* lobe (*cf.*
Fig. 36) which is a C-curved structure extending completely around the
diencephalon.

A small area of cortex remains which may not be considered as being
part of any one particular lobe. This is the insular cortex which is overgrown by the frontal, temporal and parietal lobe and thus comes to lie
in the deep sulcus lateralis (Sylvian) on the lateral surface (see also Figs.
37, 38). Its functional relations appear to be somewhat concerned with
the viscera. The cortex overlying the insula is frequently called the *operculum*. There is a part of the telencephalon which is deep to the surface
cortex and underlying white matter and seen only in sections. It is
referred to as the basal nuclear complex and consists of the *caudate
nucleus*, *putamen*, *globus pallidus*, *claustrum* and *amygdala* (*cf.* Fig. 39). These
nuclei appear in many planes of section and vary somewhat in configuration in each.

The function of the subdivisions may be loosely described as follows.

5.1.1 Frontal lobe

The function of the frontal lobe (**1**) concerns voluntary motor function,
the organization of the motor units necessary for expressive speech or
language communication, and some contribution toward what may be
called 'original' thinking or evaluation of ideas. The cortical localization
of these 'functions' may be more precisely stated (Fig. 85). Thus, the
cortex of the precentral gyrus (area 4) forms a primary motor area with a
relatively specific separation into smaller areas for different regions of the
body. The face is represented on the lower third of the gyrus, with an
upright orientation; the hand, with a large proportion of the cortex
concerned with thumb movements, occupies the middle third, followed
by the trunk and hip in the upper third. The localization of a motor
cortex for the lower leg in area 4 is on the rostral portion of the para-
central lobule on the medial surface.

A premotor area, which exists just rostral to the primary motor cortex,
occupies the caudal part of three horizontally oriented frontal gyri
(area 6). Associated with this is a so-called frontal eye field (corresponds
to the inferior part of area 8) located in about the middle or caudal end

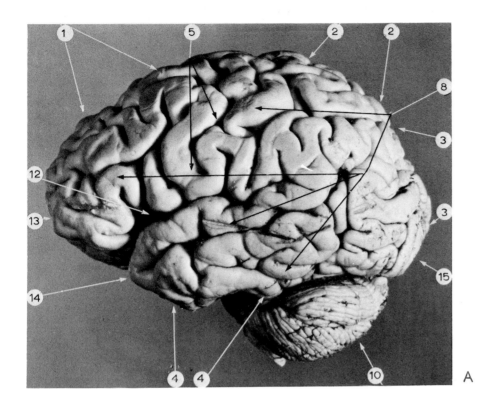

A

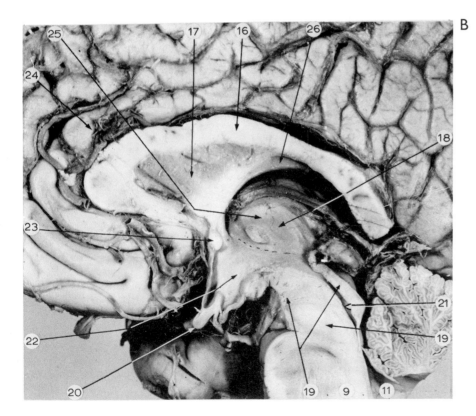

B

Fig. 34. A, lateral, and B, midsagittal view of the brain.
5, sulcus centralis; 8, cerebral gyri; 9, pons; 10, cerebellum; 11, ventriculus quartus; 12, sulcus lateralis; 13, polus frontalis; 14, polus temporalis; 15, polus occipitalis; 16, corpus callosum; 17, septum pellucidum; 18, 25, thalamus; 19, mesencephalon; 20, chiasma opticum; 21, aqueductus cerebri; 22, hypothalamus; 23, commissura anterior; 24, gyrus cinguli, 26, fornix.

of the middle frontal gyrus. Stimulation of various areas of the motor cortex has elicited motor responses of specific structures usually in the contralateral side of the body. Stimulation of the frontal eye field has induced eye and head turning movements to the opposite side. The more rostrally located cortex has been considered by some to be involved with processes relating to 'original' thought, though how one defines 'thought' has been subject to considerable disagreement. A region of interest clinically and functionally is in the inferior frontal gyrus. This is the *pars opercularis* (area 44), which in the left hemisphere appears concerned with the organization of the motor units involved with speech. Stimulation of this region may induce vocalization, but not true speech. If speech is in progress at the time of stimulation, there will be an arrest of speech.

5.1.2 Parietal lobe

The function of the parietal lobe (2) may be summarized as reception of somatic sensations, memory in regard to language and learning and a role in spatial organization. The lobe contains one gyrus at its rostral aspect which parallels the motor cortex of the precentral gyrus. This is the postcentral gyrus, or primary sensory cortex (areas 3, 1 and 2). A localization comparable to that observed in the motor cortex has been mapped, largely by direct stimulation of the exposed cortex during

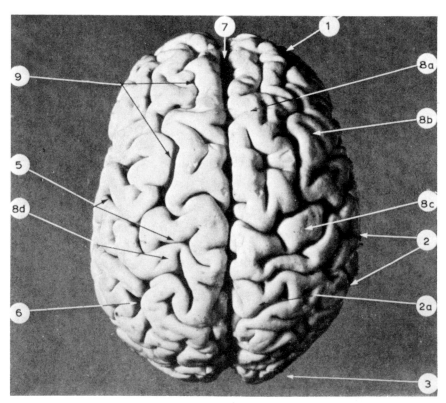

Fig. 35. A, dorsal aspect of cerebral hemispheres.
5, sulcus centralis; **6,** sulcus interparietais; **7,** fissura cerebri longitudinalis; **8a,** gyrus frontalis superior; **8b,** gyrus frontalis medialis; **8c,** gyrus precentralis; **8d,** gyrus postcentralis.

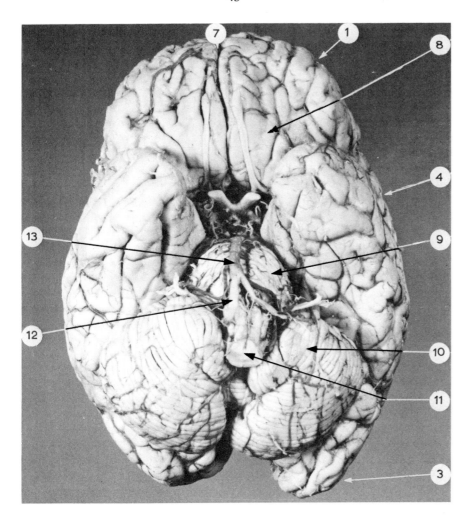

Fig. 35. B, ventral aspect of brain.
8, gyri et sulci orbitales; **9,** pons; **10,** cerebellum; **11,** medulla oblongata; **12,** arteria vertebralis; **13,** arteria basilaris.

neurosurgical procedures. It might be pointed out that the primary sensory and motor areas overlap each other. The remainder of the parietal lobe may be divided into a superior and inferior parietal lobule. Areas 5 and 7 in the superior lobule appear concerned with the correlation of different modalities of somatic sensory information to provide for conscious appraisal of the weight, texture, size and contour of an object. The ability to recognize these modes of sensation would appear related to the less closely defined function of 'hand dexterity' which has been applied to the region. The inferior parietal lobule (supramarginal and angular gyri) appears closely related to speech mechanisms in that lesions in the left hemisphere in this area lead to speech disturbances of a receptive nature.

The role of the parietal lobe in spatial organization has been less extensively studied. However, there does appear to be a defect in spatial judgement in patients with right parietal lobe lesions. A similar defect may occur with lesions of the left parietal lobe, but the speech defect which occurs is of such a magnitude as to make any evaluation impractical.

5.1.3 Occipital lobe

This is the primary center for vision. The occipital lobe (3) has long been recognized as the part of the cortex concerned with vision. A primary visual cortex along the calcarine sulcus (area 17) is recognized. Adjacent to it is a 'psychic' or interpretive visual area (18) which is believed to assemble the signals received by area 17 into an image. Patients with lesions in area 18 see, but do not recognize objects. Area 19 surrounds area 18 and blends with the adjacent associative parietal cortex. It is at this level in the visual cortex that the significance of what is seen appears to be appreciated. Irritation of this area triggers hallucinations and dreamlike images. One might note that the so-called psychic areas (19, 42, 5 and 7) all have an interpretive or associational role in comprehending information. Furthermore, they all surround the inferior parietal lobule or contribute to it. Thus, it is perhaps not too difficult to understand why left hemispheric lesions in the center of this confluence of 'psychic' cortical areas have such a global effect on the understanding of those symbols used in communication. Why this is almost always related to the left hemisphere (dominant hemisphere) still remains uncertain, since it apparently has little relationship to the cortical dominance which influences 'handedness'.

5.1.4 Temporal lobe

This part of the brain (4) deals with reception of auditory sensation, a participation in speech through auditory monitoring, and also plays some role in spatial recognition and memory. The transverse temporal gyrus (area 41) has been long recognized as the primary auditory center. A small area (42) surrounding this gyrus has been described as a psychic or interpretive auditory area. This region, as a psychic auditory area, appears according to Krieg[75] to be too small. He observes that stimulation of most of the temporal lobe, particularly along the middle temporal gyrus, induces a sensation which the patient describes as an auditory response. Patients with lesions in the temporal lobe in the 'psychic area' may lose appreciation of tones.

Area 22, in the left hemisphere, has also been associated with speech inasmuch as lesions in this region result in individuals who are unable to comprehend tne spoken word. They act as if they are unable to monitor the words they hear or speak. There is also some evidence that the temporal lobe is associated with 'vestibular' sense inasmuch as stimulation of the caudal part of the superior temporal gyrus in conscious patients induces vertigo and a sensation of rotation. Deep lesions in the temporal lobe often compromise the lowermost fibers of the optic radiations arising from the lateral geniculate body and thus produce visual defects. This should not be considered as being related to the function of the temporal lobe cortex, however. The temporal lobe has also been variously claimed to be concerned with memory and dreams. The deeply placed amygdala, adjacent cortex and the hippocampus and parahippocampal gyrus are functionally a part of the 'limbic' system.

5.1.5 Limbic lobe

Fig. 36. The structures forming this lobe are as follows: *area subcallosa, gyrus cinguli, isthmus gyri cinguli, gyrus parahippocampalis* and *uncus hippocampi* with an underlying nuclear structure, the *corpus amygdaloideum* and the *diagonal band of Broca*. Some information of an olfactory nature may enter the limbic system *via* the projections arising from the olfactory bulb which traverse the olfactory tract and lateral olfactory stria which reach the prepyriform area and amygdala. The function of this lobe, which contains components of the frontal, parietal and temporal lobes is more complex. It involves behavioral reactions of the individual toward the external environment as a result of receiving information through all the sensory modalities. In addition, the response may be influenced by the internal environment, which may alter the excitability of the nervous system (circulating levels of hormones, electrolytes, availability of glucose, etc.). It seems to operate in preserving the individual (feeding, fleeing or fighting) or the species (reproduction). These responses are mediated through lower centers of the diencephalon. Some relation to the olfactory sense also seems apparent in that stimulation or lesions of the hippocampal region are associated with odors, usually unpleasant.

The above assessment of functional areas of the cerebral cortex is at best sketchy, and certainly inconclusive. Our concepts of localization of function in the cortex have been changing rapidly and we have, with time, become less positive in our attempts at cortical localization. Furthermore, numerous secondary areas have been described and we have observed a considerable overlap in the described 'functional' areas.

The concept of 'silent' areas (regions in which stimulation produced

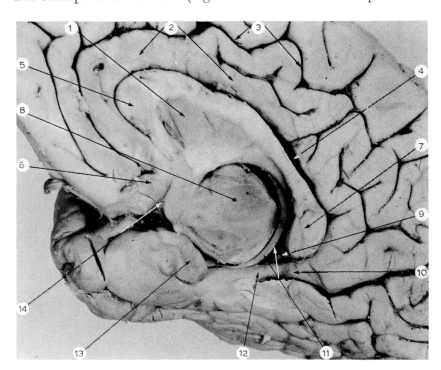

Fig. 36. Sagittal view showing the superficial components of the limbic system.
1, septum pellucidum; **2,** gyrus cinguli; **3,** sulcus cinguli; **4,** sulcus corporis callosi; **5,** genu corporis callosi; **6,** area subcallosa; **7,** splenium corporis callosi; **8,** thalamus; **9,** gyrus fasciolae; **10,** isthmus gyri cinguli; **11,** fornix; **12,** gyrus parahippampalis; **13,** uncus; **14,** diagonal band of Broca.

no specific result) has been discarded as our methods of measurement have improved. Attempts to associate specific regions of the cortex with the more abstract types of function, such as thought, have become less popular and we now tend to consider that most of the cortex may be concerned with such activities.

The deep nuclear masses (caudate nucleus, etc.) are a part of what might be termed the primitive or phylogenetically older sensory-motor system which predominates in lower species. In primitive forms the *striatum* is the highest center for correlation of all sensory impulses. In reptiles the striatum can be subdivided into a paleo- (old) and a neo- (new) striatum. The paleostriatum corresponds to the human globus pallidus, while the neostriatum corresponds to the caudate nucleus and putamen. The paleostriatum in reptiles, as in mammals, is predominantly motor in function while the neostriatum is sensory. This primitive sensory-motor complex appears to be associated with stereotyped instinctual behavior. In mammals, this has been superseded by a newer system arising from the cerebral cortex which provides for greater flexibility. These older levels of neural integration have not been discarded and function in coordination with the newer system. Furthermore, the nuclear regions representative of the primitive sensory-motor system may have undergone additional modifications in man. This seems likely since surgical lesions destroying the newer motor units in man and mammals are not accompanied by a paralysis or a return to a stereotyped form of motor response.

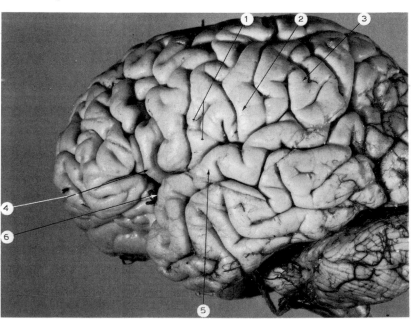

Fig. 37. Fronto-parieto-temporal operculum (see p. 42).
1, gyrus precentralis; **2,** gyrus postcentralis; **3,** gyrus supramarginalis; (**1 + 2 + 3,** frontoparietal operculum); **4,** gyrus frontalis inferior (frontal operculum); **5,** gyrus temporalis superior (temporal operculum).

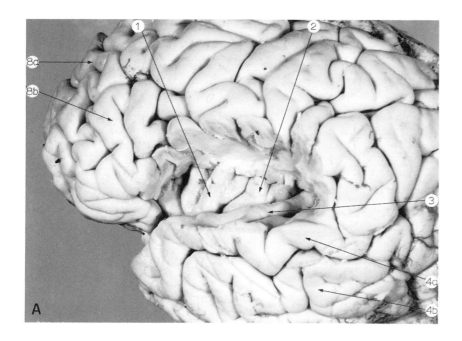

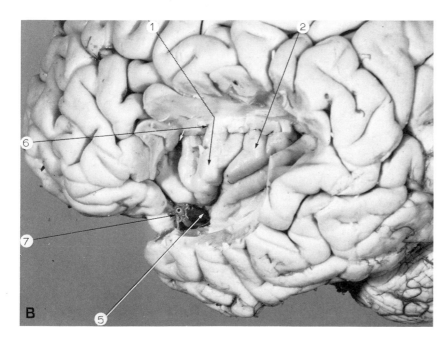

Fig. 38. **A** and **B**, lateral exposures of insula (see p. 42).
1, gyri breves insulae; **2,** gyri longi insulae; **3,** gyri temporales transversi; **4a,** gyrus temporalis superior; **4b,** gyrus temporalis medialis; **5,** limen insulae; **6,** sulcus circularis insulae; **7,** arteria cerebri media; **8a,** gyrus frontalis medialis; **8b,** gyrus frontalis inferior.

Fig. 39. The corpus callosum (22) is a large white bundle of fibers which connects the two cerebral hemispheres to each other. Experiments[93, 124] have demonstrated that the function of this large commissural bundle appears concerned with transfer of information from one hemisphere to the other.

In various types of training experiments it appeared that learning in one hemisphere is usually inaccessible to the other hemisphere if the connections between the hemispheres are missing. The obvious conclusion is that the corpus callosum has the important function of allowing the two hemispheres to share learning and memory. From a wide variety of experiments involving one-side training and testing of various eye-limb correlated functions and other combinations, Sperry[125,127] provides the following picture of the function of the corpus callosum:

– correlation of images in the left and right halves of the visual field;
– integration of sensations from paired limbs, or for learning that requires motor co-ordination of the limbs;
– unification of cerebral processes of attention and awareness. It has also been shown that its absence slows down the rate of learning.

Similar results were reported for a few patients, when the corpus callosum was cut for therapeutical reasons. In general, the impairments of brain function from such neurosurgery did not show up in the normal activities of daily life but were detected under special testing conditions. Other patients with a damaged corpus callosum have shown significant disturbances in the normal behavior. Most notable are such effects as

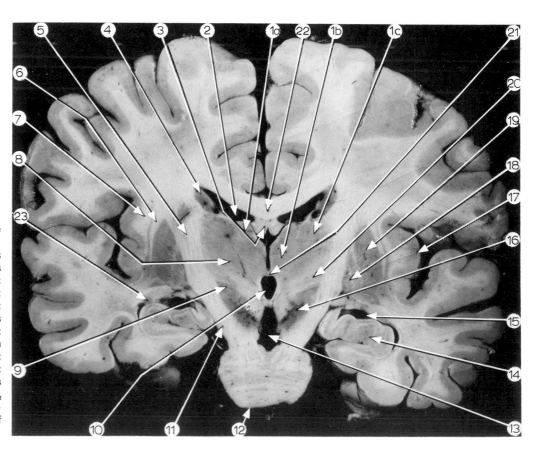

Fig. 39. Coronal section of brain at the midthalamic level.
1a, nucleus anterior thalami; **1b,** nucleus medialis thalami; **1c,** nucleus lateralis thalami; **2,** ventriculus lateralis; **3,** fornix; **4,** nucleus caudatus; **5,** capsula interna; **6,** capsula externa; **7,** capsula extrema; **8,** nucleus ventralis thalami; **9,** nucleus subthalamicus; **10,** ventriculus tertius; **11,** crus cerebri; **12,** pons; **13,** fossa interpeduncularis; **14,** pes hippocampi; **15,** ventriculus lateralis, cornu inferius; **16,** substantia nigra; **17,** insula; **18,** globus pallidus; **19,** putamen; **20,** H_1 and H_2 fields of Forel; **21,** adhesio interthalamicus; **22,** corpus callosum; **23,** cauda of nucleus caudatus.

word-blindness, word-deafness and faulty communication between the left and right limbs.

Thus, this fiber bundle is not just a connection, but an important system for the transfer of learning mechanisms.

It has been stated above that the cerebral hemisphere, or at least the outer cellular cortex has some function in speech other than to act as a source of motor nerve fibers concerned with the movement of muscles involved with speech. These losses in speech, which are termed *aphasias*, may be classed as being primarily motor (expressive) or sensory (receptive). As indicated, the area of cortex involved forms literally a half ring of tissue around the caudal aspect of the left sulcus lateralis. The *motor* or *verbal* aphasia is related to degeneration in the region of the pars opercularis of the frontal lobe. A similar loss of cortex in gyrus temporalis medialis of the temporal lobe causes an auditory aphasia where the patients appear to be unable to correctly monitor speech with their auditory system.

Degeneration of cortex or underlying white matter in the parietal lobe (gyrus supramarginalis and angularis) produces a receptive speech defect in which the patients appear unable to remember the names of objects (*nominal* aphasia) or fail to recognize the significance of words (*semantic* aphasia).

The auditory, nominal and semantic aphasias comprise the sensory receptive group. Many subclassifications have been suggested which may be useful in clinical practice although the excessive subdividing into areas 'specific' for different variations of aphasia is often confusing.

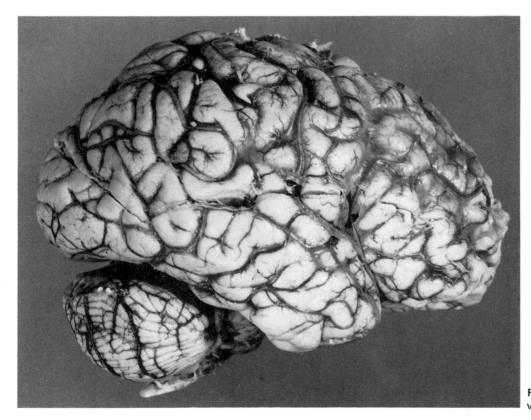

Fig. 40. Lateral view of brain with vessels and leptomeninges intact.

5.2 Diencephalon

Fig. 41. The *diencephalon* may be subdivided into five regions, more or less interdigitated with each other. These are dorsal thalamus (**1**), metathalamus, hypothalamus (**3**), epithalamus (**4**) and subthalamus (**5**).

5.2.1 Dorsal thalamus

The dorsal thalamus (**1**) contains many separate nuclear regions with different and sometimes overlapping functions. (The term nucleus, when used grossly in neuroanatomy refers to an aggregation of cells, frequently having a common function. However, the usual meaning of the term still applies to the nuclear chromosomal center of the cell). In conjunction with the metathalamus, the dorsal thalamus serves to relay sensory information to the cerebral cortex. Certain nuclear masses provide for projection of specific forms of information to specific cortical areas (Fig. 41**B**). These are as follows: the ventral posterior region of the dorsal thalamus (nuclei ventralis thalami posterior medialis **6**, and lateralis **7**) relays discriminative touch sensations from the opposite side of the face and body to the postcentral gyrus of the parietal lobe. A region just rostral in the dorsal thalamus (nucleus ventralis thalami intermedialis) relays impulses arising from the cerebellum to the primary motor area of the precentral gyrus. These energies are concerned with modifying the nature of motor stimuli being sent to the musculature so that the message which reaches the lower nerve cells will produce an organized response. The most rostral of this ventral lateral group is *the nucleus ventralis*

Fig. 41. Diagrammatic representations of, **A**, the principal hypothalamic nuclear masses, and the components of the epithalamus; **B**, the nuclear masses present at the diencephalic-mensencephalic junction indicating some degree of overlap of nuclear groups.
1, dorsal thalamus; **3**, hypothalamus; **3a**, sulcus hypothalamicus; **4a**, corpus pineale; **4b**, habenula; **4c**, stria medullaris thalami; **5**, nucleus subthalamicus; **6**, nucleus ventralis thalami posterior lateralis; **7**, nucleus ventralis thalami posterior medialis; **8**, nucleus centralis thalami medialis; **9**, nucleus lateralis hypothalami; **10**, nucleus ruber; **11**, substantia nigra; **12**, nucleus interpeduncularis; **13**, corpus mammilare; **14**, adenohypophysis; **15**, neurohypophysis; **16**, fasciculus longitudinalis medialis; **17**, aqueductus cerebri; **18**, fornix; **19**, septum pellucidum; **20**, chiasma opticum; **22**, mesencephalon; **23**, nucleus posterior hypothalami; **24**, commissura anterior; **25**, nucleus paraventricularis; **26**, nucleus supraopticus; **27**, nucleus ventromedialis hypothalami; **28**, corpus callosum; **29**, colliculus superior; **30**, colliculus inferior; **31**, lemniscus medialis; **32**, tractus corticospinalis; **33**, fibrae pontis transversae; **34**, nucleus dorsomedialis hypothalami; **39**, tuber cinereum.
see also Fig. 42.

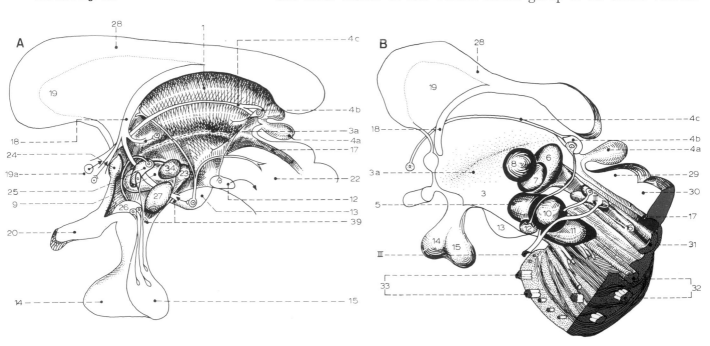

thalami anterior which relays impulses arising from the basal nuclear masses to the premotor cortex. One further nucleus which may be considered as a specific projection center to a specific cortical area is the *nucleus anterior thalami*. This is the most rostral and dorsal of the thalamic nuclei. It relays information arising from the corpus mammillare to the rostral part of the gyrus cinguli. Thus, it in a sense is a thalamic part of the limbic system in that interconnects two important anatomical components of the system.

Other nuclei have an associational role, acting in conjunction with the relay nuclei of the dorsal thalamus and with the cerebral cortex. These would include the *pulvinar, postero-lateral* and *dorso-lateral* nuclear masses.

A third group of nuclei form less discretely organized structures. These consist of cells scattered amongst the fibers which act to form capsular elements *(nuclei intralaminares thalami)* around the major thalamic nuclei (7). This also includes some cells in the subthalamus, and two centrally placed nuclei *(nucleus centralis medialis thalami* (8), and *nucleus centralis thalami lateralis)* and the cells of the midline nuclear groups *(adhesio interthalamica)*. These are the *non-specific projection nuclei* which differ from the first group in that they do not project to those highly specific areas of cortex which are concerned with particular functions. Instead they serve to project brain stem influences diffusely to the limbic cortex. They are in a sense the most rostral component of a scattered collection of cells (sometimes in discrete nuclei) and fibers which extend up the central core of the brain stem from the medulla. This is the *reticular formation*, and these are the thalamic reticular nuclei.

5.2.2 Metathalamus

The *metathalamus* contains two nuclear regions, the *nuclei corporis geniculati medialis* and *lateralis*. The term geniculate (genu = knee) is appropriate since the course of the fiber pathways of which these nuclei form a part, bends at the location of these nuclei, which thus form a knee or bend in the tracts. The lateral geniculate body is concerned with relaying visual information while the medial geniculate body is in the pathway which transmits auditory information.

5.2.3 Hypothalamus

The *hypothalamus* (3) which is just ventral to the dorsal thalamus (1) is the most rostral element of the visceral (autonomic) nervous system. It is concerned with salt regulation, sleep, blood pressure and respiration, temperature regulation, water conservation, hunger and satiety, the regulation of the endocrine systems through its ability to control the adenohypophysis *via* releasing or inhibiting factors, and apparently provides some contribution for emotional expression.

5.2.4 Epithalamus

The *epithalamus* (**4**) includes the *corpus pineale* (**4a**) and *habenular nuclei* (**4b**) medially adjacent to the dorsal thalamus (Fig. 41**A**). It has anatomic connections with the limbic system and the reticular core of the mesencephalon, and may serve to link them. Its connections with the limbic system arise from the septal area. Some fibers from the visual system in certain lower mammals whose reproductive functions are light oriented project into or near the septal area. Impulses may then reach the habenular-pineal area *via* the *stria medullaris thalami* (**4c**), which is also included in the epithalamus. Inasmuch as recent studies of the pineal body suggest that it may produce an anti-ovarian factor in some species, one is tempted to define a function for the epithalamus, particularly the pineal, as being in the realm of controlling gonadal maturation or the cyclic nature of reproductive function in these species. How this could be accomplished remains to be demonstrated, though the possibility of septal associations to the pineal are most interesting, particularly since the septal area possesses hypothalamic connections which may stimulate gonadal function, but autonomic connections appear more promising.

The habenular nuclei have also recently been shown to have projections which reach the hypothalamus and dorsal thalamus. It has again been suggested that these connections serve to help interconnect the limbic system with the diencephalon.

5.2.5 Subthalamus

Fig. 42. The *subthalamus* (**5** in Fig. 41**B**) includes a nuclear mass of the same name (*nucleus subthalamicus*, **5a**) plus several less discrete nuclear areas and some fiber bundles arising from the basal nuclear masses of the telencephalon. It appears functionally interconnected with the *nucleus ruber* (**10** in Fig. 41**B**) and *substantia nigra* (**11** in Fig. 41**B**) of the mesencephalon. This in a sense indicates that its function is correlated with that of the basal nuclear masses which constitute the primitive sensory-motor system.

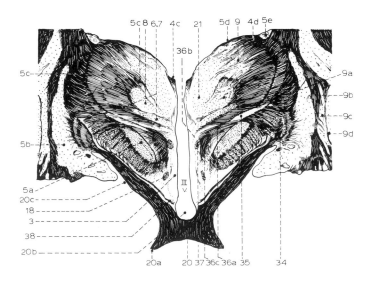

Fig. 42. A diagrammatic representation of the subthalamic structure as seen in a section through the diencephalon parallel to the optic tract (about 15° from the horizontal).
4c, stria medullaris thalami; **4d,** stria terminalis; **5a,** nucleus subthalamicus (Luys); **5b,** putamen; **5c,** lamina medullaris thalami externa; **5d,** stratum zonale; **5e,** nucleus caudatus; **6, 7,** nucleus ventralis thalami posterior, lateralis et medialis; **8,** nucleus centralis medianus thalami; **9,** nucleus lateralis thalami; **9a,** capsula interna; **9b,** capsula externa; **9c,** claustrum; **9d,** capsula extrema; **18,** fornix; **20,** chiasma opticum; **20a,** nervus opticus; **20b,** recessus opticus; **20c,** tractus opticus; **34,** globus pallidus; **35,** zona incerta; **36a,** fasciculus lenticularis (H₂); **36c,** tegmental field of Forel (H); **37,** fasciculus mammillo-thalamicus; **38,** commissura supraoptica.

5.3. Mesencephalon

The *mesencephalon* or midbrain extends caudally from a plane which passes through the *commissura posterior* dorsally and just caudal to the *corpus mammillare* ventrally and ends at the *isthmus rhombencephali* caudally. The posterior commissure is a large bundle just dorsal to the rostral end of the cerebral aqueduct. It is also located just ventral to the pineal. The isthmus rhombencephali represents the position of a constriction by the same name which is between the 2nd and 3rd primary vesicles (Fig. 5). It is a somewhat artificial landmark in the adult brain, as there are few structural landmarks. However, the decussating fibers of the IVth cranial nerve (trochlear) do exit from the dorsal surface of the brain stem in this plane.

The midbrain can be subdivided into three major components the *tectum, tegmentum* and the *crus cerebri*. The roof plate or *tectum mesencephali* is situated dorsally. It is comprised of 4 elevations, the two *superior* and two *inferior colliculi*. Both are concerned with reflex functions. The colliculus superior is a laminated nuclear structure involved in visual and total body reflexes, like those of the 'startle' reflex. The colliculus inferior is a component in the auditory circuit and consequently its reflex functions are related to sound.

The *tegmentum mesencephali* is anterior or ventral to the colliculi. The aqueductus cerebri exists in a longitudinal plane between the tectum and tegmentum. The tegmentum contains many descending and ascending fibers systems pertaining to somatic sensation and the primitive motor systems. Several nuclear regions are also present. Thus there are the nuclei of origin of the 3rd and 4th cranial nerves, as well as the *nucleus ruber* and several smaller tegmental nuclear aggregations associated with the reticular formation. The tegmentum may in a sense be regarded as a central core of motor and reticular nuclei, with related systems which extend from the diencephalon caudally to the lowermost extent of the myelencephalon (medulla oblongata). In the metencephalon this core will be termed the tegmentum pontis. A large paired fiber bundle, the basis pedunculi, or crus cerebri is ventral or anterior to the tegmentum mesencephali. These bundles contain primarily the large descending motor fibers arising from the cerebral cortex which will transmit efferent, motor impulses to the cranial nerve and pontine nuclei *(tractus cortico-bulbaris or tractus corticonuclearis)* and to the spinal cord motor nuclei *(tractus corticospinalis)*. Between the prominent fiber bundles on the anterior surface of the midbrain and the tegmentum is a large nucleus of pigmented cells (containing melanin). This group of cells which form the *substantia nigra* is usually considered to be an anatomical component of the basis pedunculi, but functionally it should be considered along with the red nucleus and reticular nuclei of the midbrain as being a part of the motor system. The substantia nigra is ventro-lateral to the nucleus ruber and just caudal to the subthalamic nucleus (Fig. 41**B, 5, 10**).

5.4 Metencephalon

Fig. 43. This rostral portion of the embryonic rhombencephalon contains three essential parts. On the anterior (ventral) surface is a large swelling, the *pons* or *pars basilaris pontis* (**1**). This contains many scattered nuclear groups as well as the descending fiber tract system passing through the basis pedunculi. These nuclei of the pons send their fibers contralaterally to the cerebellar cortex and act as relay stations, informing the cerebellar cortex as to the nature of the impulses sent *via* the corticobulbar and spinal tracts to the lower motor cells. The *pars dorsalis pontis*, on the other hand, contains brain stem nuclei for cranial nerves (V, VI, VII and part of VIII) as well as reticular nuclei and ascending (sensory) and descending fiber (primitive motor) systems. The pars dorsalis pontis is also referred to as the tegmentum pontis.

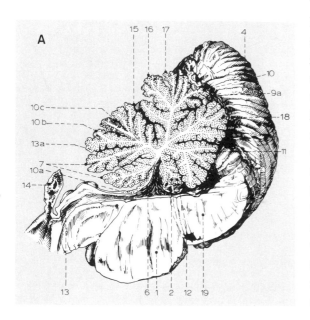

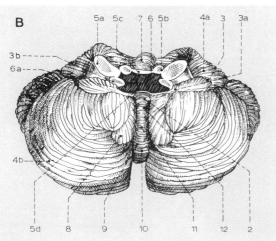

The largest component of the metencephalon is the cerebellum (**4**). This much convoluted structure has an interesting phylogenetic history. It develops from the rhombic lip of the neural tube where it is in close apposition with the vestibular (equilibratory) nuclei. The rhombic lip forms as a zone of cells intermediate between the alar plate and roof plate at the pontine flexure. The cells in this region give rise to both the cerebellar cortex and the deep cerebellar nuclei which relay the cerebellar influence to both higher and lower centers. The cells of the alar plate in the region of the medulla give rise to the pontine and inferior olivary nuclei which project to the cerebellar cortex. When the pontine flexure occurs, the rhombic lip is flared out laterally, giving rise to what will eventually be the lateral foramina of Luschka. That part of the rhombic lip just rostral to the lateral recess or foramina (**6a**) is believed to form the flocculonodular lobe (**3**) of the cerebellum. The adjacent alar plate gives rise to vestibular nuclei which are closely associated functionally with the flocculonodular lobe of the cerebellum. The more rostral portion of the rhombic lip gives rise to the rest of the cerebellum, including both the central vermis (**10**) and lateral hemispheres (**4**).

Edinger introduced the terms *paleocerebellum* and *neocerebellum* in 1909. The paleocerebellum would include all the *vermis* except the nodulus, while the neocerebellum denotes the cerebellar hemispheres and *nucleus dentatus* (**4d**). This, however, represents somewhat of a simplification as there have been many evolutionary stages in the development of the cerebellum. The earliest stage (*cf.* Fig. 44) is represented by two commissures which bridge the fourth ventricle (**6**), (*ventriculus quartus*). This may be represented by the form of the cerebellum in the newt *(Triturus)* in which there is the lateral commissure interconnecting the two auricles of the lateral line vestibular system[81, 82]. The second commissure arises from the trigeminal nerve and decussating fibers of the spinocerebellar system. Cells migrating from the alar plate pass along these commissures to form the cerebellar plate or basis cerebelli. This, in conjunction with the flocculi (derived from the auricle), represents the most primitive cerebellar cortex or *archicerebellum*. In the further development, the vermis (paleocerebellum) makes its appearance before the lateral hemispheres (neocerebellum). The hemispheres start to become apparent in lizards. Birds have a well developed flocculonodular lobe and vermis, but only a small unfoliated lateral hemisphere. Furthermore, the pons and pontine fibers of birds are only rudimentary. The hemispheres appear clearly in mammals and are most fully developed in primates. With the enlargement of the lateral hemisphere, there is an accompanying enlargement of the nucleus dentatus. The lateral hemispheres become divided into an anterior and a posterior lobe by a deep fissure seen best in the midsagittal plane (*fissura prima*, **15**). The flocculonodular lobe (**2, 3**) may be seen to be divided from the rest of the cerebellum by the fissura posterolateralis (**12**), also seen in the midsagittal plane.

The function of the anterior lobe may be described, from experiments on lower mammals, as dealing with tonus of muscle groups and the posterior lobe as being concerned with synergic regulation of opposing muscle groups. These distinctly different functions for the two lobes are not completely demonstrated clinically. Indeed the cerebellum has been removed from patients who have eventually recovered from their tonic and synergic dysfunction. Animals and man have been born lacking a part of a cerebellar lobe or with complete agenesis without marked impairment of function. This does not necessarily mean that the cerebellum is not needed. What is suggested is that there may be other means of sub-

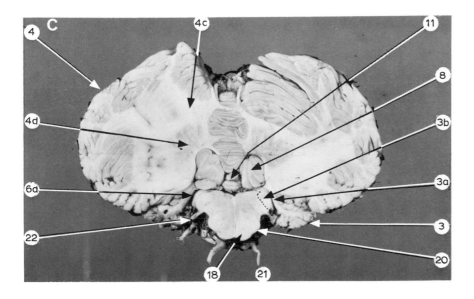

Fig. 43. **A**, the cerebellum in midsagittal plane; **B**, ventral or anterior surface of cerebellum; **C**, section through coronal plane of brain stem and cerebellum.
1, pons; 2, nodulus; 3, flocculus; **3a**, stalk of 3; **3b**, pedunculus cerebellaris inferior; 4, hemispherium cerebelli; **4a**, lobus anterior; **4b**, lobus posterior; **4c**, corpus medullare; **4d**, nucleus dentatus; **5a**, brachium pontis; **5b**, pedunculus cerebellaris superior; **5c**, velum medullare anterior; 6, ventriculus quartus; **6a**, recessus lateralis ventriculi quarti; 7, lobus centralis; 8, tonsilla cerebelli; 9, pyramid; 10, tuber vermis; **10b**, culmen; **10c**, arbor vitae; 11, uvula; 12, fissura posterolateralis (prenodular); 13, aqueductus cerebri; 14, corpus pineale; 15, fissura prima; 16, declive; 17, folium; 18, pyramis; 19, medulla oblongata; 20, nucleus olivaris inferior; 21, nervus abducens; 22, nervus vagus.

serving these same functions which the cerebellum ordinarily supersedes in the intact or normal animal.

Imbedded within the deep white matter of the cerebellum are several nuclei. The first and most primitive is the medially located nucleus fastigii. As one goes laterally, new deep nuclear masses have been added with development of the cerebellum. Thus, one finds, progressing laterally, the *nucleus globosus, emboliformis* and *dentatus* (Fig. 43**C, 4d**).

Large fiber bundles project into or leave the cerebellum. The fibers from the nuclei of the pons which project to the contralateral cortex have been mentioned. The fiber bundle is called the *pedunculus cerebellaris medialis* and it is afferent. The restiform body or *pedunculus cerebellaris inferior* (**3b**) is also afferent, transmitting information from the spinal cord concerning the whereabouts of the limbs and state of tonus of the muscles. There is also a large contribution of fibers arising from the *nucleus olivaris inferioris* (**20**) of the medulla which enter the contralateral restiform body. These olivocerebellar fibers appear anatomically to be in a position to provide information to the cerebellum concerning the nature of motor activity being initiated through the fibers of the primitive motor system. Other contributions are made to the inferior peduncle from the reticular formation. The *pedunculus cerebellaris superior* contains most of the efferent fiber systems of the cerebellum, projecting the cerebellar influence to the brain stem, diencephalon and cerebral hemispheres. In a cybernetical system, the cerebellum may be considered as the little black box which regulates and assists in coordinating motor activity. Thus, it receives information from the cord pertaining to the position

Fig. 44. A, midsagittal aspect of human cerebellum.
1, pars basilaris pontis; **1a,** mesencephalon; **1b,** tectum mesencephali; **2,** nodulus; **3c,** corpus callosum; **3d,** thalamus; **3e,** hypothalamus; **4,** cerebellum; **6,** ventriculus quartus; **7,** lobus centralis; **7a,** tractus spinocerebellaris; **7b,** tractus cerebellotegmentalis; **9,** pyramis; **9a,** fissura prepyramidalis; **9b,** fissura postpyramidalis; **10,** tuber vermis; **10a,** lingula cerebelli; **10b,** culmen; **11,** uvula; **13a,** recessus fastigii; **14,** corpus pineale; **15,** fissura prima; **16,** declive; **17,** folium vermis.

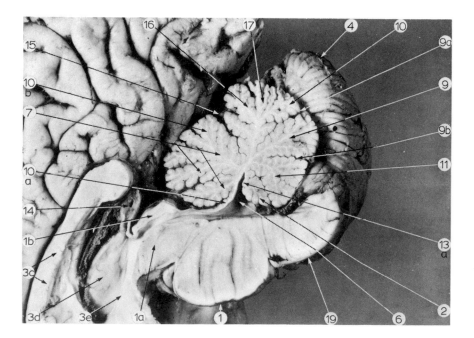

and tonus of muscles, individually and in relation to each other. The new motor system, concerned with 'voluntary' motor function, provides information to the cerebellum *via* fibers terminating directly on the nuclei of the basis pontis. Collaterals arising from the fibers running to the neurons which actually initiate the motor act also contribute through their connections with the nuclei of the basis pontis. The primitive motor system which appears primarily concerned with associated or background motor function in man (arm swinging in walking or other automatic motor sequences initiated by striated muscle fibers) is also provided with a cerebellar component.

A large bundle of fibers running in the tegmentum mesencephali and pontis arises from neurons of the *substantia grisea centralis* (periaqueductal grey) of the midbrain, *zona incerta* of the subthalamus, basal ganglia and *nucleus ruber*. It appears to effect its cerebellar connections *via* its terminations in the inferior olive. The olive then serves to relay such information to the cerebellar cortex. Having received input regarding position and tonus of muscles and of the intended motor act *via* new and older motor pathways, the cerebellum appears to act to modify (intensify or depress) the intended motor sequence in order to promote the most coordinated response through its superior peduncle or efferent limb. This it may achieve by connections with the midbrain reticular nuclei or by projections to the dorsal thalamus which relays the cerebellar influence to those parts of the cerebral cortex which originally initiated the motor sequence.

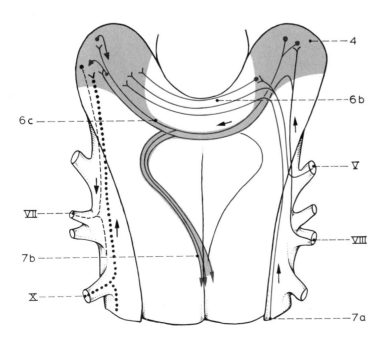

Fig. 44. B, primitive cerebellum with nerve roots of a newt *(Triturus).*

5.5 Myelencephalon

Fig. 45. The myelencephalon or *medulla oblongata*, like the metencephalon contains a tegmental core of nuclear groups and associated fiber systems. Thus, it is a center for the nuclei of origin of part of VIII and of IX, X, part of XI and of the XIIth cranial nerves. It assists the pons in the regulation of respiration. It is also concerned with the reflex control of the cardiovascular system, emetic reflexes and equilibrium. The latter is mediated through the vestibular division of the VIIIth cranial nerve. A long nuclear and fiber tract component of the Vth nerve descends through the dorsolateral aspect of the medulla and is reported to reach as far caudal as the 4th cervical cord segment. Long ascending and descending tract systems are also present in the medulla. Thus, the prominent descending corticospinal tracts are observed ventrally as the *pyramids* (**23b**), named for their morphologic shape. Dorsolaterally are the ascending sensory bundles (**8**, pedunculus cerebellaris inferior) arising partly from the spinal cord which project information concerned with position of body parts and muscle tonus to the cerebellum. Running through the medulla are tracts for pain, temperature and light touch (incorporated together as a single bundle, the *lemniscus spinalis*), and a larger bundle, the *lemniscus medialis* arising from cells at the caudal dorsal aspect of the medulla. This latter system is more gnostic than the spinothalamic and may be said to be concerned with discriminative sensation, position and vibratory sense.

Fig. 45. Medulla oblongata and pons, **A**, in dorsal or posterior view; **B**, in lateral view; **C**, in ventral or anterior view.

1, lingula; **2**, velum medullare anterius; **3**, eminentia medialis; **4**, fovea superior; **5**, pedunculus cerebellaris superior; **6**, pedunculus cerebellaris medialis; **7**, colliculus facialis; **8**, pedunculus cerebellaris inferior; **9**, tuberculum acusticum; **10**, striae medullares (ventriculi quarti); **11**, taenia ventriculi quarti; **12**, trigonum nervus hypoglossi; **13**, trigonum nervus vagi; **14**, area postrema; **15**, obex; **16**, tuberculum nuclei cuneati; **17**, tuberculum nuclei gracilis; **18**, funiculus lateralis; **19**, sulcus lateralis posterior; **19a**, sulcus lateralis anterior; **20**, funiculus cuneatus; **21**, sulcus intermedialis posterior; **22**, funiculus gracilis; **23**, sulcus medianus posterior; **23a**, pons (basilaris); **23b**, pyramis; **23c**, oliva; **23d**, decussatio pyramidalis; **24**, crus cerebri; **25**, colliculus inferior; **25a**, brachium colliculi inferioris; **25b**, colliculus superior.

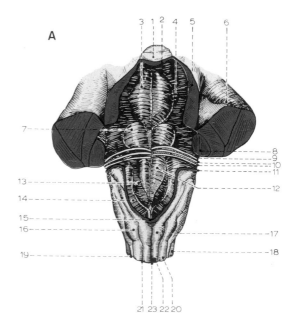

5.6 Reticular substance

Reference has been made to a reticular formation in the previous sections. This may be described as a mixture of cells and fibers with multiple interconnections between cellular units. It extends from the medulla to the diencephalon into which it has nuclear extensions and fibrous projections. It may be considered as white reticular formation if the white myelinated fibers predominate or grey reticular formation if cell bodies and poorly myelinated fibers predominate. While a reticular formation is not usually described in the spinal cord, the central nuclear grey core of the cord is more or less continuous with the reticular formation of higher levels. Furthermore, a series of short longitudinally running axonal units (*fasciculi proprii*) which surround this grey matter of the cord and which serve to interconnect the various spinal segments, connect in all probability with the reticular formation of the medulla. The functions of the reticular formation are as yet ill defined. The 'centers' for cardiovascular and respiratory control of the medulla and pons appear to be in regions defined as reticular. Emetic control also appears in this domain. Ascending activation of higher elements (diencephalon and cortex) appears as another highly important role for this system.

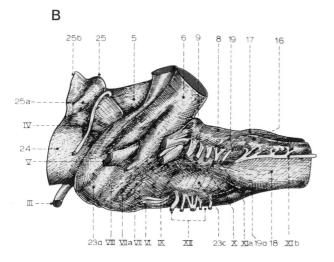

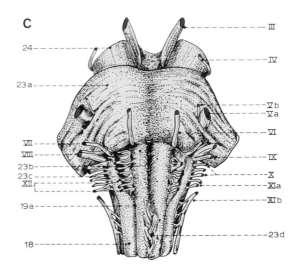

62

5.7 Spinal cord

Fig. 46. The spinal cord contains the cells of origin for the nerves supplying the somatic musculature of the body. These, and other cells form a central cellular core around the central canal. On cross section the cellular area has the shape of the letter H. Thus, the grey matter of the cord may be defined as having posterior and anterior horns and an intermediate as well as a commissural component. The posterior horn (**5**) is predominantly sensory in function, containing cells which relay the sensory input toward higher centers or to the ventrally placed motor cells for reflex response. The anterior horn (**12**) provides the motor cells which innervate the muscles. These motor cells, as well as the cells of the cranial nerve nuclei, were described by Sherrington[119] as forming the 'final common pathway'. This appears appropriate since all descending or segmental reflex connections which will produce a motor act do so as a result of the summation of their activities on these cells. The intermediate zone of the cord contains cells which interconnect the sensory and motor units.

Fig. 46. Diagrammatic representation of a horizontal (coronal) section through the spinal cord, showing its principal components.
1, sulcus medialis posterior; **2**, funiculus posterior; **3**, fasciculus dorsolateralis (Lissauer); **4**, substantia gelatinosa; **5**, cornu posterius (sensory); **6**, nucleus proprius of **5**; **7**, funiculus lateralis; **8**, substantia intermedia centralis; **9**, commissura anterior spinalis; **10**, cornu laterale (sympathetic); **11**, substantia intermedia lateralis; **12**, cornu anterius; **13**, funiculus anterior; **14**, fissura mediana anterior.

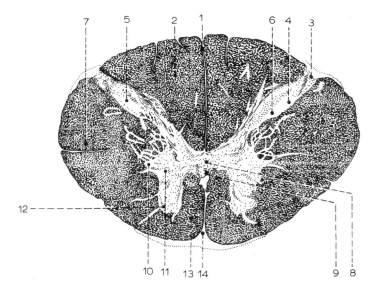

A fifth cellular zone extends from the 1st thoracic to about the third lumbar segment of the cord. It projects laterally and is intermediate between the dorsal and ventral horns. This is the intermediolateral cell column (**10**, *cornu laterale*) which contains motor cell elements of the autonomic system (in this instance sympathetic). These units are concerned with the innervation of glands, muscles of piloerection and the smooth muscles in the walls of arteries, arterioles and visceral organs.

Surrounding the grey core (**8**) of the cord is a white mantle of ascending and descending myelinated fiber systems. These will transmit ascending sensory information which may reach conscious levels in the cortex, terminate earlier for reflex responses, or both. Various types of descending tracts provide motor information for the ventral horn cells. There are also the short fiber systems *(fasciculi proprii)* which ascend and descend to interconnect the various segmental units of the cord.

During the third fetal month, the spinal cord extends the entire length of the spinal canal. In the succeeding months before birth, the vertebral column grows in length faster than does the cord, so that at birth the spinal cord descends in the spinal canal only as far as the third lumbar level (ascensus medullae). This differential in growth rate continues during the first few years after birth, soon reaching the adult state in which the cord extends only to the lower border of the first lumbar vertebra. The result of this differential rate in growth is that the roots of the spinal nerves descend in the spinal canal after leaving the cord before exiting through their proper foramina. The extent of this is most marked in the caudal segments where the roots of the lower thoracic, lumbar and sacral nerves descend a considerable distance before leaving the spinal canal. The caudal end of the cord, which is bluntly tapered, is termed the *conus medullaris*. The nerve roots of the lower cord which descend past the conus medullaris are held together within the meningeal sheaths, forming the *cauda equina*. A fine fibrous thread formed by a prolongation of the pial investment of the cord extends caudally from the conus medullaris to become attached distally to the periosteum of the coccygis. This filament, which anchors the cord at its distal end, is the *filum terminale*. Since the cord ends at the lower border of the first lumbar vertebra in adults, the subarachnoid space surrounding the nerve roots forming the cauda equina is a relatively safe place in which to insert a needle (lumbar puncture) for the purpose of withdrawing spinal fluid or injecting materials for diagnostic or anesthesia purposes.

5.8 Blood vessels

5.8.1 Arterial supply

Fig. 47. The arterial supply of the brain is derived from two primary sources. The *arteriae carotis internae* (**1**) supply the rostral end of the brain and the two vertebral arteries which fuse beneath the medulla to form the *arteria basilaris* (**13**) supply the caudal end. A pair of communicating vessels (**8,** *arteriae communicantes posteriores,* or the proximal stems of the posterior cerebral arteries) interconnect the rostral carotid and caudal basilar arterial systems beneath the diencephalon. A further communicating trunk develops between the two *arteriae cerebri anteriores* (**5**) which arise from the carotid vessels. This is the *arteria communicans anterior* (**4**) which completes the arterial ring *(circulus arteriosus cerebri)* beneath the diencephalon.

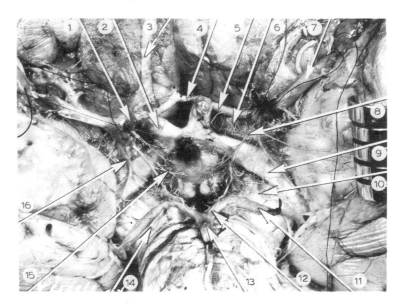

Fig. 47. Ventral surface of the brain illustrating the circulus arteriosus cerebri. **1**, arteria carotis interna; **2**, nervus opticus; **3**, tractus olfactorius; **4**, arteria communicans anterior; **5**, arteria cerebri anterior; **6**, medial perforators of **5**; **7**, arteria cerebri media; **8**, arteria communicans posterior; **9**, tractus opticus; **10**, crus cerebri; **11**, arteria cerebri posterior; **12**, mesencephalic stem of **11**; **13**, arteria basilaris; **14**, rami ad tectum mesencephali; **15**, diencephalic perforators of **8**; **16**, arteria choroidea anterior.

Subdivisions of the arteria carotis interna (**1**). This large vessel which nourishes the rostral part of the brain becomes divided into 4 primary vessels, the *arteria cerebri anterior* (**5**), *the arteria cerebri media* (**7**), the *arteria choroidea anterior* (**16**) and the proximal stem of the arteria cerebri posterior (**8**, *arteria communicans posterior*). The two anterior cerebral vessels are then linked together by the *arteria communicans anterior* (**4**).

Each of these four vessels gives off a series of perforating arteries to the deep nuclear masses before breaking up into a cortical network from which arise additional perforators to supply the cortex. The final small arterial units of these perforators serve as functional 'end arteries' to the neuronal groups they supply. Thus, an occlusion of one of these vessels results in the death of the neurons in the area supplied. Occlusion of at least some of the rami within the surface network of vessels, however, need not necessarily result in serious cortical damage, as there is a considerable degree of collateral anastomosis accomplished through the network (see also Figs. 48–50).

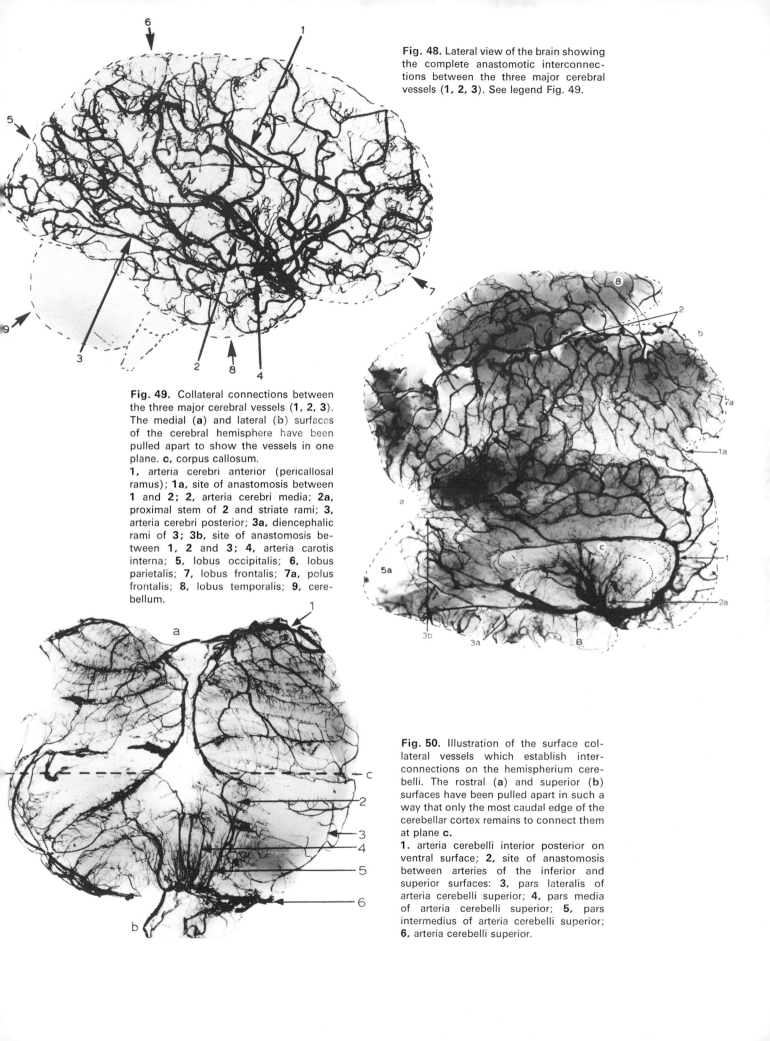

Fig. 48. Lateral view of the brain showing the complete anastomotic interconnections between the three major cerebral vessels (**1, 2, 3**). See legend Fig. 49.

Fig. 49. Collateral connections between the three major cerebral vessels (**1, 2, 3**). The medial (**a**) and lateral (**b**) surfaces of the cerebral hemisphere have been pulled apart to show the vessels in one plane. **c**, corpus callosum.

1, arteria cerebri anterior (pericallosal ramus); **1a,** site of anastomosis between **1** and **2**; **2,** arteria cerebri media; **2a,** proximal stem of **2** and striate rami; **3,** arteria cerebri posterior; **3a,** diencephalic rami of **3**; **3b,** site of anastomosis between **1, 2** and **3**; **4,** arteria carotis interna; **5,** lobus occipitalis; **6,** lobus parietalis; **7,** lobus frontalis; **7a,** polus frontalis; **8,** lobus temporalis; **9,** cerebellum.

Fig. 50. Illustration of the surface collateral vessels which establish interconnections on the hemispherium cerebelli. The rostral (**a**) and superior (**b**) surfaces have been pulled apart in such a way that only the most caudal edge of the cerebellar cortex remains to connect them at plane **c**.

1. arteria cerebelli interior posterior on ventral surface; **2,** site of anastomosis between arteries of the inferior and superior surfaces: **3,** pars lateralis of arteria cerebelli superior; **4,** pars media of arteria cerebelli superior; **5,** pars intermedius of arteria cerebelli superior; **6,** arteria cerebelli superior.

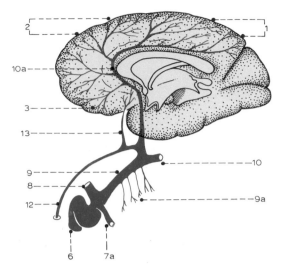

Fig. 51. Diagrammatic representation of the distribution of the arteria cerebri anterior.

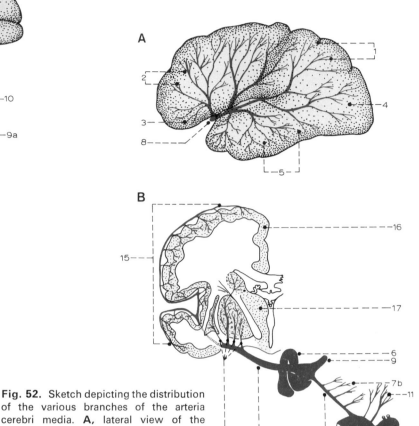

Fig. 52. Sketch depicting the distribution of the various branches of the arteria cerebri media. **A,** lateral view of the cerebral hemisphere illustrating the distribution of the cortical rami of the arteria cerebri media; **B,** coronal section through the cerebrum to demonstrate the deep nuclear distribution of vessels arising from the artery.

Legend for Figs. 51, 52, 53, 54.
1. rami parietales; **1a,** rami parieto-occipitales; **2,** rami frontales; **3,** rami orbitales; **4,** rami occipitales; **5,** rami temporales; **6,** arteria carotis interna; **6a,** arteria choroidea anterior; **6b,** ramus of **6a** to choroid plexus, medial division of globus pallidus, nucleus intermedius thalami and the nuclei intralaminares thalami; **7,** arteria cerebri posterior; **7a,** proximal stem of **7** (arteria communicans posterior); **7b,** diencephalic perforators of **7a**; **7c,** choroidal diencephalic artery giving rise to arteria choroidea posterior (**7e**) as well as diencephalic ramus: **7d,** ramus of **7e** to choroid plexus of ventriculus lateralis; **7e,** ramus to choroid plexus of ventriculus tertius; **8,** arteria cerebri media; **8a,** rami striati of **8** (lenticulostriate arteries); **9,** arteria cerebri anterior; **9a,** proximal perforators of **9** to preoptic area; **10,** arteria communicans anterior; **10a,** pericallosal stem of **10**; **11,** posteromedial perforators to tegmentum mensencephali; **12,** ramus centralis of **9** (arteria striata medialis of Heubner); **13,** ramus of **12** to septal area; **14,** arteria basilaris; **15,** rami corticales; **16,** cortex cerebri; **17,** diencephalon; **17a,** pulvinar.

Figs. 51, 52. The lateral perforating vessel of the arteria cerebri anterior (**9**) is the *ramus centralis* (**12,** arteria striata medialis of Heubner) which supplies the *corpus striatum*. Medial perforators of this vessel supply the preoptic areas. The medial perforators of the arteria cerebri media arise from the proximal stem of the artery. They pass dorsally through the *substantia perforata anterior* to supply the *putamen* and *globus pallidus* (lenticular nucleus) and the body of the *nucleus caudatus*. While these perforators are known as the *rami striati* (**8a**) of the arteria cerebri media, they are more commonly referred to as the lenticulostriate arteries. The proximal stem of arteria cerebri posterior provides perforating vessels to the rostral diencephalon and the arteria choroidea anterior provides proximal perforating vessels to the *corpus amygdaloideum* (**d**), to the *nucleus intermedius* (**b**) and to the *lateral reticular nuclei* of the thalamus as well as providing arteries for the choroid plexus of the cornu inferius of the ventriculus lateralis and the medial aspect of the globus pallidus.

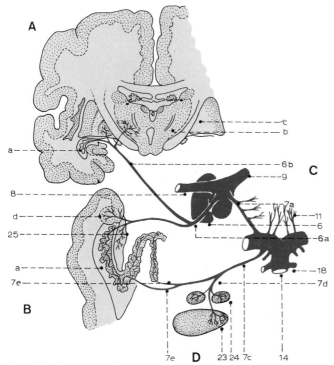

Fig. 53. Diagrammatic representation of the distribution of the various branches of the arteria choroidea. **A,** coronal section through the brain at the level of the nucleus intermedialis thalami; **B,** horizontal section through the temporal lobe to demonstrate the vascular branches of the artery to the amygdala (**d**), the choroid plexus in the inferior horn of the ventriculus lateralis (**a**), and the para-hippocampal gyrus (**25**); **C,** arterial stems for vascular supply; **D,** thalamus.
a, inferior horn of lateral ventricle with choroid plexus; **b,** nucleus intermedius thalami: **c,** medial division of globus pallidus; **d,** amygdala.

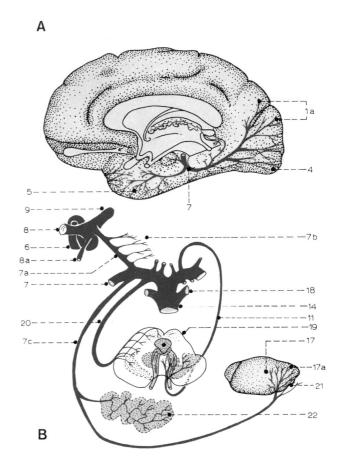

Fig. 54. Diagrammatic representation of the distribution of the arteria cerebri posterior.
A, midsagittal view of cerebral hemisphere; **B,** arterial stems for vascular supply.

Fig. 53, 54. The *arteria cerebri posterior* (**7**) appears to develop embryo-logically from a vessel arising from the arteria carotis interna. This vessel, which becomes the proximal stem of the arteria cerebri posterior (arteria communicans posterior) in the adult (**7a**), fuses with the terminal rostral vessel *(arteria mesencephalica)* of the arteria basilaris at about 6- to 7-mm stage. From this time on, most of the blood which will be directed to the posterior aspect of the cerebral hemisphere will *usually* come through this mesencephalic ramus of the arteria basilaris. Over the years, this mesencephalic stem from the basilar artery has come to be considered the origin of the arteria cerebri posterior, although it has assumed this role secondarily. Near the origin of the mesencephalic stem, but distal to the point where the proximal stem joins it, there arises the large lateral perforating ramus of the arteria cerebri posterior (choroidal diencephalic artery) which is directed to supply the caudal third of the thalamus and the metathalamus. It also supplies the plexus choroideus of ventriculus tertius.

Subdivisions of the vertebral–basilar arterial group

Fig. 55. The two arteriae vertebrales join together just beneath the medulla oblongata to form the arteria basilaris. Just prior to this junction, each gives off a small medially directed artery. These anastomose to form the *arteria spinalis anterior* (**27**) which descends along the anterior aspect of the medulla spinalis, providing perforating vessels for the ventral aspect of the spinal cord.

Another important vessel usually arises from the arteria vertebralis. This is the *arteria cerebelli inferior posterior* (**26a**). However, the vessel may also arise from the arteria basilaris (**14**), or from a common stem vessel which divides into anterior and posterior branches of the inferior cerebellar artery (**14a, 26a**). This stem vessel may itself arise from either the vertebral (**26**) or basilar vessel (**14**). The arteria cerebelli inferior anterior usually arises from the arteria basilaris. One further cerebellar vessel arises from the rostral end of the basilar vessel. This is the *arteria cerebelli superior* (**18**). The arteria basilaris then bifurcates into the two mesencephalic arteries which initially supplied the midbrain, but which have come to be mesencephalic stem arteries for the arteria cerebri posterior.

Two of the major cerebellar arteries (Fig. 55, **18, 26a**) provide deep perforating vessels to the deep cerebellar nuclei. All are then peripherally distributed in a much branched anastomotic cortical network from which arise the cortical perforators. The cortical rami of the posterior inferior vessel supply the posterior inferior surface of the cerebellar hemisphere. There is, however, an additional group of perforators from this vessel which supply the dorsolateral aspect of the medulla oblongata. The anterior inferior artery provides the cortical rami for the anterior inferior cerebellar surface and usually gives rise to the *arteria labyrinthi* (**14b**) which enters into the *meatus acusticus internus* to reach the inner ear. This vessel occasionally has an independent origin from the arteria basilaris. The superior cerebellar artery (**18**) supplying the superior cortical surface, usually becomes subdivided into three major rami: the *pars media, intermedialis,* and *lateralis* (**18c, b, a**). All of these cerebellar vessels establish anastomotic connections with each other in the surface cortical network (*cf.* Fig. 50).

Fig. 55. Diagrammatic representation of the distribution of the cerebellar arteries. **A,** medulla-pons, with left side of medulla cut away; **B,** ventral and **C,** dorsal aspect of the cerebellum.
a, nervus trigeminus; b, pons; c, pedunculus cerebellaris medius (brachium pontis); d, pedunculus cerebellaris superior (brachium conjuctivum); e, pedunculus cerebellaris inferior (restiform body); **7**, arteria cerebri posterior; **14**, arteria basilaris; **14a**, arteria cerebelli anterior inferior; **14b**, arteria labyrinthi; **18**, arteria cerebelli superior; **18a**, pars lateralis of **18**; **18b**, pars intermedialis of **18**; **18c**, pars media of **18**; **26**, arteria vertebralis; **26a**, arteria cerebelli inferior posterior; **26a′**, is **26a** after giving off rami to the medulla; **27**, arteria spinalis anterior; **27a**, rami vasorum corinalium from **27**.
Arabic numerals correspond with those in Figs. 51, 52, 53, 54.

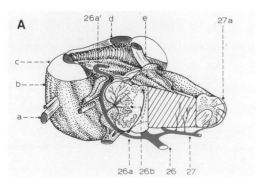

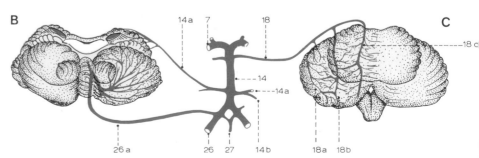

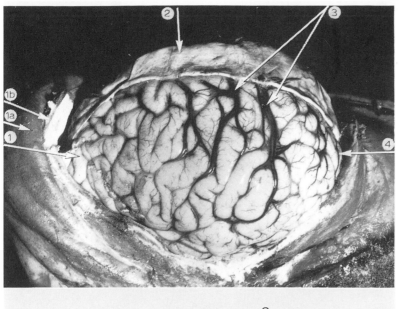

Fig. 56. Dorsolateral view of the brain at autopsy showing several congested venae cerebri superiores (**3**).

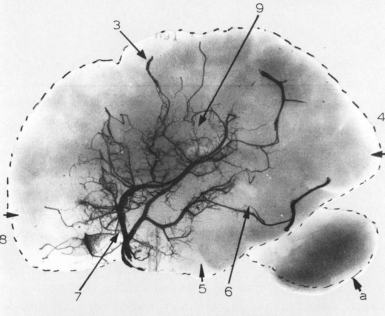

Fig. 57. Lateral aspect of the brain illustrating the venous drainage around the sulcus lateralis **a**, cerebellar hemisphere.

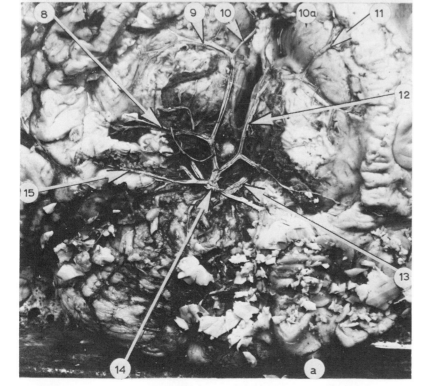

Fig. 58. Dorsal (posterior) aspect of the complete dissection illustrating the components concerned with the formation of the vena cerebri magna (Galen). **8**, vena subependymalis posterior; **9**, vena subependymalis media (vena thalmostriata); **10**, vena subependymalis anterior (vena septi pellucidi); **10a**, caput of nucleus caudatus; **11**, vena subependymalis; **12**, vena cerebri interna; **13**, vena basalis (Rosenthal); **14**, vena cerebri magna (Galen); **15**, vena cerebri occipitalis; **a**, cerebellum.

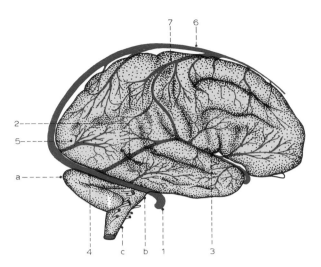

Fig. 59. Lateral view of the brain showing the various large collecting and anastomotic veins. **a,** cerebellum; **b,** pons; **c,** medulla; **1,** origin of sinus sigmoideus; **2,** vena anastomotica inferior (Labbé); **3,** vena cerebri media superficialis; **4,** sinus transversus; **5,** vena cerebri inferior; **6,** sinus sagittalis superior with venae cerebri superiores draining into it: **7,** vena anastomotica superior (Trollard).

The terminal mesencephalic stem vessels of the arteria basilaris each give off an important cluster of vessels, the *posteromedial perforators*, which pass through the *substantia perforata posterior* of the fossa interpeduncularis to supply the *tegmentum mesencephali* (Fig. 54). A second important group of vessels arise from this mesencephalic stem somewhat lateral to the tegmental perforators. These vessels encircle the mesencephalon, giving off perforating arteries to the lateral and superior surface areas. These are the *rami ad tectum mesencephali*, or tectal arteries.

5.8.2 Venous drainage

Figs. 60, 61. The rostral components of the CNS are drained by superficial and deep venous systems. The superficial system consists of those veins which drain the cerebral cortex and which empty into the intradural sinuses. Thus, there are the *venae cerebri superiores* (**4**) which drain into the *sinus sagittalis superior* (**3**) and *venae cerebri inferiores* which empty into the *sinus transversus* (**2**). A *vena cerebri media superficialis* (**9d**) runs rostrally along the lateral edge of the sulcus lateralis and then becomes medially directed around the polus temporalis. It finally empties into the *sinus cavernosus*. This large vein receives blood from the inferior parietal and frontal lobes and from the superior surface of the temporal lobe. One large vein frequently extends from the sinus sagittalis superior to the vena cerebri media superficialis. This is the *vena anastomotica superior*. A second anastomotic vein *(vena anastomotica inferior)* frequently extends between the vena cerebri media superficialis and the sinus transversus. Both of the anastomotic veins receive tributaries during their course (see Figs. 56, 57 and 58). Medial cortical veins dorsal to the corpus callosum drain into the *sinus sagittalis inferior* (**17**).

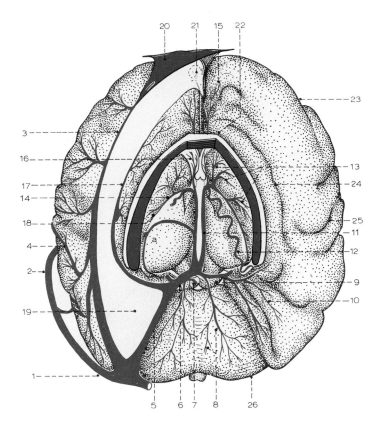

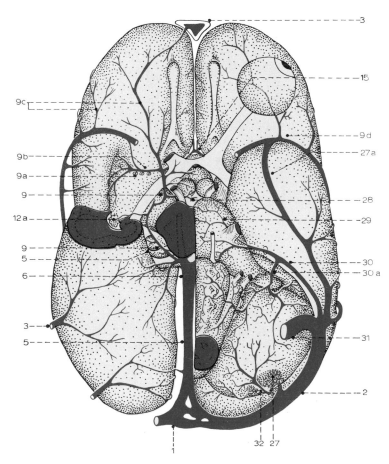

Fig. 60. Diagrammatic sketch of the brain in dorsal view, demonstrating the deep collecting venous system and its association with the superficial venous drainage *via* the vena cerebri magna (**6**) and the sinus rectus (**5**). The two hemispheres have been pulled apart dorsally and the bulk of the corpus callosum (**22**) removed.

Legend for Figs. 60, 61.
1, confluens sinuum; **2**, sinus transversus; **3**, sinus sagittalis superior; **4**, vena cerebri superior; **5**, sinus rectus; **6**, vena cerebri magna (Galen); **7**, vena mesencephali draining into **6**; **8**, venae cerebelli superiores; **9**, vena basalis; **9a**, vena striata inferior; **9b**, vena cerebri medialis profunda; **9c**, venae orbitales; **9d**, vena superficialis medialis cerebri; **10**, venae occipitalis draining into **9**; **11**, vena cerebri interna; **12**, vena choroidea; **12a**, plexus choroideus in ventriculus lateralis and vena choroidea anterior; **13**, vena subependymalis; **14**, vena subependymalis media (vena thalamostriata); **15**, vena cerebri anterior; **16**, vena subependymalis anterior; **17**, sinus sagittalis inferior; **18**, vena subependymalis posterior; **19**, falx cerebri; **20**, dura mater; **21**, crista galli; **22**, corpus callosum; **23**, lobus frontalis; **24**, sulcus cinguli; **25**, sulcus centralis; **26**, cerebellum; **27**, sinus in tentorium cerebelli; **27a**, anastomotic vein between vena cerebri media superficialis and sinus transversus; **28**, venae interpedunculares; **29**, venae pontes; **30**, sinus petrosus superior; **30a**, vein draining into **30** (vena cerebelli anterior); **31**, vena jugularis interna; **32**, vena cerebelli posterior.

Fig. 61. Newborn venous system in ventral view.

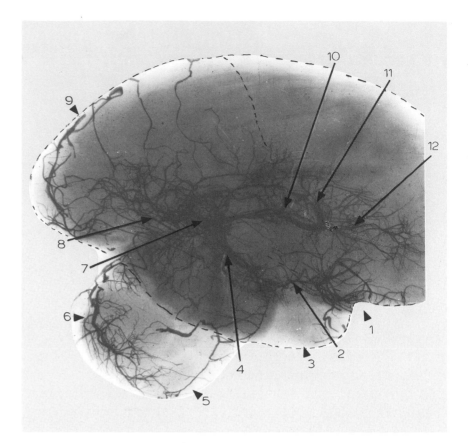

Fig. 62. Lateral aspects of the brain illustrating the components of the deep venous drainage system.

1, vena cerebri anterior; **2,** vena basalis (Rosenthal); **3,** lobus temporalis; **4,** vena basalis, lateral to mesencephalon; **5,** cerebellum; **6,** venae cerebelli superiores; **7,** venae cerebri magna (Galen); **8,** vena cerebri occipitalis; **9,** sinus sagittalis superior; **10,** vena cerebri interna; **11,** vena subependymalis media (vena thalamostriata); **12,** vena septi pellucidi.

Fig. 62. The deep draining veins consist of two principal groups, the veins which are basal and those which are dorsal to the diencephalon and basal nuclei. The dorsally located veins are made up of a number of subependymal vessels: the anterior or *vena septi pellucidi* (receiving veins draining the septum pellucidum and rostral part of the nucleus caudatus), and the middle and posterior subependymal veins which are usually united to form a single *vena thalamostriata* (**11**) which drains the nucleus caudatus. The last is the *vena choroidea* of the choroid plexus of the ventriculus lateralis (*cf.* Figs. 60, 61, **12, 12a**). The septal, thalamostriate and choroidal veins coalesce at the dorsal aspect of the *foramen interventriculare* (area of the roof plate in the primitive neural tube) to form the *vena cerebri interna* (**10**), which runs caudally along the roof of the ventriculus tertius. The two internal veins then become directed superiorly, passing just lateral to the pineal and extend up under the splenium of the corpus callosum. At this point they fuse, forming the *vena cerebri magna* (**7**, great vein of Galen) which empties into the *sinus rectus* (Fig. 60, **5**). A series of thin walled vessels (essentially possessing only an endothelium and a basement membrane) extend between the veins of the cerebral cortex and the subependymal veins. These have been called the transcerebral veins by Kaplan and Ford[70] (see Fig. 64, **5**).

Fig. 63. Ventral aspect of the brain stem illustrating the superficial collecting veins of pons and medulla.
1, large pontine collecting vein; **2,** crus cerebri; **3,** anastomosis between the pontine veins and mesencephalic veins which empty into vena basalis; **4,** hemispherium cerebelli; **5,** medulla; **6,** surface collecting vein for the medulla.

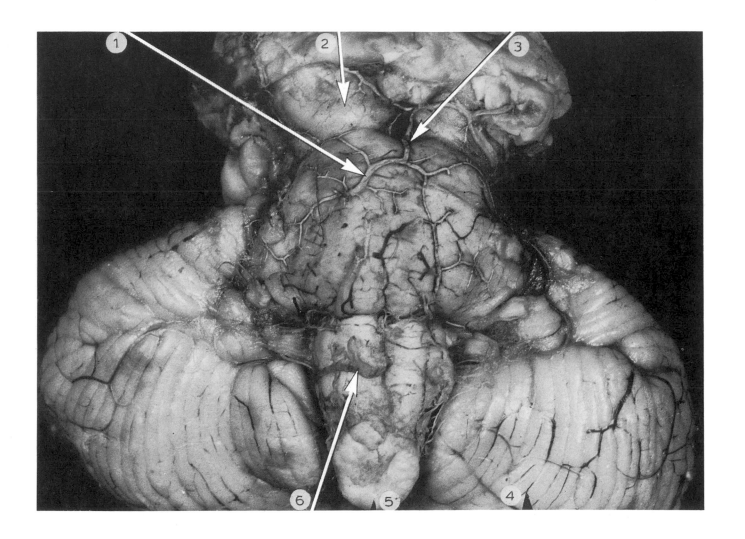

Fig. 65. The basal draining veins are extremely thin walled and difficult to see unless they are congested. The *vena cerebri media profunda* (**1**) and the *vena cerebri anterior* (**2**) join in the region of the *substantia perforata anterior*. These veins are more deeply placed than the arteries forming the *circulus arteriosus cerebri*. The deep middle cerebral veins drain the lenticular nuclei and the anterior vein drains the area of the corpus striatum as well as some cortical areas of the inferior medial margin of the lobus frontalis.

The new vein just formed is the *vena basalis* (**4**). It runs caudally collecting tributary veins draining the diencephalon and midbrain tegmental regions *via* veins exiting through the substantia perforata posterior. The basal vein then passes dorsally around the mesencephalon, and finally empties into the vena cerebri magna in conjunction with veins draining the medial occipital cortex and the medial rostral superior cerebellar surface. As this basal vein passes around the mesencephalon it receives tectal and caudal diencephalic tributaries and probably some choroidal draining veins as well (Figs. 60 and 61).

The veins draining the pons and medulla course across their ventral surfaces (Fig. 63) and empty into the *sinus petrosus superior* (Fig. 61, **30**) rostrally or caudally into the veins of the spinal cord. They may also anastomose with the vena basalis.

The cerebellar cortex (*cf*. Figs. 60, 61) is drained by surface networks directed both rostrally and caudally. The medial surface veins drain rostrally into the *vena cerebri magna* (**6**) while posterior medially placed vessels are frequently observed draining caudally into the *sinus rectus* (**5**) or into the *confluens sinuum* (**1**). The lateral aspects of the rostral margin of the cerebellum drain *via* lateral cortical veins into the *sinus petrosus superior* (**30**). The caudal lateral cortex has veins emptying into the *sinus transversus* (**2**).

Legend for Figs. 64, 65.
1, vena cerebri media profunda; **1a,** venae striati draining base of basal nuclei into **1**; **2,** vena cerebri anterior; **3,** diencephalic collecting veins; **4,** vena basalis (Rosenthal); **5,** transcerebral veins; **6,** lobus temporalis; **7,** lobus frontalis; **7a,** gyri orbitales of **7**; **8,** lobus occipitalis; **9,** septum pellucidum; **10,** caput nucleus caudatus; **11,** capsula interna; **12,** nucleus lentiformis; **13,** tuber cinereum; **14,** medulla oblongata; **15,** pons.

Fig. 64. Coronal section of the brain through the caput of the nucleus caudatus showing the distribution of the transcerebral veins along the radiating fibers of the corona radiata.

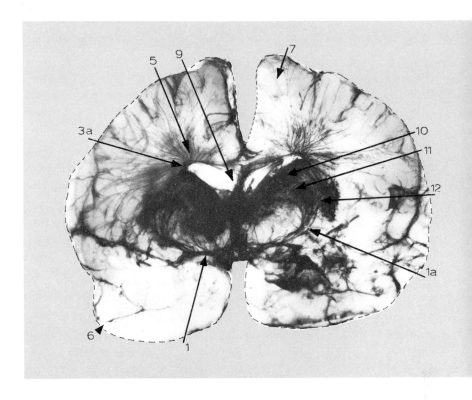

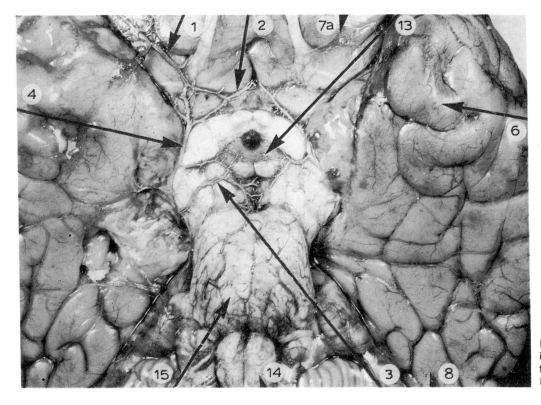

Fig. 65. Ventral aspect of the brain stem illustrating the disposition of the veins forming the vena basalis (vein of Rosenthal).

5.8.3 Vascular supply for the spinal cord

Figs. 66, 67. The arterial supply for the medulla spinalis (spinal cord) is provided by the *arteria spinalis anterior* (**9,** derived from the arteriae vertebrales) and by the *arteria spinalis posterior* (**5**) which may arise from either the arteria cerebelli inferior posterior or the arteria vertebralis. The posterior vessels descend along the dorsum of the cord as two interconnected plexiform vessels while the anterior vessel descends in the vicinity of the fissura mediana anterior. A surface network arises from these posterior and anterior arteries with numerous encircling *'vasocoronal'* vessels (**8**). Both the posterior and anterior arteries receive additional blood supply from the segmental arteries arising from the ventral intercostal and lumbosacral vessels. These have been termed the segmental medullary arteries (**4, 7**). Rami are also given off to supply the dorsal root ganglia. Perforating vessels from the anterior and posterior spinal arteries supply the internal grey matter, while the white matter (**11**) seems to rely on perforators arising from the vasocoronal vessels (**8**).

The venous drainage of the medulla spinalis is accomplished *via* an anterior longitudinal venous trunk and a series of posterior longitudinal veins. These vessels are interconnected by a well developed anastomotic plexus of veins around the surface of the cord. This surface plexus is itself drained by medullary veins which empty into the segmental veins and into an extensive epidural plexus (**17, 18**). This plexus establishes a venous drainage connection caudally with the veins draining the prostate and penis. Rostrally, the epidural plexus becomes associated with the occipital veins.

Fig. 66. Diagrammatic representation of the arterial supply of the spinal cord. **a,** vertebral body; **b,** transverse process of **a; c,** spinal process of **a.**

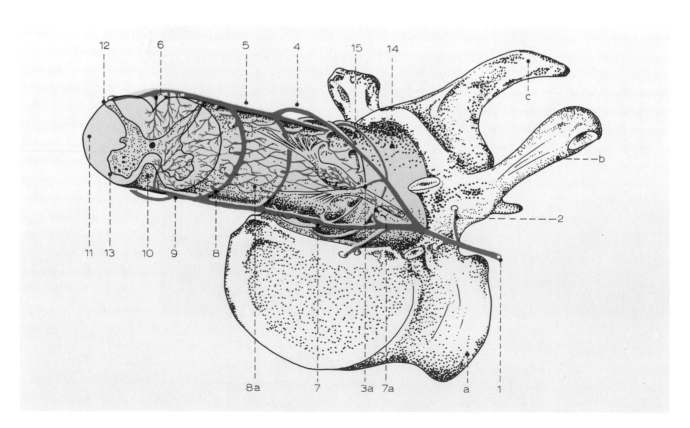

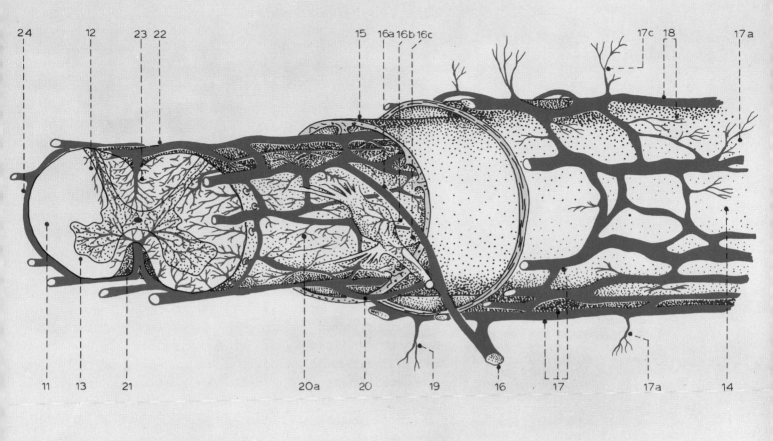

Fig. 67. Diagrammatic representation of the venous drainage of the spinal cord.

5.8.4 Blood–brain barrier

Figs. 68, 69. In 1885 Ehrlich observed that certain aniline dyes injected intravenously stained all tissues of the body except the brain. Since then many investigators have noted that a wide variety of substances penetrate into the brain parenchyma less readily than in other tissues. In time a concept was formulated to the effect that there was some sort of a blood–brain barrier which prevented many blood-borne compounds from entering the brain. Ideas concerning the nature and purpose of this barrier have had an extremely varied history.

When considering the nature of the barrier, one must first consider the anatomy of the brain structures which could function in this manner, particularly in relation to other tissues. The first anatomical unit which could influence the penetration of materials into the brain is the capillary (**5b**). The endothelial cells of the capillaries in the brain are interdigitated with each other and possess no evidence of pores except in the median eminence and area postrema (which are not thought to possess a barrier). Furthermore, there is no large perivascular space outside the basement membrane which overlies these cells, except around the vessels in the median eminence and area postrema. This in general differs from what is observed in most of the rest of the body, particularly in the liver which is the organ most often compared with the brain and in which endothelial cells do not interdigitate and in which there is a well developed perivascular space. In brain, this space is small by comparison, being only about 200 Å units in width. This is similar to the extracellular spaces of brain, and like them varies considerably in different brain areas.

The next unit between the neuron (**8**) and the blood is the astrocyte (**9**) which has feet-like processes which ensheath all but about 15% of the capillary area. These astrocytes then extend between the capillary and the neuron, where another cell membrane is encountered. Thus, in the brain there are a number of membranes which exist between the cytoplasm and the blood, each of which may contribute to whether or not a particular solute may reach a neuron. The absence of a large perivascular space in the brain into which the fluid component of blood and its dissolved solutes can pool, may also influence the exchange of materials between the blood and the tissue.

Having conceded that there is an anatomical substrate which by its position must influence the movement of materials from the blood to the neuron and that all the different membranes of these cellular units may contribute, one should consider other factors which may have an influence on whether a particular substance may reach neurons or not. Considering the various substrates which might or might not enter the brain, Lajtha[80] has recently classified them into three categories.

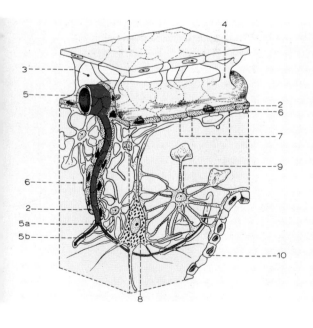

Fig. 68. Sketch illustrating the relationship of the leptomeninges (pia and arachnoid) to the outer glial limiting membrane on the surface of the cerebral hemisphere. The relationship of the arteries and capillaries to the meninges, glia and nerve cells is also indicated.
1, arachnoid; **2,** pia; **3,** subarachnoid space; **4,** arachnoid trabecule; **5,** artery; **5a,** arteriole; **5b,** capillary; **6, 7,** glial feet; **8,** neuron; **9,** astrocyte; **10,** ependyma.

1. Substances which do not penetrate the various membranes at all. These could be very large molecules or materials completely foreign to the organism.

2. Substances that penetrate membranes by diffusing passively through the membranes. This group includes a large number of compounds whose ability to reach neurons depends somewhat on physical constants: lipid solubility, ionization, size or degree of binding to plasma proteins. With this group, the anatomy of the brain capillary system wherein there are essentially no large perivascular spaces and where the endothelial cells interdigitate with each other and have few or no pores probably is important in influencing the rate at which such materials can leave the blood to enter the brain.

3. Substances that penetrate membranes by carrier or mediated mechanisms. This probably includes most of the physiological substrates normally used metabolically by glia and neurons, but does not preclude other substances which might utilize the same transport systems. This category is also probably considerably influenced by the metabolic state and demands in a particular area.

Various compounds have been found which belong in each of the above categories. The fact that some compounds do not leave the brain vascular system at all is useful for utilizing such compounds as ^{131}I-serum-albumin, to measure blood volume in the brain. (This compound does undergo degradation with time with the release of some labeled material which enters the brain.) Alcohol and steroid hormones, both of which are lipid soluble, fit readily into the second category of substances. Calcium and thyroid hormones also fit into the second category and are examples of materials which are restricted somewhat in reaching the neuron by their binding to plasma proteins and probably by the absence of any perivascular space of appreciable size, wherein pooling might occur. Amino acids and perhaps the purine and pyrimidine bases appear to fall into the third category of substances in entering brain *via* a carrier system. The rate at which such materials reach the neurons may depend on the physiological requirements of the neurons (Dobbing[31], Kaplan and Ford[70]), and may in some circumstances be facilitated in their rate of entry. Thus, the blood–brain barrier phenomenon represents a complicated anatomical–biochemical–physiological system which appears to have an important role in determining which materials reach the neurons and the rate at which this occurs. Whether a particular substance reaches the neurons appears to depend on some combination of all these factors, each of which could be considered as influencing the movement of the substrate at each of the anatomical membranes existing between the blood and the neuronal cytoplasm.

Fig. 69. Diagrammatic representation of the relationship between the brain capillaries (**C**), astrocytic glial cells (**A**) and neurons (**N**). The axons are indicated by **AX** and the dendrites by **D**. The five membrane surfaces interposed between the blood and the neuronal cytoplasm are: **1**, basement membrane of the capillary, shown as a sheath around the vessel; **2**, endothelial cell walls of the capillary; **3**, cytomembranes of the astrocyte foot processes in apposition with the capillary basement membrane; **4**, cytomembranes of astrocyte foot processes in apposition with the cell wall of the neuron; **5**, neuronal cell wall.

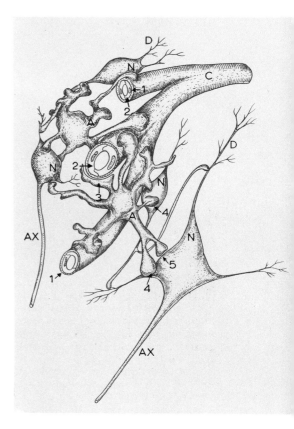

A
B

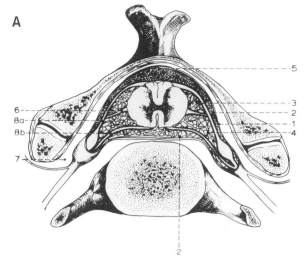
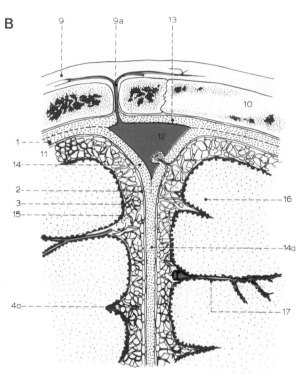

Fig. 70. **A,** the spinal cord as it would appear suspended in the spinal canal surrounded by the three protective or supporting meningeal coverings: dura mater (**1**), arachnoid (**2**) and pia mater (**3**); **B,** the two dural layers in relation to the skull and deeper meningeal layers, which are in turn related to a glial layer on the surface of the cortex.
4, arachnoid trabecules; **4a,** subarachnoid space; **5,** septum posticum; **6,** ligamentum denticulatum; **7,** epidural space; **8a,** radix dorsalis; **8b,** radix ventralis; **9,** scalp; **9a,** vena emissaria; **10,** skull bone, outer support to brain, **11,** inner support; **12,** sinus; **13,** periosteal dura; **14,** deep dural layer; **14a,** falx cerebri; **15,** glial layer of glial feet; **16,** grey matter; **17,** capillary.

5.9 Meninges

Fig. 70. The central nervous system of vertebrates is well protected, the brain being enclosed within the calivarium while the spinal cord is contained within the vertebral canal. The nerves which reach the periphery must, as a result, pass through foramina in this closely fitting bony armor (*cf.* also Figs. 71–74).

The central nervous system is further enclosed and protected by three membranes, the meninges. The outer membrane (*dura mater,* **1**) is tough, being composed of fibrous connective tissue. In the skull cavity, the dura fuses to the periosteal lining (**13**) of the inner surface of the bone except where the large veins draining the brain become enclosed between the periosteal membrane and dura. In the vertebral canal, the dura is separated from the periosteum by an accumulation of fat and an epidural venous plexus. In the cranial cavity, the dura proper becomes reflected away from the cranial wall where the great venous sinuses draining the brain are located. These connective tissue reflections extend some distance away from the venous sinuses they enclose, forming dense connective tissue plates which separate some of the major subdivisions of the brain. One such membrane, the *falx cerebri* (**14a**), extends between the two cerebral hemispheres.

Figs. 71, 72. The *tentorium cerebelli* (**13**) extends horizontally across the posterior fossa of the skull, separating the cerebellum from the cerebrum. There is a notch in the anterior margin of the tentorium, the *incisura tentorii* (**e**) through which the brain stem passes. Another reflection of the dura *(diaphragma sellae)* helps to enclose the pituitary gland in the *sella turcica.* A further reflection, the *cavum trigeminale,* exists in relation to the ganglion and divisions of the trigeminal nerve.

The *arachnoid* which surrounds the brain and spinal cord is a rather thin spider web sort of membrane of white fibrous and elastic tissue found just deep to the dura. It is separated from the dura by what is termed the subdural space. This space does not exist under normal circumstances. It is what is frequently called a 'potential space'. Normally, the arachnoid is in contact with the dura and no space exists, although no physical structure attaches them to each other. However, the arachnoid bounds an inner cavity (subarachnoid space) filled with cerebrospinal fluid which is under a slight pressure. In all likelihood, this pressure would expand the arachnoid envelope outwards, keeping it in close apposition with the dura in the cranial cavity. The arachnoid is connected to the deepest meningeal layer, the *pia mater,* by thin trabeculae. The fluid-filled subarachnoid space (Fig. 68, **3**) separates these two membranes.

The pia and arachnoid are frequently considered together as the *leptomeninges* (Fig. 68). The pia differs from the arachnoid in being firmly adherent to the surface of the brain and spinal cord at all points, being actually bound to a surface layer of astrocytes which, together with the pia, form what is termed the *pial-glial membrane.* In some areas the subarachnoid space is considerable. It is then called a cistern.

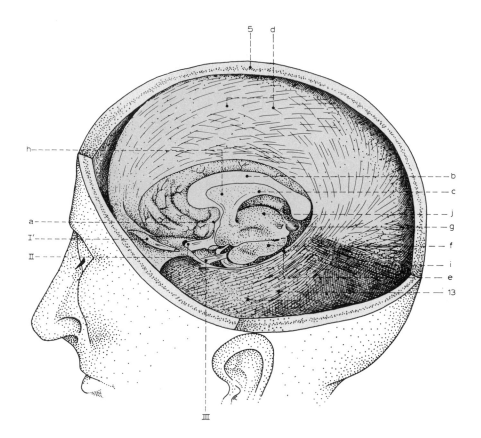

Fig. 71. Diagrammatic sketch of the brain stem in relation to the incisura tentorii (**e**) of the tentorium cerebelli (**13**). **I**, tractus olfactorius; **II**, nervus opticus; **III**, nervus oculomotorius; **a**, commissura anterior; **b**, corpus callosum; **c**, fornix; **d**, falx cerebri; **e**, incisura tentorii; **f**, mesencephalon; **g**, corpus pinealis; **h**, septum pellucidum; **i**, region of sinus rectus; **j**, thalamus; **5**, skull; **13**, tentorium cerebelli.

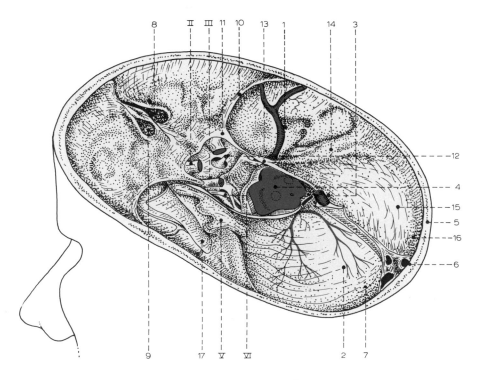

Fig. 72. Diagrammatic sketch of the floor of the skull with telencephalon and diencephalon removed. The left side of the tentorium cerebelli has also been removed and a flap of the dura mater (**17**) pulled back to demonstrate the three sub-divisions of the trigeminal nerve (**V**) just prior to their exit from the cranial cavity. **II**, nervus opticus; **III**, nervus oculomotorius; **V**, nervus trigeminus; **VI**, nervus abducens; **1**, arteria meningea media; **2**, arteria cerebelli superior; **3**, vena cerebri magna (Galen); **4**, mesencephalon; **5**, skull; **6**, confluens sinuum; **7**, superior surface of cerebellum; **8**, crista galli; **9**, cavity in the anterior cranial fossa for the bulbus olfactorius; **10**, ala minor of os sphenoidale; **11**, processus clinoideus anterior; **12**, infundibulum projecting through diaphragma sellae; **13**, incisura tentorii; **14**, pars petrosa of os temporale; **15**, tentorium cerebelli; **16**, sinus transversus; **17**, dura over cavum trigeminale reflected superiorly.

Fig. 73. Sketch of a dissection of the interior of the floor of the skull. The telencephalon has been completely removed as has the left half of the rest of the brain. The major venous sinuses of the left side have been opened.

II, nervus opticus; **III,** nervus oculomotorius; **IV,** nervus trochlearis; **V,** nervus trigeminus; **VII,** nervus facialis; **VIII,** nervus cochleovestibularis; **IX,** nervus glossopharyngeus; **X,** nervus vagus; **XI,** nervus accessorius; **1,** cut edge of tentorium cerebelli; **2,** sinus sigmoideus; **3,** sinus petrosus superior; **4,** sinus cavernosus exposed after reflection of dura; **5,** arteria meningea media; **6,** region of the lamina cribrosa and bulbus olfactorius; **7,** crista galli; **8,** processus clinoideus anterior; **9,** arteria carotis interna; **10,** sinus sagittalis superior (opened); **11,** arachnoid granulation; **12,** region of the foramen magnum; **13,** mesencephalon; **14,** vena cerebri magna (Galen); **15,** falx cerebri; **16,** sinus rectus; **17,** confluens sinuum; **18,** sinus transversus; **19,** posterior cranial fossa.

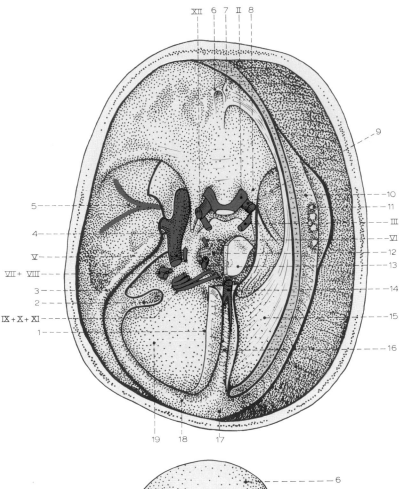

Fig. 74. The menigeal envelopes of the medulla spinalis.

1. ligamentum denticulatum with process projecting laterally through **2; 1a,** ligamentum denticulatum attached to dura spinalis; **2,** arachnoidea spinalis; **3,** radix dorsalis with accompanying sleeve of pial-arachnoid tissue; **3a,** radix dorsalis passing through dura spinalis; **3b,** rami dorsales passing through the arachnoid; **4,** nervus spinalis; **5,** ganglion spinale; **6,** dura mater spinalis; **6a,** dura mater reflected laterally; **7,** pia mater spinalis with arteria spinalis posterior.

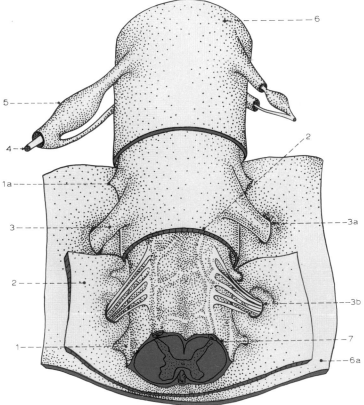

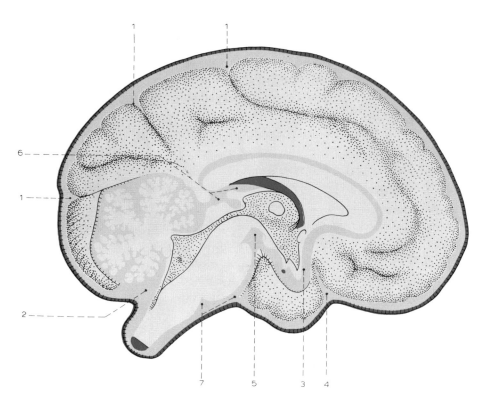

Fig. 75. The cisternae of the cavum sub-arachnoideale.
1, subarachnoid cisterna (an expanded portion of the cavity where the arachnoid bridges any depression of the surface of the brain). A term applying to all cisternae.
7, cisterna of pons.

Additional reinforcements for support are provided for the spinal cord by two membranes: These are the *denticulate ligaments* which extend from the pia laterally to the dura, and the *septum cervicale intermedium* which extends longitudinally along the posterior surface between the pia and arachnoid membranes in the cervical region.

5.10 Cisternae

Fig. 75. Since a cisterna occurs whenever the pia is widely separated from the arachnoid membrane, such a space is present in relation to every sulcus or fissure and could be named accordingly. However, only the largest of these enlargements of the subarachnoid space are named. They are as follows: *cisterna cerebellomedullaris* (**2**) or cisterna magna, which is just below the caudal inferior aspect of the cerebellum and just above the surface of the medulla. This is the largest of the cisterns. The *cisterna chiasmatis* (**3**) is the enlargement of the subarachnoid space between the optic chiasm and the rostrum of the corpus callosum. The *cisterna fossae lateralis cerebri* (**4**), as the name implies, is within the lateral fissure, while the *cisterna interpeduncularis* (**5**) is between the crura cerebri. The *cisterna venae magnae cerebri* (**6**) constitutes the extension of the sub-arachnoid space posteriorly from the crus cerebri around the lateral margins of the mesencephalon up over the tectum mesencephali and then rostrally over the roof of the *ventriculus tertius*. This final rostral extension of the cistern is just under the splenium and the truncus corporis callosi.

A pial layer covers the roof of the third ventricle, the under surface of the corpus callosum and the medial edge of the fornix. The space between these two pial layers is filled with loose leptomeningeal tissue containing many blood vessels. This whole double pial layer is often termed the *velum interpositum*. The enlarged subarachnoid spaces without specific names which contain small localized accumulations of cerebrospinal fluid are termed the *cisternae subarachnoidales* (**1**).

Small specialized outgrowths of the arachnoid membrane, capped with epithelial cells, project through the dura in various places into the intradural venous sinuses. These are the arachnoid granulations through which at least some of the cerebrospinal fluid (CSF) filling the subarachnoid spaces may drain into the blood stream. There is also a fine plexus of vessels of capillary dimension in the pia which also serves to absorb some of the CSF. The largest accumulation of the arachnoid granulations is in association with the sinus sagittalis superior though granulations may be found in association with all the other intradural sinuses as well.

5.11 Ventricular system

Figs. 76, 77. As is apparent from the embryology, the vertebrate nervous system develops as a hollow tubular structure from which the cerebral vesicles evaginate. As these hemispheric dilations arise from the neural tube, the hollow cavity of the primitive tube extends into them. As a result of the flexures within the neural tube, the development of hemispheric structures, the growth of the alar and basal plates which progressively decrease the diameter of the neural canal, the myelinization of the fibers of the white matter and the growth of the corpus striatum on

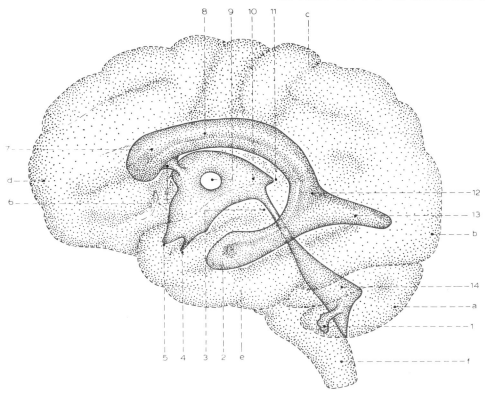

Fig. 76. Diagrammatic representation of the ventricular cavities of the brain in relation to the surface structures.
a, cerebellum; **b,** lobus occipitalis; **c,** lobus parietalis; **d,** lobus frontalis; **e,** lobus temporalis; **f,** medulla oblongata; **1,** apertura laterales ventriculi quarti (foramen of Luschka); **2,** ventriculus lateralis, cornu inferior; **3,** aqueductus cerebri; **4,** recessus infundibularis; **5,** recessus opticus; **6,** foramen interventriculare; **7,** ventriculus lateralis, cornu anterior; **8,** ventriculus lateralis, central part; **9,** adhesio interthalamica (massa intermedia); **10,** ventriculus tertius; **11,** recessus pinealis; **12,** antrum of ventriculus lateralis; **13,** ventriculus lateralis, cornu posterior; **14,** ventriculus quartus.

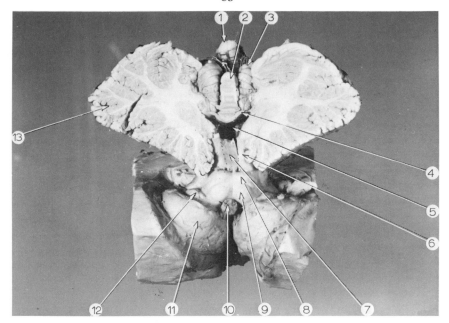

Fig. 77. Section through the metencephalon passing through the fastigial recess of the fourth ventricle.
1, medulla; **2**, uvula; **3**, tonsil; **4**, velum medullare posterior; **5**, recessus fastigii; **6**, pedunculus cerebellaris superior; **7**, velum medullare anterior; **8**, colliculus inferior; **9**, colliculus superior; **10**, pineal; **11**, pulvinar; **12** corpus geniculatum mediale; **13**, cerebellar folia.

the medial floor of the telencephalon, the ventricular cavities, cerebral aqueduct and the various foraminae of the ventricular system attain their adult configuration. A pair of openings exists at the caudal end wherein the space of the ventriculus quartus connects with the cavum subarachnoideale. These are the paired *apertura laterales ventriculi quarti* (foramen of Luschka). At the most caudal end of the roof of the ventriculus quartus there is an area where the roof is greatly thinned or open through which some of the cerebrospinal fluid filling the ventricular cavities may escape. This is the foramen of Magendi.

The ventricular cavities and the cerebral aqueduct which connects the ventriculus tertius and quartus are lined throughout with ependymal cells. This ependymal lining provided the original germinal epithelium of the primitive neural tube. In the fully formed brain these cells become ciliated and lose most of their germinative qualities. However, in many species mitotic divisions have been observed in this lining membrane at all ages. Furthermore, these cells are capable of uncontrolled multiplication any time after birth, producing intraventricular tumor masses. The cilia of the ependyma have been observed to beat in waves in such a manner that a current is produced in the cerebrospinal fluid which progresses from the lateral to the third ventricle and then to the cerebral aqueduct and finally to the fourth ventricule and the foramen of Luschka[149]. This should apparently aid in directing the flow of the cerebrospinal fluid to the draining foramen of the ventricular system.

The ependymal lining cells undergo histological modification in various areas. Thus, the cells are tall columnar elements over grey matter (*i.e.*, caudate nucleus and thalamus), almost squamous over white matter (corpus callosum) and highly modified in at least one area to form a pseudostratified columnar epithelium (subcommissural organ) beneath the *commissura posterior* at the rostral end of the aqueductus cerebri).

5.12 Cerebrospinal fluid

The fluid filling the ventricular system and subarachnoid space is a clear, almost cell free fluid which is slightly alkaline and isotonic with blood plasma. It normally contains very little protein (15 to 45 mg%), which varies from individual to individual and with age, being lower in children, and higher in adults. The fluid also normally contains small amounts of sugar, calcium, potassium, sodium, chloride, magnesium, lactic acid, amino acids, creatinine, uric acid, urea and cholesterol. A few cells may also be present (5/ml), which are mostly lymphocytic elements.

The formation of cerebrospinal fluid appears to be largely due to the secretion of a hypertonic saline by the choroid plexus which is then brought to isotonicity by diffusion of water through the ependymal cells lining the ventricle. Increases in blood pressure increase the rate of formation of fluid, possibly by increasing the secretion of the hypertonic saline. The choroid plexus also appears capable of secreting other materials into the cerebrospinal fluid.

5.12.1 Circulation of the cerebrospinal fluid

Fig. 78. The greatest proportion of the cerebrospinal fluid (CSF) is formed in the lateral ventricles while lesser amounts are formed in the other ventricles which contain choroid plexuses. Diffusion of water may occur, however, across all the ependymal linings, in areas where there is no choroid plexus. Resorption of water and certain compounds (amino acids, ions) of the CSF may occur back across all the ependymal linings into the brain parenchyma. The general direction of flow is caudally toward the foramen of the ventriculus quartus. This would seem to be largely due to the fact that there is a 'head of pressure' at the rostral end of the system caused primarily by the rate of formation here which causes it to flow caudally toward the lateral foramen of Luschka. This flow may be aided by the cilia of the ependymal cells. Current ideas as to the amount of CSF produced appear to be in the range of 50 to 100 ml/day to maintain a total volume of CSF in the entire ventricular-subarachnoid system of about 135 ml (range of 75 to 150 ml). Thus, almost as much must be resorbed each day as is produced. While some resorption may occur within the ventricular system *via* the ependymal cells, most of this occurs after the CSF has left the ventricular cavities *via* the foramen of Luschka. CSF leaves the subarachnoid space at many points. Arachnoid granulations associated with the intradural venous sinuses and with epidural venous plexuses of the spinal cord appear to have a valve-like function

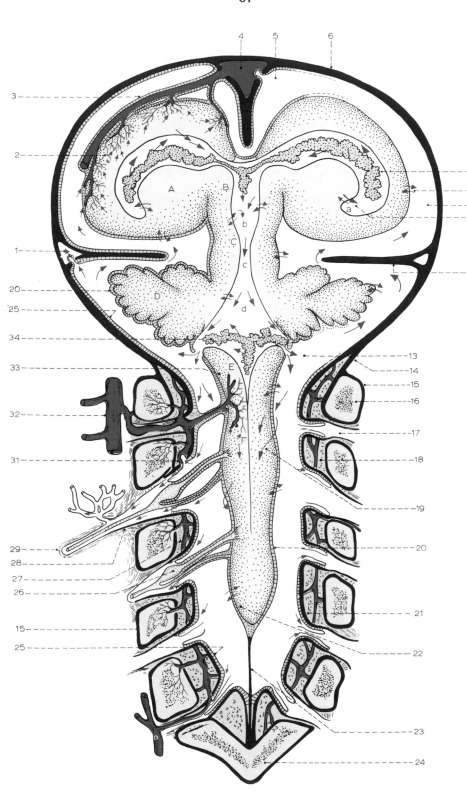

Fig. 78. Diagrammatic scheme indicating the various sources for formation of the cerebrospinal fluid and the sites where resorption will return it to the venous system. The size of the arrows indicates the magnitude of formation, resorption and direction of flow.

A, telencephalon; **B,** diencephalon; **C,** mesencephalon; **D,** cerebellum; **E,** medulla oblongata; **F,** medulla spinalis; **a,** ventriculus lateralis; **b,** ventriculus tertius; **c,** aqueductus cerebri; **d,** ventriculus quartus; **1,** sinus transversus with arachnoid granulation; **2,** resorption into small pial vessels which drain into the venae cerebri superiores; **3,** vena cerebri superior; **4,** sinus sagittalis superior; arachnoid granulation projecting into sinus sagittalis superior; **6,** dura and skull periostium; **8,** plexus choroideus; **9,** exchange of fluid between brain parenchyma and fluid within the subarachnoid cavity (**10**); **10,** cavum subarachnoideale; **11,** exchange of fluid between brain parenchyma and fluid within the ventricular cavity; **12,** tentorium cerebelli; **13,** CSF leaving the ventricular space via the apertura lateralis ventriculi quarti; **14,** point of junction of dura mater spinalis with the periostium of the cranial bones at the foramen magnum; **15,** vertebral periostium; **16,** vertebra; **17,** foramina intervertebralis; **18,** epidural space; **19,** arrow indicating flow of CSF down the posterior aspect of the medulla spinalis; **20,** pia mater spinalis; **21,** dura mater spinalis; **22,** exchange of fluid between the parenchyma of medulla spinalis and the cavum subarachnoideale; **23,** filum terminale; **24,** os coccygis; **25,** arachnoidea spinalis; **26,** ganglion spinale; **27,** epidural space; **28,** dural sheath of nervus spinalis blending with epineurium; **29,** nervus spinalis showing perineuronal space; **31,** small arachnoid granulation projecting into an epidural vein; **32,** vein from the plexus venosi vertebrales externi; **33,** CSF entering small venules within the pia; **34,** plexus choroideus.

which allows CSF to drain into the venous system when CSF pressure exceeds venous pressure. Some is also apparently resorbed through the extensive plexus of small pial venules which eventually drain into intra-dural sinuses and segmental veins. Water and some ions also appear to be able to pass through the pial-glial membrane covering the surface of the CNS. Presumably this fluid and contained solutes may then reach small venules within the brain parenchyma *via* glial pathways.

5.12.2 Function of the cerebrospinal fluid

The CSF surrounds the brain with an aqueous cushion which presumably may help in protecting the brain from outside shocks. It has also been suggested that it may help in the removal of waste products from the brain *via* a neuron-glia-ependymal-ventricular cavity pathway.

Hydrocephalus is a condition which occurs when abnormal amounts of CSF collect. This may be caused by overproduction in the ventricles or more commonly by a pathologic process which blocks the normal flow and escape of CSF from ventricular cavities to subarachnoid spaces as might occur if the foramen of Luschka or the ventriculus tertius were blocked by an inflammatory process. Another possibility could be atresia or pathologic occlusion of the aqueductus cerebri. In both of the above examples, drainage of CSF from the ventricular cavities rostral to the site of occlusion is restricted without impairment of CSF formation. This leads to dilation of the ventricular cavities to accommodate for the increasing amount of CSF present and eventually causes a serious compromise in the functional integrity of the brain.

6. Distribution of cells

The organization of the cells within the CNS shows various special arrangements in different regions. In the broadest sense, cell bodies may assemble together into a cluster of cells with a related function, forming a nucleus, or they may be distributed in layers, as in the cerebral and cerebellar cortex, each layer contributing in a specific way to the functional integrity of the structure and each layer having characteristic types of cells. The cellular zones make up the grey matter. Fibers, myelinated or 'unmyelinated' (*cf.* p. 94) are found in varying degrees in all these areas of cell body localization. Interspersed among the nerve cells are numerous nerve cell processes (axons and dendrites) as well as the cell bodies and processes of the supporting glial cells. These processes, in conjunction with vascular elements, constitute the *neuropil*. The axonal-dendrite relationship in this neuropil is very close. It has been estimated, for example, that the activity of one fiber reaching the visual cortex may activate an area of 0.1 mm³ and that its impulses may be dispersed among 5000 neurons. This pattern of a diffusion of effect may also be reversed in that a single cortical motoneuron may have several thousand synaptic endings from other neurons terminating on its dendrites, perikaryon and axon hillock. This may be illustrated by the Purkinje cells of the cerebellar cortex each of which has a dendritic area of about 250,000 μ^2 on which there are estimated to be 200,000 synaptic terminals. In other regions, there are no nerve cell bodies, just fibers and supporting glial cells. The areas in which such fiber accumulations predominate constitute the white matter. Fig. 84 shows four examples of different organizations of white matter intermixed with the grey neuron-rich areas. Fig. 83**A** of the spinal cord illustrates a region where grey and white matter are distinctly separate.

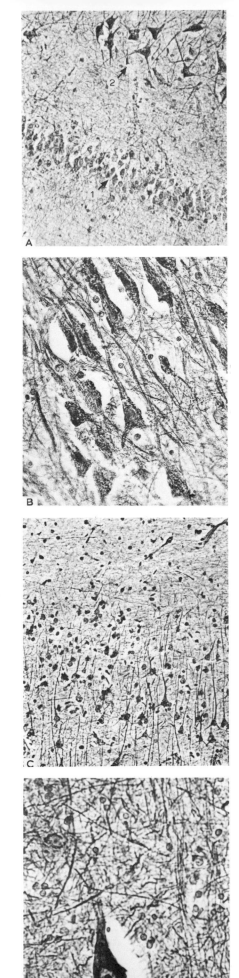

Fig. 79. **A** and **B,** hippocampal cortex; **A,** showing the pyramidal cell layer (**1**) and the polymorphic cell layer (**2**). **B** shows only the pyramidal cell layer. **C** and **D,** neocortex; only the 3 superficial cortical layers are shown in **C,** which has the same magnification as the cortex in **A. D** shows a large pyramidal cell of the primary motor cortex (area 4).

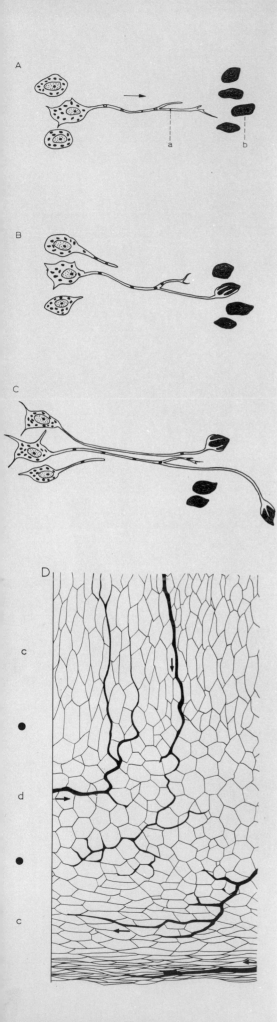

6.1 Structural organization

Fig. 80. In the adult animal no such simple pattern as is seen in the embryonic neural tube exists. Neurons have migrated, associations have been made and cells of similar function aggregated. What induces these changes?

It has been shown that the axon of a neuron is established as a direct protoplasmic extension. At a given point on the cell body, presumably at some break in the surface membrane, a short thread of cytoplasm is extended. Since these sprouts in embryonic nerve cells appear to arise from the same side of all members within a given group of neuroblasts, some degree of polarization seems likely, either from within the cell or from the environment. The sprout continues to elongate by virtue of forces within the cell body. It has no rigid skeleton, no sheath and according to Harrison[60] advances in an amoeboid manner. As the growing tip advances, it leaves a filamentous protoplasmic thread behind it. This amoeboid advance, powered by some sort of 'pumping action' within the cell continues until the sprout becomes permanently attached to a peripheral receptor or effector cell. The cell body remains anchored during this process.

Further elongation of the fiber after the tip becomes attached to its terminal end organ appears somewhat passive, the fiber being towed out by the tissues into which it has insinuated itself. During the early course of free advance, the position of a nerve fiber is dependent on the path taken by the roving free tip. This early 'pioneer' fiber establishes the course followed by subsequent fibers which terminate in the same end organ. The subsequent passive process followed by the 'pioneer' and adjacent fibers as they are carried along by the tissue to which they attach is called 'towing'[145].

Fig. 80. Diagrammatic representation of a 'pioneer' neuron seeking out the peripheral target which it will innervate. Other neurons then follow the path established by the neuron. Subsequent growth of the target away from the central axis of the organism tows the nerve fibers behind it.
A, pioneering; **a,** growing axon tip; **b,** target organ; **B,** application to target with younger nerves following the pioneer; **C,** towing: peripheral shift of target pulls nerve fiber after it; **D,** advance of fibers in fibrous media; **c,** organized network; **d,** disorganized network.

How the first pioneer fiber arrives at the proper place of termination represents a further question. Many varieties of 'tropism' have been mentioned in the past (chemical, electrical, mechanical or undefined physiological). Weiss[143] presents a concept in which the outward growth of peripheral nerves proceeds along facial planes. Such interfaces are numerous in the body. All fibrous units (fibrils, fibers, filaments) that exist in the liquid spaces between cells and tissues, forming the solid components of 'ground substance', or the interfaces between a solid and a liquid or two immiscible liquids have been suggested by Weiss as providing adequate facial planes for directing the course of outwardly growing neurons. Fig. 80**D** illustrates how a nerve fiber would advance in media with differing arrangements of fibrous components. This mode of advance whereby growing pioneer neuronal tips proceed along inter-facial planes is termed 'contact guidance'. The rate of free growth of such a system appears to be a function of the rate of protein synthesis, etc., in the neuron itself plus the configuration of the pathway system. The rate of growth as it occurs has been observed to be irregular, consisting of alternating spurts and delays. The more irregular the substrate into which a fiber grows, the more frequent will be the delays in growth. Thus, growth is fastest along straight pathways. During regeneration of an injured axon this would be achieved by following the old de-generated myelinated tube of the previous axon. Thus, the nerve fiber grows out toward its final termination, guided apparently by the im-mediate surroundings which shape its course. What it is which induces nerve fibers from specific areas of the neural tube to seek out certain terminal targets remains another question. The concept of 'contact guidance' as described by Weiss may help to explain the course taken by an outgrowing axonal tip, but it does not explain why certain targets are selected in preference to others. Perhaps, as summarized by Detwiler[29], embryonic nerve growth may be actively routed toward centers of active growth. This too appears as an over-simplification. More recent observa-tions by Sperry[127] have been based on optic fiber systems which will terminate in the superior colliculus. Fibers redirected to the inappropriate colliculus altered their course of growth so as to terminate at their normal site. Even when anchored in a path directing them to the wrong colliculus, the growing visual system fibers were capable of making such adjust-ments in growth direction as to eventually lead them to the proper target. Such observations are in contradiction to growing nerve tips being attracted to centers of active growth or of simply following along contact fiber systems and reintroduce concepts of inducers or some form of nerve target specificity. Obviously much remains to be done before we will understand how nerves arrive at their final adult configuration.

6.2 Architectural arrangements within the CNS

What is occurring centrally in regard to migration and final position of the cells in relation to each other and the various fiber systems is more complex. In the cerebral cortex, for example, studies with ^{3}H-thymidine-labeled cells in rodents have shown that the deeper layers of the cortex are established first[5]. The cells of the more superficial layers then migrate through the deeper layers presumably establishing some sparse collateral connections at the same time. Such connections must be very scanty at best, since the extensive dendritic aborizations which develop are not established until much later[36]. The penetration of ascending projecting fibers from lower centers into these cortical layers also appear to occur later.

Why the cells in the cerebral hemisphere come to be superficially placed instead of deep as they are in the spinal cord cannot be easily answered. From experiments with rodents[125] it would appear that the proliferation of cells in the telencephalon is much greater than in the cord, forming a relatively thick mantle layer. A thin superficial marginal layer is still present, however (molecular layer of the adult cortex). In subsequent development, when the neuroblasts form corticofugal axonal processes, those which would terminate on the cells of what will be the basal nuclei and thalamus are directed medially toward the deep nuclei instead of sweeping out into the molecular layer, as occurs in the spinal cord. Such a path would also provide the shortest route for those fibers descending to even lower centers to activate motor neurons. Later, when these axons become myelinated, the white matter which subsequently results would naturally be deep to the cortical cells of origin. Whether one can assume that developing neurons will follow what appears to us as the shortest and most logical path is, however, another matter.

Fig. 81. In the developing cerebellar cortex, a somewhat different situation exists. In the adult we find an inner much branched core of white (lamina albae vitae), a layer of small densely packed cells (the granule cell layer), a layer of scattered larger cells (the Purkinje cell layer) and an outer layer rich in fibers with only a few nerve cells (the molecular layer). In the developing embryo one finds, however, an outer granule layer on the surface. These cells, after migrating all the way to the surface from the germinal epithelium lining the central canal, finally migrate internally to end up with the cells of the inner adult granule layer. They also give rise to the stellate and basket cells of the molecular layer. It has been presumed that such behavior on the part of these neurons enables them to better establish axonal-dendritic connections with the dendrites of the Purkinje cells. Whether the last assumption is true or not remains to be proven.

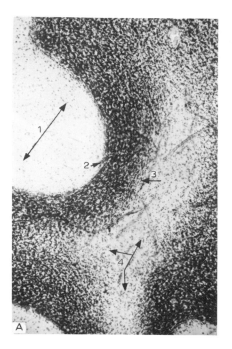

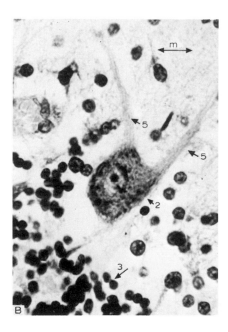

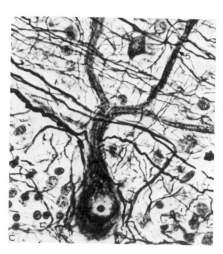

Fig. 81. **A,** low power view of the cerebellar cortex, illustrating the molecular (**1**), Purkinje (**2**) and granule cell (**3**) layers as well as the deep white matter (**4**) (Gallocyanin stain); **B,** Purkinje cell (**2**) showing its two prominent dendrites (**5**) and relationship to molecular **m** and granule cell (**3**) layers (Thionin stain); **C,** Purkinje cell stained with a neurofibrillar stain (Cajal's). Illustrates the basket-like plexus of fibers which are formed around its cell body. Its large dendritic tree (**5**) can be observed branching into the molecular layer.

6.3 Structural localization

What now remains is to briefly indicate some of the structural modifications which occur within the CNS. These modifications form a virtual gross topographic mosaic of functionally specialized regions. Such specializations may in a sense be shared with other areas in that there are similarities in cell type and nuclear organization among the motor nuclei supplying somatic muscles, although they may be in different locations within the neural axis. However, the structural peculiarities of various other nuclei are frequently not shared by others (*i.e.*, the cells of the supraoptic and paraventricular nuclei in the diencephalon are highly specialized units which produce the polypeptide endocrine hormones of the neurohypophysis). Just how the physicochemical properties of these neuronal aggregates promote the functional specificity frequently demonstrated is not clear. Whatever the microconnections are which enable such regional specialization, apparently considerable individual variation exists in the manner in which such connections are effected as well as a considerable potential for substitution within such centers.

6.3.1 Spinal cord

Fig. 82. Throughout the cord, the nerve cell bodies and their supporting tissue (glial cells) form a central H-shaped core around the central canal. Large multipolar cells with prominent masses of Nissl substance (RNA and protein) predominate in the ventral part of the cellular core (Fig. 82**A**, **B**). These cells constitute the elements which activate the somatic muscles. Some degree of functional localization occurs with these units (Fig. 82**C**). Considerable secondary splitting into groups of cells for particular functions (*i.e.*, pronation, supination) also occurs. Particular localizations for cell groups giving rise to such specific nerves as the phrenic and the spinal component of the XIth cranial nerve have been noted[142].

Fig. 82. A, distribution of Nissl substance in the cell bodies and dendrites (**1**) of spinal cord ventral horn cells, and its absence in the axon hillock (**2**) and axon (**3**); **B,** the highly complex neuropil of the spinal cord grey matter is well illustrated in a silver preparation counterstained with Luxol Fast Blue; **C,** diagram illustrating localization of ventral horn cells into specific groups for specific functions. (After *C. U. Ariëns Kappers*). **4,** ventromedial nucleus (neck and trunk); **5,** ventrolateral nucleus (shoulder girdle and upper arm); **6,** dorsolateral nucleus; **7,** retrodorsolateral nucleus (intrinsic muscles of forearm and hand); **8,** dorsomedial nucleus (neck and trunk); **9,** posterior median septum; **10,** posterior funiculus; **11,** lateral funiculus; **12,** flexors, adductors; **13,** extensors, abductors.

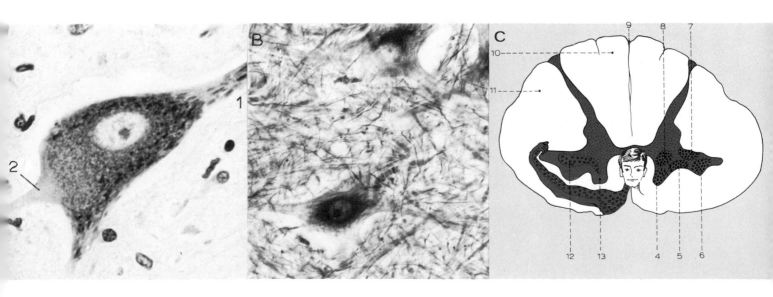

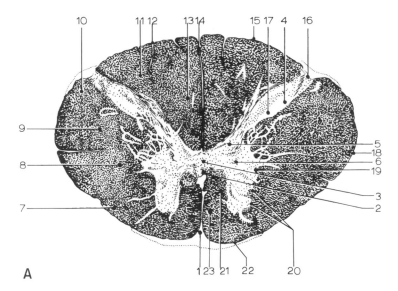

A

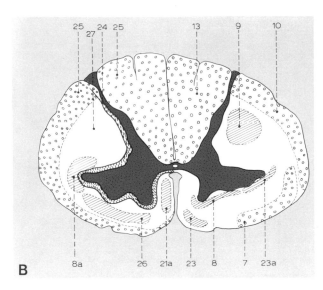

B

Fig. 83. A, upper thoracic part of spinal cord (Weigert-Pal staining); **B,** distribution of fiber systems within the white matter of the spinal cord. Note that ascending sensory fibers (circles) are more peripheral than descending motor fibers (hatched). Also note that considerable overlap occurs and that adjacent fiber systems usually blend with each other. **1,** fissura mediana anterior; **2,** anterior white commissure; **3,** substantia intermedia centralis around canalis centralis; **4,** substantia gelatinosa (of cornu posterior); **5,** nucleus dorsalis (thoracicus); **6,** substantia intermedia lateralis; **7,** fasciculus anterolateralis (tractus spinothalamicus anterior et lateralis, tractus spinoreticularis et spinotectalis); **8,** tractus reticulospinalis; **8a,** tractus reticulospinalis lateralis (**8** and **8a** are indirect motor tracts); **9,** tractus corticospinalis lateralis (direct motor tract); **10,** tractus spino cerebellaris (anterior et posterior); **11,** fasciculus cuneatus; **12,** sulcus intermedius posterior; **13,** fasciculus gracilis; **14,** sulcus medianus posterior; **15,** funiculus posterior; **16,** fasciculus posterolateralis; **17,** cornu posterior; **18,** funiculus lateralis; **19,** cornu laterale; **20** cornu anterior; **21 (A), 21a (B),** tractus corticospinalis anterior (direct motor tract); **22,** funiculus anterior; **23,** tractus tectospinalis medialis; **23a,** tractus tectospinalis lateralis; **24,** fasciculus proprius; **25,** circles indicate sensory tract systems; **26,** tractus vestibulospinalis medialis et lateralis; **27,** white and numbered hatched areas indicate motor tract systems.

Fig. 83. A group of smaller motor cells of the autonomic motor system extends in a column from T_1 to L_2 or L_3. This group of cells between the posterior and anterior cornu forms the intermediolateral cell column or the *cornu laterale*. Just medial to it is a more deeply placed column of cells, the intermediomedial column.

The dorsal horn is also subdivided by the type of neuron present in various areas (*i.e.*, stellate cells of substantia gelatinosa; larger cells with scattered stellate cells in the nucleus proprius, or cells with eccentric nuclei and long ascending axons in the nucleus dorsalis or nucleus thoracicus found medially at the base of the dorsal horn). The dorsal horn can also be subdivided by function. The cells of the substantia gelatinosa are concerned with pain and temperature plus proprioception and tactile sense, and the nucleus dorsalis is concerned only with proprioception. Thus, cells may be grouped somewhat by morphological appearance or by function.

The periphery or marginal layer in the spinal cord contains the ascending or descending nerve fibers arising from the cord neurons plus fibers from many higher centers which terminate on the cord cells. These fibers are of many sizes and degrees of myelination. Some have extremely little myelin (posterolateral fasciculus). The peripheral white mass can be grossly subdivided into three large bundles or funiculi, the posterior, lateral and anterior. Some ideas of the subdivisions within these funiculi into specific tract systems are demonstrated in Fig. 83**B.**

6.3.2 Medulla oblongata

Fig. 84. In this and the more rostral components of the brain stem, the relatively simple arrangement seen in the cord is lost. Certain bundles of fibers as might be found in the marginal layers remain (pyramids and the spinocerebellar tract). The fibers of the posterior funiculus of the cord which are virtually all ascending sensory units have synapses in nuclear masses at the caudal posterior end of the medulla. The secondary ascending fibers arising from these nuclei have not continued in their superficial pathway, but have decussated and entered into the deep parenchymal mass of the medulla, breaking up the nuclear masses with intersecting fiber bundles. This mixing of cell masses with fibers continues throughout the brain stem. It gives rise to a reticular formation which contains specific nuclei for cranial nerves as well as less well circumscribed nuclei such as those concerned with respiration, cardio-vascular control, emetic centers, etc.

6.3.3 Metencephalon

At this level, the massive fiber mass of the pars basilaris pontis has been added at the ventral aspect of the rostral reticular extension from the medulla. In the metencephalon, the *crus cerebri* which lies on the anterior surface of the mesencephalon, has penetrated into the pars basilaris and broken up into many fascicles. Intermingled with these fascicles are clusters of cells which form the nuclei of this part of the pons. These descending fibers contribute to the descending corticospinal path and are in a position comparable to that of the pyramids of the same system in the medulla. Convenient subdivisions of the neural tube into ependymal, mantle and marginal layers are not easily made in these regions.

6.3.4 Cortex of the metencephalon

In the cerebellum (Fig. 81), the final distribution of cells is such that the nerve cells reside in what may be termed the outer edge of the mantle layer. The zone of cortical nerve cells can be subdivided into a thick inner layer of small granule cells and a thin outer layer of flask-shaped Purkinje cells. Superficial to those cells is what may be considered a zone analogous to the primitive marginal layer. It contains few neurons and many nerve fibers deficient in myelin. This is the molecular layer. Deep to the outer cellular cortex is the white matter, while still deeper are large nuclear accumulations of cells upon which terminate the axons of the cortical Purkinje cells. The axons arising from the deep nuclei provide for the fibers which transmit cerebellar influences to higher or lower centers.

Fig. 84. Diagrammatic representation of the distribution of cells and fibers in **A**, the rostral mesencephalon; **B**, the caudal mesencephalon; **C**, the medulla and **D**, the pons. The lighter zones indicates areas rich in nerve cell bodies or unmyelinated fibers. Myelinated fibers have been drawn in black to conform with the image seen in the standard preparations stained for myelin.

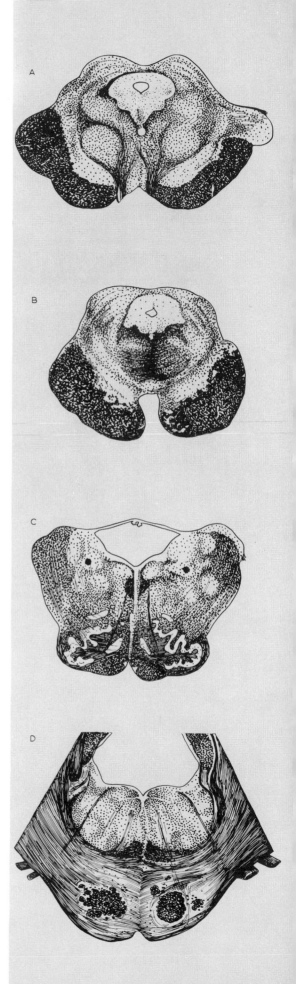

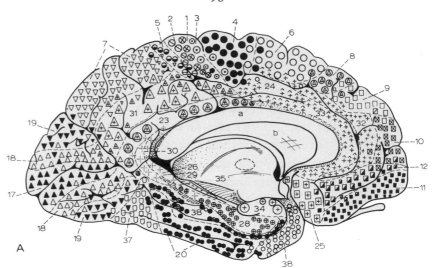

Fig. 85. Modification of the Brodmann numbering system for the cerebral cortex. There is an overlap of adjacent areas and the symbols used have been selected to suggest a similarity between adjacent regions rather than a dissimilarity. **A,** the midsagittal surface; **B,** the lateral surface.
a, corpus callosum; **b,** septum pellucidum.

6.3.5 Telencephalic cortex

The cerebrum, as we have seen, also has a cortical arrangement of cells on the surface, with an underlying fibrous white matter containing the fibers leaving and entering the cortex (see also Fig. 87). A series of deeper nuclear cell aggregations is also present which projects to and receives fibers from the cortex and lower centers. The cerebral cortex has a more complicated structure than that of the cerebellum. There are six layers in most of the cortex (isocortex) of man though the region of the hippocampus (phylogenetically older) has only three layers (allocortex). Other areas of cortex (cortex of uncus and rostral hippocampal gyrus), which arise more recently phylogenetically and which are adjacent to the hippocampus, are also included under the classification of allocortex. Although there are six layers, like the isocortex, they are differentiated from it on the basis of there being fewer cell types.

These six cortical layers vary from one region of the cerebral hemisphere to another. Thus, the granular cortex of the medial surface of the occipital lobe (visual receptive center), which contains many small cells, appears quite different from the agranular cortex of the precentral gyrus (motor cortex) of the frontal lobe where there are many sizes of cells including giant pyramidal (Betz) cells. These variations in cortical structure provide the basis for the study of architectonics, in which such variations have been classified and the location of each type of cortex mapped. Pre-eminent among the cortical mappers are the names of Brodmann, Vogt, Von Economo, Bailey and Von Bonin. These investigators have not only mapped the cortex, but provided numbering schemes for the future identification of these areas. That of Brodmann is perhaps the one most commonly used. Unfortunately, there is a considerable variation in numbering systems. This has raised questions as to whether or not one can truly map differences in cellular architecture so conclusively.

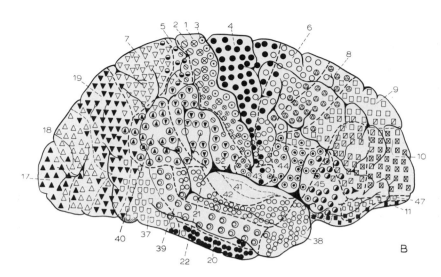

Clark[21] calls attention to the inexactness of architectural science in the brain. He cites that the descriptive terms used have not generally been well defined, (*i.e.*, what may be a medium sized cell to one investigator may be a small one to somebody else). Thus, since the many numbering systems disagree on several points and since varying criteria for definitions of regions have been used, the current use of such numbering has little sound anatomical basis. Nevertheless, these numbering schemes have proved a useful 'short hand' for referring to various regions. Other investigators have attempted, with varying degrees of success, to provide some functional localization in the cortex using physiological techniques or by electrically stimulating the exposed human cortex during neurosurgical procedures. While such localizations of functions to particular gyri, or parts of gyri have been demonstrated, one must not assume that all human brains would have these functional localizations parcelled out identically. The over-all pattern may well be similar but the specific interrelationships between neurons may vary.

Fig. 85. An attempt has been made to correlate some of the more generally accepted functional regions with the Brodmann numbering scheme. The regions, as numbered by Brodmann, have been outlined with the dashed lines. The symbols for each area overlap and are in a general way related to each other to suggest that the cortical architecture, at least as far as 'boundary lines', may not be too dissimilar. Thus, all the motor and premotor areas are indicated by circles, as are the sensory areas whose function is integrated with the motor areas. The visual cortex (areas 17, 18 and 19) is all indicated by similar symbols which extend into the parietal lobe as an overlapping of the circle symbol from the adjacent sensory field. This is intended to indicate the relation of the parietal lobe to the primary sensory areas (3, 1 and 2) and visual cortex in serving to store information from both regions. For a similar reason, the circle motif was used in the temporal lobe which physiological and clinical research have indicated has some role, like the parietal lobe, in memory. The square used for the frontal pole is intended to suggest that its function may be unrelated to the more caudal motor areas except in that it may 'direct' them. The plus symbol has been used for the limbic system. The symbols for the adjacent areas are frequently overlapped with the '+' to indicate this region which appears to have some role in behavior may be interrelated with these areas and may influence the manner in which they mediate their response.

Fig. 87. There is another type of functional localization which occurs in the cortex. This depends on the function of the various lamina of the six layered cortex. The names applied to these layers are indicative of the cell type (Fig. 86). Therefore, there is an outer molecular layer composed of a few horizontal and granule cells, but being mainly made up of fibers which are the terminals of apical dendrites, ascending axons and collaterals of descending axons. This is layer I. Layer II is the external granule layer made up of small pyramidal cells and granule cells. The axons of these cells end in layers III, V and VI. Layer III is the external pyramidal layer which can be subdivided into two major subdivisions based on the size of the pyramidal cells. Those adjacent to layer II are medium size while those next to layer IV are larger. Layer III has cells whose axons end in other deeper cortical layers or enter the underlying white matter and pass to a nearby cortical area as association fibers. It also receives some of the fibers arising from the thalamus. Layer IV is the internal granule layer which is made up of small granule cells and a few small pyramids. Apical dendrites reach layer I and basilar dendrites end in layer IV. The axons may ascend to more superficial layers, pass to deeper layers, or enter the subcortical white matter as association fibers after giving off collaterals in layers V and VI. Layer V, the internal pyramidal layer or ganglionic layer, contains large pyramidal cells, particularly in the precentral gyrus which constitutes the primary motor cortex. Some pyramids here are extremely large. These are the giant Betz cells. Axons usually enter the white matter as association, commissural or projection fibers. Layer VI is characterized by having many kinds of cell shape, hence the term polymorphic layer. Fusiform or spindle-shaped cells are included in this region. The VIth layer contains many cells whose axons pass back to the surface of the cortex or enter the white matter as long or short association fibers to adjacent gyri.

Thus, the cells in layer V have fibers which are predominantly corticofugal and leave the cortex as commissural or projection fibers. Some few axons of the deeper part of lamina III of the motor cortex (area 4) pass as projection fibers to the subcortical and spinal centers. Layers I, II, III and IV receive thalamic and association projections. Layer III provides primarily for intracortical projections or short associational fibers; layer II has cells whose axons also end in the neighboring deeper cortical layer while layer I contains primarily the apical dendritic ending

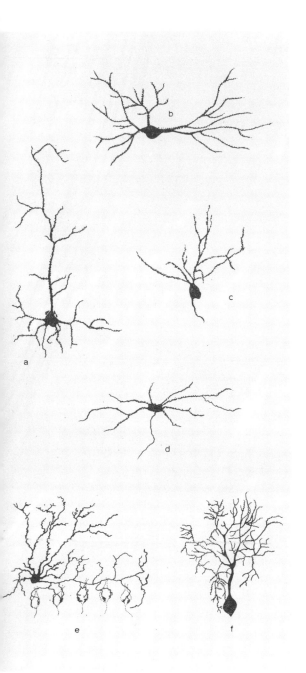

Fig. 86. Various neuronal cell types. **a,** pyramidal cell; **b,** double pyramidal cell of hippocampus; **c,** granule cell of dentate gyrus; **d,** fusiform cell; **e,** basket cell; **f,** Purkinje cell.

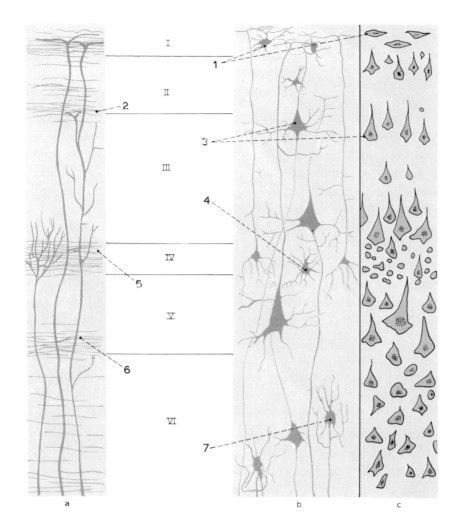

Fig. 87. Sketch of cerebral cortex comparing the appearance following stains for nerve fibers with those for cell bodies (Golgi) or Nissl substance.
a, afferent fibers; **b,** cell types seen in Golgi preparations; **c,** Nissl cytoarchitecture.
1, horizontal cells; **2,** stripe of Kaes; **3,** pyramidal cells; **4,** stellate cell; **5,** external stripe of Baillarger; **6,** internal stripe of Baillarger; **7,** modified pyramidal cell.

of pyramidal cells in the deeper layers plus the endings of associational and collateral axons of deeper layers. Associational and commissural axons give off collaterals to cells in layers V and VI as well as the more superficial layers. One may, in a sense, therefore, speak of the efferent cortical layers V and VI, and afferent layers III and IV within the cortex. Layer III appears to have a function concerned with intracortical association as well as playing some role *via* short associational fiber connections which enter the white matter. The above discussion obviously represents an extreme simplification of the available facts.

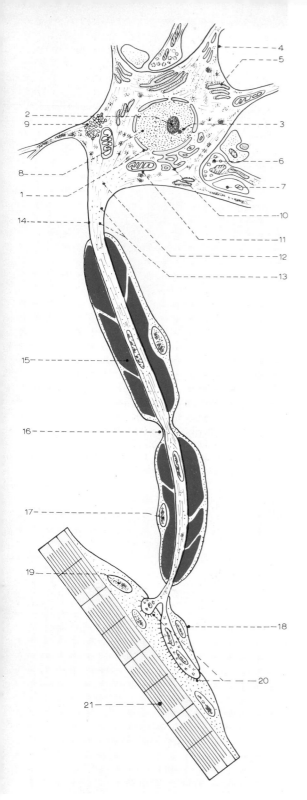

7. The nerve cell

Fig. 88. The neuron, as a cell, consists of a cell body with from one (pseudo-unipolar) to several (multipolar) processes.

Nerve cells possess the particular property of being able to conduct and transmit impulses. They synthesize neurotransmitters such as acetylcholine, catecholamines and indolamines and must provide for their own maintenance (aided by glial cells). Thus, they are also involved in lipid, carbohydrate and protein synthesis. A turnover of both DNA and RNA[42, 66, 74] is known to occur normally. Some specialized cells are even capable of forming a protein product (octa-peptide) which is stored and secreted as an endocrine hormone (antidiuretic hormone, vasopressin and oxytocin[33, 34, 115]). Other neurons, in the basal hypothalamus elaborate the so-called releasing factors which influence the function of the adenohypophysis. The thyroid hormone releasing factor has been identified as a tri-peptide. All neurons have a high metabolic rate and they require a constant supply of O_2 and glucose as well as other nutritional components.

The processes of nerve cells have been classified as being of two sorts. One, the dendrite (afferent), transmits generally an impulse toward the cell body or soma and the other, the axon (efferent), transmits an impulse away from the soma under normal conditions. The surface area of the dendrites, which receives the 'messages relayed through the axons' of other neurons, is greatly enlarged by the existence of small projections. In the case of the Purkinje cell this area enlargement may be as much as 250,000 μ^2.

Bodian, realizing that the conventional terminology of neuron structure was lagging behind current functional concepts, has re-examined the terminology of the generalized vertebrate neuron. The unique value of his contribution deserves an extensive quotation from his paper. He defines the following major neuronal divisions, emphasizing impulse origin rather than cell-body location as the focal point:

Fig. 88. Sketch illustrating the major components of a neuron.
1, nucleus; **2,** nucleolus; **3,** perinucleolar satellite; **4,** dendrite; **5,** endoplasmic reticulum with RNA granules (Nissl substance; red dots); **6,** synaptic ending; **7,** astrocyte foot; **8,** DNA granules; **9,** lipofuscin; **10,** Golgi apparatus; **11,** mitochondrion; **12,** axon hillock; **13,** neurofibrils, **14,** axon; **15,** myelin sheath; **16,** node of Ranvier; **17,** Schwann cell nucleus; **18,** telodendroglia; **19,** muscle cell nucleus; **20,** myoneural junctions; **21,** muscle.

Fig. 89. *Dendritic zone* (**a**), the receptor membrane of a neuron, either consisting of a set of tapering cytoplasmic extensions (dendrites) which receive synaptic endings of other neurons (**C, D**) or differentiated to convert environmental stimuli into local-response-generating activity (**A, B**). Mitochondrial concentrations may be present.

Axon (**b**), a single, often branched and usually elongated, cytoplasmic extension morphologically and perhaps uniquely differentiated to conduct nervous impulses away from the dendritic zone. It is characteristically uniform in caliber and ensheathed by neuroglial or neurilemma cells. Sheath differentiation and axon caliber are related to speed of conduction.

Perikaryon (**c**), the 'cell body' or nucleated cytoplasmic mass, which is usually characterized by the presence of chromidal substance. This portion of the neuron is the focal point of embryonic outgrowth of dendrites and axon, and of axon regeneration.

Axon telodendria, the usually branched and variously differentiated terminals of axons which show membrane and cytoplasmic differentiation related to synaptic transmission or neurosecretory activity. Mitochondrial concentration, 'synaptic vesicles', or secretory granules are commonly present in bulb-like terminals.

The cytoplasmic contents of the cell body and the dendrites, which would include the RNA and its associated endoplasmic reticulum, should be considered as providing for those synthesizing mechanisms which maintain the integrity of the outer cell and fiber membranes and permit them to transmit an electrical impulse.

The cell bodies of neurons are fundamentally the same as all other cells. They are enclosed within a cell membrane and contain a nucleus and nucleolus, mitochondria, lipochondria (Golgi substance), endoplasmic reticulum and ribosomes, fibrils (neurofibrils) (Fig. 88), as well as neurotubules, dense bodies, and microvesicles. It should be noted that, in the neuron, the endoplasmic reticulum and the ribosomes are associated together to form a chromophilic structure recognized by light microscopy as Nissl substance. The volume of neurons varies as greatly as do their shapes, the range for cell bodies being from 600 to 700 μ^3 for granule cells of the cerebellum and up to 70,000 μ^3 for some anterior horn cells. Cells of the cerebral cortex may be as large as 20,000 μ^3 and as small as 500 μ^3 [115]. In terms of dry weight, a nerve cell is about 80% protein and 20% lipid. The carbohydrate content of the whole CNS is very low, being about 10% of the wet weight, while values for glycogen vary from 0.4 to 0.14%, depending on species (*cf.* for extensive reviews of the chemical anatomy of the neuron: Hydén[66]).

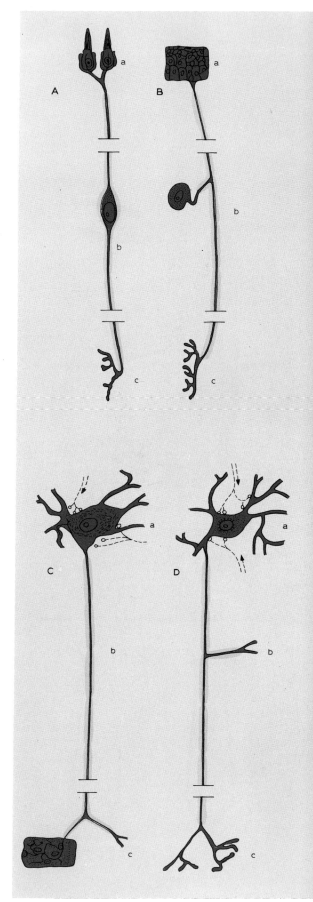

Fig. 89. The generalized vertebrate neuron (modified after Bodian). **A,** auditory receptor neuron; **B,** cutaneous receptor neuron; **C,** motoneuron; **D,** interneuron. **a,** dendritic zone; **b,** axon; **c,** telodendria.

7.1 Cell membrane

Fig. 90. Until the advent of the electron microscope, very little was known of the structure of this membrane. It now appears to be a continuous double membrane extending over the entire cell body, axonal and dendritic surface. However, the axon has in addition a series of elaborate lipoprotein lamellae wrapped round it which are provided by Schwann cells peripherally and oligodendroglia centrally. The cell membrane consists of two electron-dense layers which are separated by a structureless interzone. Thus, it is in a sense a triple-layered membrane. The total thickness of this triple-layered membrane is about 90–100 Å in which the two dense layers are separated by a structureless interzone[123]. These surface membranes appear to be geometrically asymmetric with a thicker opaque electron-dense layer at the inner cytoplasmic surface and a thinner layer at the outer peripheral surface. Such double electron-dense membranes are also seen within the cell. The nuclear wall, the endoplasmic reticulum, the Golgi complex and the mitochondria are all composed of double membranes. The membranes of the Golgi complex and the mitochondria are more symmetrical than the outer cell membrane and frequently contain stainable material in the middle 'light' layer. Axon-Schwann membranes, mesaxons associated with myelin peripherally and synaptic membranes are also double (or triple if one considers the structureless light interzone a true layer). The term mesaxon refers to the point where the edges of a Schwann cell cytoplasmic membrane come together around an embedded axon to form a paired membrane structure. The axon is in a sense suspended within a fold of the Schwann cell cytoplasmic membrane in a manner analogous to the mesenteric suspension of the intestine in the vertebrate coelom[54]. Some modification of the cell membrane occurs between the axoplasm and sarcoplasm of muscle at the motor end plates. At this point, the central region between these membranes is occupied by a dense material, thickening the total axo-sarcoplasmic membrane structure to 500 to 700 Å. Robertson[109–111] has referred to this as the synaptic membrane complex since it is not clear as to exactly which layers should be included by the term, cell membrane.

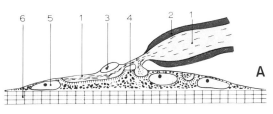

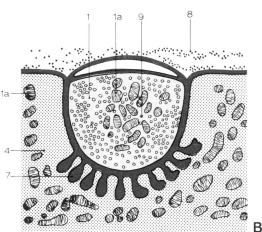

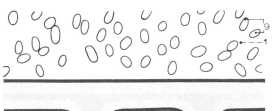

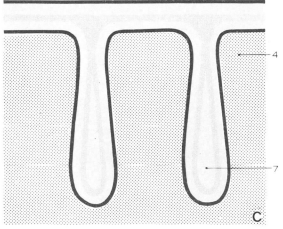

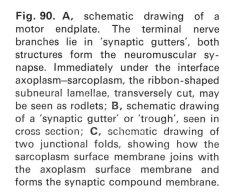

Fig. 90. A, schematic drawing of a motor endplate. The terminal nerve branches lie in 'synaptic gutters', both structures form the neuromuscular synapse. Immediately under the interface axoplasm–sarcoplasm, the ribbon-shaped subneural lamellae, transversely cut, may be seen as rodlets; **B**, schematic drawing of a 'synaptic gutter' or 'trough', seen in cross section; **C**, schematic drawing of two junctional folds, showing how the sarcoplasm surface membrane joins with the axoplasm surface membrane and forms the synaptic compound membrane.

1, axoplasm (with, as shown in **B**, mitochondria); **1a**, mitochondria; **2**, myelin sheath; **3**, telodendroglia (terminal Schwann cells); **4**, sarcoplasm with, as shown in **A** and **B**, mitochondria; **5**, muscle nucleus; **6**, myofibrils; **7**, junctional fold; **8**, collagen fibrils; **9**, vesicles.

In the earlier days of electron microscopy a 'unit membrane' hypothesis was proposed. This hypothesis assumed that all cellular membranes share a common structural pattern and that on this basis, all the membrane structures within a cell may be derived from the outer cell membrane as illustrated in Fig. 91. The hypothesis is based largely on the view that all of the double-layered membranes are of equivalent dimension and symmetry. Since investigations[123] illustrate the dissimilarity in membrane structure between mitochondria, the Golgi membranes, and α-cytomembranes, the unit membrane hypothesis appears to be of only historical interest. The rejection of the unit membrane hypothesis must, of course, induce further investigations to determine the source and manner of formation of the membrane-contained structures within the cell. While the manner of origin of the membrane system is in doubt, the presence of canals within the endoplasmic reticulum has been generally accepted. They are believed to communicate with the extracellular space and might be conceived of as providing for a cellular 'circulatory system' which facilitates entrance of nutrients or the escape of secretions or wastes. The endoplasmic reticulum has also been observed to be attached to the outer layer of the nuclear membrane. Furthermore, the spaces or pores in the nuclear membrane appear to provide a path for exchange of materials between the nucleoplasm and the cytoplasm. The combination of endoplasmic reticulum and RNA granules which occurs in neurons (Nissl substance) would appear to be comparable to the 'rough endoplasmic reticulum' described in other cells. While many RNA granules are associated with the endoplasmic reticulum to form Nissl substance, it is characteristic of neurons that there are great numbers of these granules, sometimes in clumps or rosettes which are not associated with the endoplasmic reticulum. These granules appear to be particularly numerous in the dendrites and cell body.

7.2 Nucleus

Fig. 91. The neuron, while it is a postmitotic cell, possesses a large *nucleus* (**1**) which is by comparison with nuclei of other cell types rather chromophobic. Since it has virtually as much DNA as do liver, kidney, spleen, muscle and pancreatic cells (2.3 × 10⁻¹²g) this lack of basophilia could be due to its dispersion in the relatively large nucleus. No visible sign of chromosomes can be seen in the adult nucleus by either light or electron microscopy. The double-layered membrane of the nucleus, as visualized by electron microscopy, seems to possess many openings or pores which may permit some exchange between the nucleoplasm and cytoplasm as noted above. Perhaps these pores can provide for the entrance of RNA newly formed in the nucleus which will become incorporated into the Nissl substance (**5**) of the cytoplasm.

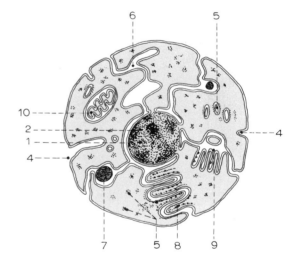

Fig. 91. Sketch based on the concept of Robertson that all the cell intracytoplasmic organelles are derived from the outer cell membrane.
1, nucleus; **2**, nucleolus; **4**, caveola; **5**, endoplasmic reticulum, Nissl substance; **6**, intraneuronal space continuous with extracellular space; **7**, secretion; **8**, ribosome; **9**, Golgi apparatus with secretory drops; **10**, mitochondrion.

A highly basophilic *nucleolus* (2) is characteristically present in neurons. It contains a large amount of RNA as well as diffuse coating of DNA. In man, it stains vividly with Luxol fast blue (positive for choline-containing lipids). A relationship between the nucleolus and the synthesis of ribonucleotides whenever a neuron is required to synthesize protein seems relatively clear from numerous studies. The significance of the Luxol fast blue reaction is, however less apparent.

Hydén[66] stated that the nucleolus is central in regard to cellular activity, particularly to nucleic acid and protein production. Tewari and Bourne[129] also observed that the nucleoli of spinal ganglion cells (rat) were centers of extreme metabolic activity and were possibly involved in the synthesis of a wide range of protein enzymes. They also observed positive histochemical reactions in the nucleolus for ATP-ase, glucose-6-phosphatase, succinic dehydrogenase, alkaline phosphatase, glucose phosphorylase, 5-nucleotidase and specific cholinesterase[130]. The intensities of the histochemical reactions varied with individual cells, apparently being dependent on the nucleolar activity. The significance of these enzyme concentrations lies in their association with the respiratory, energy-producing and synthetic functions of the cell. These, of course, do not represent the only enzymes detectable in nervous tissue, but serve to relate the nucleolus to these functional attributes of the cell. The Golgi apparatus (9) and the mitochondria (10) are also highly involved in these processes.

Variations in nucleolar size are also known to occur. They may vary from being small granular bodies to a large complex body, filling almost the whole of the nucleus. Electron microscopic investigations[147] have suggested that these variations in size are related to the physiologic state of the cell. Many workers have demonstrated that the size of the nucleolus appears biochemically related to its synthetic activity. Other observations of Tewari suggest a relationship between the formation of RNA, protein, and lipids by the nucleolus and the transfer of such materials to the cytoplasm while the nucleoli are lying close to the nuclear membrane. This confirms early reports of Einarson[40, 41] to the effect that the formation of new Nissl substance (5) in neurons proceeded from the nucleolus.

Structurally, the nucleolus appears as a dense aggregation of RNA, proteins and lipids with some DNA within the nucleus. Whether or not it is a discrete structure may be debated since it lacks any sort of limiting membrane. Its constant change in size and position and in histochemical reaction in relation to change in physiologic state of the neuron are suggestive of its extreme plasticity and importance in the synthesis of new RNA and of various enzymes.

An intranuclear fibrillar lattice inclusion which appears as a saucer-shaped sheet 1.8 μ in diameter and about 0.1 μ thick has been described by various electron microscopists. No function has been ascribed to it.

7.3 Sex chromatin

In 1950 Barr[9] reported the presence in some large neurons of an accumulation of chromatin into a small oval mass 0.5 to 2.0 μ in diameter which was usually close to or in contact with the nucleolus. Its frequent association with the nucleolus provides for its convenient name of perinucleolar satellite (Fig. 88, **3**). It is especially large in neurons of female animals, which has given rise to some investigations where the presence or absence of the satellite has been used for sex determination. The satellite is most readily seen in cerebral cortical or sympathetic ganglion cells. This accumulation of chromatin, which may be related to the XX condition of female sex chromosomes as compared with the XY state of the male sex chromosome, should not be confused with an argyrophilic dot described by Cajal which is also present in the nucleoplasm.

An interesting observation made by Barr is that this satellite abandons its perinucleolar position following nerve cell stimulation and moves toward the nuclear membrane. It was also observed to increase in size during stimulation. These observations are consistent with the hypothesis that the nucleolus and its satellite are important in the process of synthesis of ribose nucleoproteins, which increases during cell stimulation[8].

7.4 Golgi complex

This structure, as described by electron microscopists, includes a system of fairly closely packed double-layered membranes and vesicles near or around the nucleus. By light microscopy it may appear as coarse filaments or vesicular bodies. The Golgi complex, like the nucleolus, appears to undergo cyclic changes which may reflect its functional activity. It may exist in a perinuclear arrangement or be distributed throughout the cytoplasm, passing out from the perinuclear position in waves[129,130]. It may as some believe, be associated with the endoplasmic reticulum. In relation to this, Malhatra[92] has demonstrated irregular basophilic masses associated with the Golgi complex in mammalian neurons. These masses, when stained with a Nissl stain, appear to have a similar location to that demonstrated by the Nissl substance in the same neurons. This suggests that since the Golgi structure and Nissl substance are both formed in part by double-layered membranes, there may in some way be a relationship between the two structures.

The Golgi complex frequently contains spheres of a partly lipid or phosphatide nature which has led to the term lipochondria for this structure. Histochemical studies have also indicated the presence of a mucopolysaccharide.

7.5 Mitochondria

These small cytoplasmic inclusions usually appear rodlike by light microscopy. Their distribution within a cell may be perinuclear or spread throughout the cytoplasm with particular accumulations at synaptic end bulbs. They are found in the dendrites and are often in close contact with the endoplasmic reticulum. In the axons they appear as very elongated rods parallel to the axonal axis. During periods of active synthesis as might occur if an axon were to be cut, the number of mitochondria is increased. Cytochrome oxidase and succinic dehydrogenase as well as other respiratory enzymes are associated with these small bodies.

Fig. 92. Numerous mitochondria and synaptic endings with synaptic vesicles in the cerebral cortex (× 25 000).
1, mitochondria; **2**, synaptic vesicles.

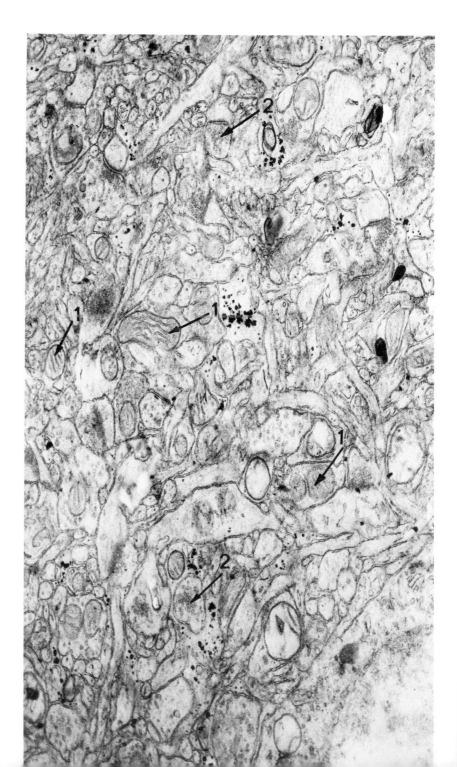

Figs. 92, 93. Electron microscopy has given us a different image of the mitochondria. They have been shown by Palade[98] and Sjöstrand[122] to be limited by double membranes and that double-membraned crista sometimes run partially across the structure between the inner limiting membranes. Palade[98] believed the crista to be derived from the inner layer of the mitochondrial membrane while Sjöstrand[123] believed them to be separate (Fig. 93). The membranes which make up the mitochondria resemble those of the cell surface. However, they are much thinner, measuring only about 50 Å according to Sjöstrand[12?]. How these structures, with membranes resembling those of the cell membrane and Golgi membranes, etc. came to be formed is still unresolved. Since there are dissimilarities between the various membrane systems suggesting differences in molecular architecture, the concept of a common derivation with the other membrane structures (unit membrane hypothesis) seems untenable.

The mitochondria are believed to be of extreme importance in cell respiration. Highly purified samples of brain mitochondria show a high rate of oxidation of glutamate, succinate, α-ketoglutarate, pyruvate and oxalacetate. Lower rates of oxidation were recorded for glycerol 1-phosphate, fumarate, glucose-6-phosphate, β-hydroxybutyrate, isocitrate, citrate and γ-aminobutyrate. However, while there is general agreement that brain mitochondria carry out citric acid cycle oxidations and oxidative phosphorylation, their role in glycolysis has not been clearly resolved, due in part to the difficulty in preparing completely pure samples. Thus, while some authors feel that there is a clean relationship between brain mitochondria and glycolysis other workers feel that only 10% or less of the total brain glycolysis can be ascribed to mitochondria. While previous notions on the functioning of brain mitochondria have implied a difference when compared with mitochondria from other tissues, the studies of Løvtrup and Svennerholm[89] emphasize the similarities.

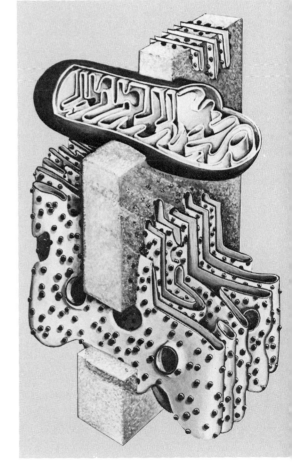

Fig. 93. Reconstruction of a small piece of the neuroplasma showing a mitochondrion (above) and part of the endoplasmic reticulum (below). (× 500 000).

7.6 Neurofibrils and neurotubules

Various histological techniques demonstrate the presence of fine sharply defined fibers within the axon. Such fibers extend into the cell body and dendrites. They have been seen in living cells and by electron microscopy. These fibrils often cross one another or anastamose into dense networks. David *et al.*[23] have presented data suggesting that the neurofibrils as seen by light microscopy may represent the endoplasmic reticulum of nerve cells after having been treated with certain histologic fixatives and silver precipitation procedures. This observation remains to be confirmed. What is apparent is that neurofibrils are commonly found in all parts of the neuron. Their function is completely unknown, although they become clumped together in bundles in hibernating lizards and mammals exposed to cold. Neural tubules with a diameter of about 200 Å have also been described in neurons by electron microscopists. The function of these tubules is also unknown.

7.7 Nissl substance

A characteristic feature of neurons is the presence of masses of basophilic material in their cytoplasm. These clumps have been named Nissl substance, after their discoverer. Investigations utilizing histochemical and electron microscopic techniques have shown that these masses consist of aggregates of narrow tubes which are often covered (but not always) with fine granules 100 to 300 Å in diameter. The tubes represent flattened cisternae, tubules or vesicles of the endoplasmic reticulum (Figs. 88, 91). The granules which may occur singly, in rows or in rosettes are comparable to the microsomes (basophilic particles) which can be isolated from the liver. They may be in apposition to the tubules, or closely adjacent. These particles represent a part of the cytoplasmic nucleic acid of neurons and are composed of ribonucleic acid plus associated protein (RNA-P). The amount of RNA per nerve cell varies with the cell type and ranges from 40 to 1550 pg per cell. All the evidence suggests that the endoplasmic reticulum with its RNA-P is concerned with synthesis of various materials, under the influence of the nucleus. Presumably, the enzymes and other proteins produced by the structure may pass down the axon, even though it may be a meter or more in length. How this is accomplished is uncertain, but labeled amino acids have been observed to be taken up by nerve cells and then passed slowly down along the axon. This process of 'axoplasmic flow' of materials appears to be supplemented by coexisting local protein synthesis in the axon distal to the cell body[38, 39]. Active movement of materials along axons has also been seen in tissue culture. The essential nature of the Nissl substance can be seen when an axon is cut. The peripheral fiber degenerates, while signs of movement of the Nissl substance within the cell body toward the axon can be seen within a few hours (in isolated neurons). *In vivo,* changes occur in the Nissl substance which suggest increased protein synthesis and new sprouts soon emerge from the proximal portion of the cut axon. It must be noted, however, that Nissl substance is not seen in the axon although segments of bare endoplasmic reticulum may be present.

Fig. 94. Nissl substance, as seen by light microscopy, is observed in the dendrites and cell body. Nissl substance has never been observed in the small zone at the origin of the axon (axon hillock) and in the axon itself (Fig. 82A). Fragments of 'bare' endoplasmic reticulum, such as might have been previously associated with ribosomes to form Nissl substance have, however, been observed in the axon. Whether or not these bare endoplasmic membranes do truly represent the skeleton of Nissl substance is not clear.

The size of Nissl particles and their arrangement within the cell varies from cell type to cell type. Thus, neurons innervating muscles have very large Nissl clumps, while sensory ganglia have much smaller particles. Cells of the nucleus dorsalis at the medial base of the posterior horn in the spinal cord have their Nissl clumps scattered along the periphery of the cell (as do neurosecretory cells), while pyramidal cells of the cerebral cortex have a more general distribution. It has also been noted that Nissl substance stains more intensely when it is near the nucleus. Variations in the appearance of Nissl substance also occur among different species. Furthermore, the Nissl substance of a cell, or its basophilia varies with cell activity. Einarson and Krogh[43] have classified the physiologic state of neurons in relation to their basophilia, which in turn depends on the Nissl substance.

There is first the *chromoneutral* cell, or normal state in which large clumps of Nissl substance would appear sharply stained in a motor cell. This represents a cell at rest or in a moderate phase of activity. *Hyperchromatic* or moderately *chromophilic* cells stain deeply. Several Nissl bodies are usually near the nucleus and the nucleolus is intensely stained and often somewhat enlarged. Many stained particles are also present in the nucleus. These cells are characterized as being in a state of slightly increased activity. This histologic picture corresponds to the biochemically observed increase in the RNA-P present in nerve cells which have been stimulated to moderate activity[65]. *Moderately chromophobic* cells show a decrease in the number and staining intensity of Nissl bodies and an increase in nuclear chromatin. The nuclear membrane stains intensely and the nucleolus is enlarged. Perinuclear caps of Nissl substance (or basophilic material) can be seen (sometimes Nissl substance is also located peripherally in the cytoplasm). This picture characterizes a cell in which the frequency of firing is believed to be increased. This would naturally be associated with increased intracellular metabolism. The nuclear caps

Fig. 94. Staining of Nissl bodies in motor neurons. **A,** toluidine blue, staining time 3 days; **B,** toluidine blue, staining time 7 days; **C,** cresylecht violet (cresyl fast violet), staining time 3 days; **D,** cresylecht violet (cresyl fast violet), staining time 7 days.

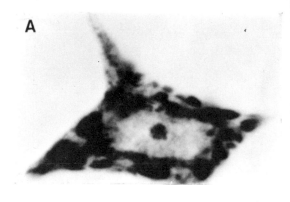
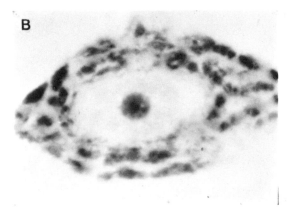
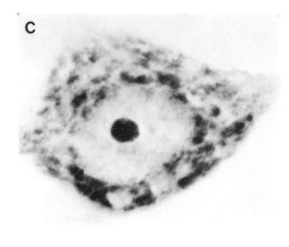
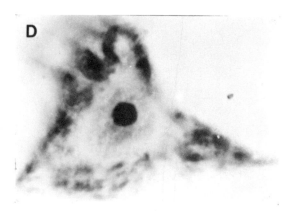

and increased nuclear chromatin staining suggest production of new nucleic acid substance which is leaving the nucleus. This stage and the following one appears to correspond to the decrease in total RNA-P reported to occur by Hydén and Pigon[69] with prolonged stimulation of nerve cells. *Extremely chromophobic* cells are pale with little stainable material in the cytoplasm or nucleus. The nucleus may be eccentrically placed, as occurs also in chromatolysis. The nuclear contour may be irregular or shrivelled. The nucleolus, in extreme cases, may lose its capacity to stain. This approaches the chromophobia of exhaustion. *Extremely chromophilic* cells stain intensely with closely packed dark Nissl bodies with a reduction of the non-basophilic substance. Cell contours are well defined and often stain for a considerable distance along the fibers. The nucleus is intensely stained, and the nuclear membrane may be hardly recognizable. The nucleolus is still discernible. This characterizes a cell which is probably not physiologically active. One might say that production of cytoplasmic nucleic acids, proteins, enzymes, etc., has exceeded the need. One might note that extremely basophilic cells have been shown to accumulate less labeled material after intravenous injection of ^{3}H-lysine than do neighboring more 'normal' appearing cells. This could be interpreted to support Einarson's concept that such cells were not as physiologically active as other cells at the time of injection. Other investigators feel that these intensely stained and shrunken cells may be artifacts. Pathologically, extreme chromophobia may proceed to complete dissolution of the cells and extreme chromophilia may proceed to cell sclerosis, cell atrophy and even complete disappearance of the cell. It may be seen that there is a wide range in the basophilic state of a neuron which can be considered. The degree of basophilia, as compared with the chromoneutral state, can give some clue as to the physiologic state of a cell. Comparable views expressing a relationship between the basophilia of a neuron and its functional state have also been expressed by other[8, 85, 139]. Indeed, such data have provided anatomical evidence for the idea that not all neurons in a 'neuron pool' need to be functionally active or active at the same time.

7.8 Dense body

For many years electron microscopists have described a 'dense' body in the neuronal cytoplasm which was extremely electron dense and is now accepted as having a closely packed lamellar structure. The cytoplasmic organelle is now recognized as being what others (Duve, 1969) called the *lysosome*. This dense granule is rich in acid phosphatase, β-glucuronidase, acid nucleases, cathepsin and a number of soluble hydrolytic enzymes with acid pH optima. It has been speculated that these bodies break down in injured nerve cells releasing their enzymes which then become involved in the dissolution of the neuronal soma.

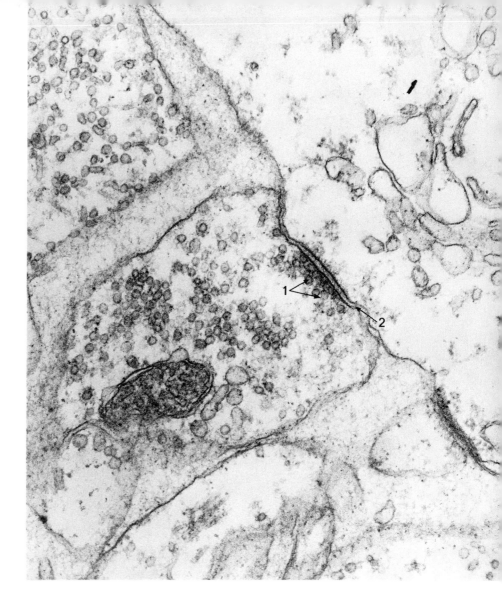

Fig. 95. Synapse in brain stem of fish. Note the accumulations of synaptic vesicles (**1**) in the presynaptic element near the synaptic cleft (**2**).

7.9 Synapse

Fig. 95. Although electron microscopy has advanced our knowledge of the structure of the nervous system in more than one area, this is particularly true for the fine structure of the synapse[144]. Progress in the understanding of many physiological mechanisms has been greatly aided by the analysis of neuronal membranes at a synaptic locus. Sherrington[119]. who coined the term synapse (derived from the Greek σνναπτω = to clasp) suggested in 1897 that the characteristic phenomena in the reflex arc may be satisfactorily explained by the properties of the close apposition of membranes of two neurons.

At a synapse the presynaptic fiber ends in an expanded terminal: the synaptic knob (also called *bouton*). This knob approaches a portion of a postsynaptic neuron very closely: this area is called the subsynaptic membrane. The distance between the two membranes, *synaptic cleft* (**2**), varies in width from approximately 150–250 Å.

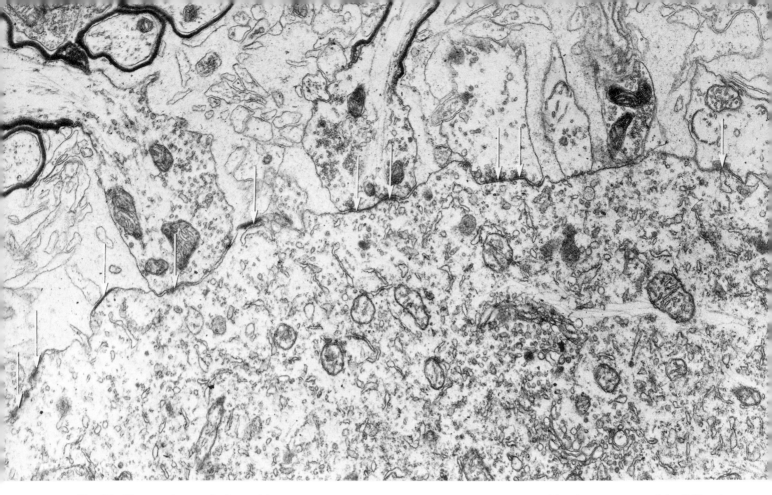

Fig. 96. Electronmicrograph of neural tissue. The arrows indicate synaptic structures; *above* presynaptic elements, *below* postsynaptic elements.

Fig. 97. Sketch based on electron microscopic studies of Gray showing the relation of mitochondria to various structures in the synapse.
1, mitochondrion; **2**, myelin; **3**, axon; **4**, presynaptic dense projections; **5**, dendrite; **6**, attachment plaque; **7**, synaptic vesicles; **8**, glial fibrils.

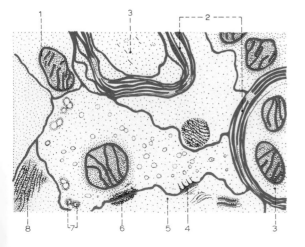

Figs. 96, 97. The synapse is characterized by the presence of the following structures:

(1) *Synaptic vesicles*, 300–600 Å in diameter, abundantly present in the presynaptic terminal[25]. In general, they are not seen in the postsynaptic cytoplasm. These vesicles may contain storage particles of the transmitter substance released at the synapse[25, 28]. It has been claimed that these vesicles open and empty their transmitter substance into the intersynaptic space (the synaptic cleft), providing for a quantal release of acetylcholine[25], or other transmitter substance[28]. Some vesicles are much larger than others and in some neurons there are both round and elongated vesicles. A further variation is the presence of vesicles containing an electron-dense material. In small vesicles this dense material has been associated with norepinephrine.

(2) A relatively high number of *mitochondria* in the presynaptic component.

(3) *Denser and thicker membranes* of both components (especially the postsynaptic one) at the locus of contact.

In addition two more structural details have been described[133, 134].

(4) Small *interlemnal elements* have been observed in the synaptic cleft. They are oriented perpendicular to the apposing membranes. A certain portion of these interlemnal elements entirely bridges the synaptic cleft, others end halfway in it. The thickness of the threads averages 70 Å, their spacing 165 Å.

(5) A *subsynaptic organelle*. This organelle is believed to exist as an agglomeration of dot- and thread-like electron-dense structures that

extend from the subsynaptic membrane for 200–670 Å into the cytoplasm of the postsynaptic neuron. It is then assumed that the so-called post-synaptic membrane thickening is not really a membrane thickening, but only seemingly so.

Other authors describe irregular spiky structures along the synaptic membrane at intervals of about 1000 Å. Gray[56] believed that these projecting processes may, like the synaptic vesicles, be involved in producing the transmitter substance at the synapse. A further variation has been described by Pappas (1966) in the habenular nucleus where a hexagonal area of electron-dense bodies was observed in the subsynaptic region. As yet the significance of these different subsynaptic organelles is unknown.

In the central nervous system there are 3 common types of synapses which are generally seen: axo-dendritic, axo-somatic and axo-axonal. A fourth type of interneuronal appositions is the dendro-dendritic junction. A fifth category recently described is the 'tight-junction'.

(1) The axo-dendritic synapse. This type can easily be recognized in electron micrographs, because it contains all characteristic features as mentioned above.

(2) The axo-somatic synapse. Here again no difficulties in recognition occur. The cell body stands out by virtue of its Nissl bodies, RNA-P granules and endoplasmic reticulum. There is however no subsynaptic organelle, but in many instances the interlemnal elements are observed.

(3) The axo-axonal synapse. Gray[56] and many others have described contacts in the spinal cord where an axon terminates on another axon near the point where it was shown to be making contact with several dendrites. This would be an axo-axonal synapse such as has also been seen in the cerebellar cortex. The discovery that synapses are super-

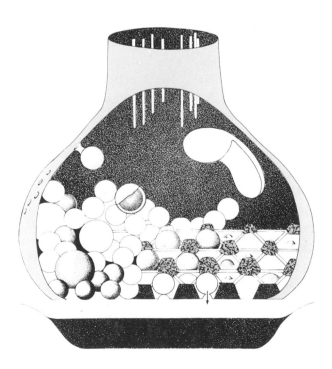

Fig. 98. Reconstruction of the molecular configuration in the presynaptic terminal. A mitochondrion and the synaptic vesicles are clearly distinguishable. The whole complex is called the presynaptic vesicular grid. (Photograph by Akert *et al.*, 1970).

imposed on presynaptic terminals has particularly contributed to our understanding of the phenomenon of presynaptic inhibition (see p. 185). Synaptic endings of axons of basket cells of the cerebellar cortex have been shown to synapse on the axon or axon hillock of the Purkinje cell to provide for presynaptic inhibition at the origin of the axonal process.

(4) The dendro-dendritic junction. In the analysis of this type of inter-neuronal contact severe problems of identification are met. In studying alternating sections with the light and electron microscope, Van der Loos[134] was able to demonstrate the characteristic features of this type of junction. There are no synaptic vesicles near the contact site, neither are there more mitochondria than can be expected on the basis of their normal distribution throughout the dendrite. Sometimes interlemnal elements are seen, whose spacing and diameter are the same as those found in the axo-dendritic synapse. Preliminary measurements have shown that the area of interdendritic apposition varies from 0.5–10 μ^2. The functional significance of the dendro-dendritic junctions remains obscure.

(5) The 'tight junction', which may be axo-dendritic or somato-somatic represents a non-humoral type of synapse in which there are no synaptic vesicles in the pre-synaptic portion. The opposing membranes appear essentially fused to each other creating a rather thickened membrane structure lacking a synaptic cleft. This type of synapse is presumed to provide for direct electrical stimulation of one nerve by an other and a 'spread' of excitation.

Investigations by Gray and by Hamlyn[59] have indicated that the axo-dendritic and axo-somatic synapses can be divided into a type 1 and type 2 synapse. The following criteria are given for distinguishing type 1 from type 2: The synaptic cleft is wider (300 Å) as against 200 Å for type 2; the postsynaptic membrane is more dense and thick and in the cleft there is a zone of extracellular material nearer to the subsynaptic membrane. The synapses on the small spines of the dendrites of the pyramidal cells in the cerebral cortex are always type 1, however, the synapses on the cell bodies of pyramidal cells are always of type 2. The suggestion has been made that the latter is the histological substrate of inhibitory action. Many of the above described types of synapses may be present on the same neuron, as occurs on the pyramidal cell of the hippocampus.

The relation of glial processes to synapses remains uncertain. Gray[56] states that no glial processes occur between the two parts of the synaptic membrane. Palay[99], however, provides evidence that such processes may intervene between synaptic surfaces.

The distance between the terminal end of an axonal fiber and the end of the myelin sheath coats on an axon undoubtedly varies. This distance may be quite short, being shown by electron microscopy to be within 2.0 μ of the synaptic membrane.

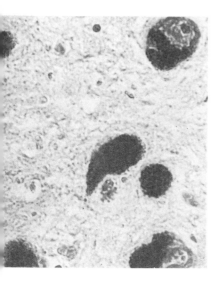
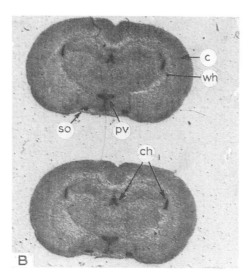
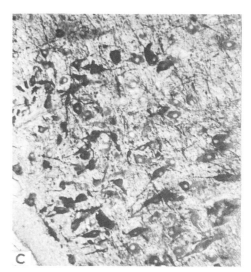

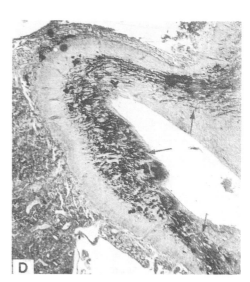

7.10 Pigments

Fig. 99, A. Amongst the various other cytoplasmic inclusions (vacuoles, glycogen, crystalloids, iron-containing granules in the substantia nigra) are certain pigments. These pigment granules are black or very dark brown. They are melanin-like granules and are normally observed in the cells of the substantia nigra, locus ceruleus and occasionally in the dorsal motor vagal nucleus, and in spinal and sympathetic ganglia. What role they play in normal neuronal function is uncertain, but it has been stated in one diseased state (Parkinson's syndrome) that there may be a decreased number of cells of the substantia nigra and other areas containing pigmented cells. This does not mean that the pigment *per se* has been involved, but that cells which contain the melanin-like pigment seem to be affected by this disorder.

The decrease in pigmented cells in the substantia nigra has been recently associated with a decrease in dopamine in this nucleus and also in the nucleus caudatus. Since both the melanin-like pigment of these cells and dopamine may be derived from tyrosine, investigators in the field have been tempted to relate the three and associate the decreased dopamine levels of the caudate with Parkinson's syndrome. Only time and additional study will determine if this relationship is justified.

Lipochrome and lipofuscin-staining granules of yellow-green, grey, brown-orange or orange-red color have also been observed in the nerve cells. Hydén[65] observed that the yellowish pigment granules first appear in the neurons of the spinal cord and medulla at seven to eight years of age. These granules increase in number with age, apparently without affecting nerve cell function, although the amount of Nissl substance present per cell is reduced.

Fig. 99. A, Cells of the substantia nigra by light microscopy showing large accumulations of melanin like pigment; **B,** Radioautographic location of ^{35}S-1-cystine in the brain of the rat. **c,** cortex; **wh,** white matter; **ch,** choroid plexus; **pv,** nucleus paraventricularis; **so,** nucleus supraopticus. Note that the supraoptic and paraventricular areas contain more of the labeled amino acid than any other neuronal area; **C,** Neurosecretory cells of the nucleus supraopticus in the dog. Many cells as well as their axons are seen filled with the neurosecretory material; **D,** The pituitary stalk of the dog, showing many axonal fibers (arrows) filled with neurosecretory material. (**C** and **D** were stained by the Gomori aldehyde fuchsin technique.)

7.11 Neurosecretions

Fig. 99, B, C, D. Some neurons have become so modified that their principal function appears to be secretory in nature. Thus, the cells of the supraoptic and paraventricular nuclei contain secretion granules which have been related to the hormones (antidiuretic hormone, vasopressin, oxytocin) of the posterior pituitary lobe (**C, D**). The secretory granules coalesce into droplets in the cell bodies and axons and may be selectively stained with Gomori's chrome alum hematoxylin phloxin and aldehyde fuchsin techniques. The stainable material does not appear to be the hormone, but a large glyco-lipo-protein carrier molecule. The hormone is rich in cystine which can be demonstrated radioautographically in the nuclear centers (Fig. 99**B**) after injection of ^{35}S-cystine into experimental animals.

The cell nuclei of the cells in the supraoptic nucleus contain many small phloxinophilic granules not seen to any great extent in the nuclei of paraventricular cells where there is predominance of small basophilic granules. Furthermore, the appearance of the peripherally placed Nissl substance differs between the two cell types, being more distinct in supraoptic cells. The observations that the cells of these two nuclear groups are not morphologically identical may correlate with observations[94] that paraventricular cells seem to be primarily associated with oxytocin while the supraoptic cells seem more associated with antidiuretic hormone and vasopressin.

7.12 Myelin formation

Fig. 100. The axons of nerve fibers are encased in a proteolipid sheath extending from just distal to the cell body to within 2 μ of the terminal synapses. This sheath is external to the limiting membrane (axolemma) of the axon, which, like the cell membrane with which it is continuous, consists of two electron-dense layers separated by one which is less dense. Nerves surrounded by such proteolipid sheaths are said to be myelinated. In the past, many peripheral nerves appeared to have no such "insulating" layer by light microscopy and were hence called 'unmyelinated'. Investigations by electron microscopy, have, however, shown that even these fibers possess a thin sheath of this material.

Microchemical studies have shown that this sheath contains cholesterol, phospholipids, certain cerebrosides and some fatty acids, plus a proteinaceous material which remains after the lipid components have been

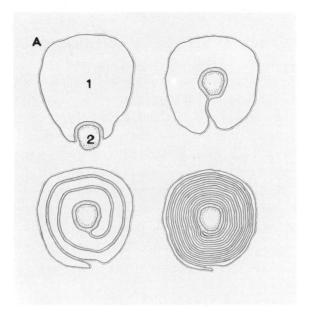

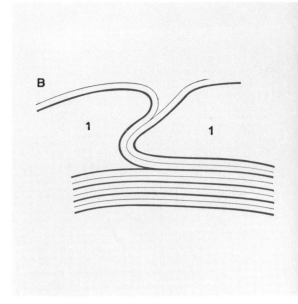

dissolved. This appears as a wavy network by light microscopy and seems to be what is referred to as neurokeratin. The chemical nature of myelin differs somewhat in the peripheral nerves from that observed in the central nervous system. This may be related to the fact that myelin is formed centrally by oligodendroglia and by Schwann cells peripherally.

The lipoprotein sheaths are not continuous, but are broken up at intervals along the fibers. These regions of discontinuity are spoken of as the *nodes of Ranvier* (Figs. 103 and 104). While the anatomical characteristics and frequency differ, such nodes appear in both the CNS and the peripheral nervous system, being most frequently observed in the peripheral nerves. Branching of nerve fibers may occur at these nodes. The nodes occur between adjacent Schwann cells, which form the myelin sheaths around the peripheral nerve fibers. A relative narrowing of the axon occurs near the termination of the myelin sheath at a node and the axon may be reduced by about one-third of its total diameter. This has been observed principally in large axons. The axon bulges slightly in the region of the node where it is bare. This bare segment varies in length from about 0.5 μ in large (10–15 μ diameter) fibers to as much as 2.5 μ in small (3–10 μ diameter) fibers. The nodal axon is, however, not completely uncovered, but is surrounded by minute finger-like processes from the two adjacent encircling Schwann cells. These Schwann processes do not actually contact the axons.

Fig. 100. A, schematic representation of the membrane theory of the origin of nerve myelin. Four stages in the engulfment of the axon (2) by the Schwann-cell (1) and the wrapping of many double layers which, after condensation, form the compact myelin; B, enfolding of Schwann-cell surface membranes to form compact myelin, after the theory of Geren. Note differentiation between inner and outer surfaces of enfolding membrane; in the double membrane, this gives rise to Finean's 'difference factor' and explains why the full repeat distance in the radial direction involves two bimolecular leaflets of lipoprotein (two membranes).

7.12.1 Myelinization peripherally

Figs. 101, 102. The Schwann cell is the cellular element responsible for the formation of myelin around peripheral nerves. In earlier descriptions, the Schwann or sheath cells were believed to wrap around the axon and then to elaborate the myelin which was deposited within the sheath cell. The outer layer of the sheath cell was left as a surface structure surrounding the myelin, dipping down at the nodes of Ranvier to contact the axon[132]. The outer sheath cell membrane of the Schwann cell was then considered to form the neurilemma.

Numerous electron microscopists[44, 54, 103, 110, 122] have confirmed that the myelin of the peripheral nerve is indeed formed by the Schwann cell. Now, however, the myelin is no longer believed to be created by an intracellular accumulation of lipid within the Schwann cell. It has instead

Fig. 101. A, cross section, rat sciatic nerve. The internodal Schwann-cell cytoplasm surrounding this large, myelinated axon contains few organelles. Both the external and internal mesaxons are apparent at the upper left of the figure. (× 29 000); **B,** cross section, myelin sheaths, rat sciatic nerve. The lamellar pattern of compact myelin consists of alternate dense and less dense lines with a period of 120–130 Å (× 195 000).

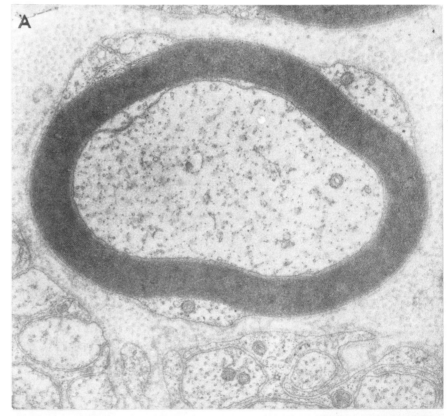

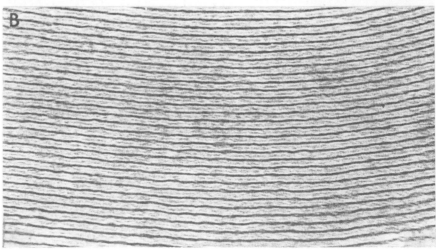

been shown to be made of a series of cell membranes which come in contact with each other as pseudopodia-like processes of a Schwann cell wrapped around an axon. These membranes are in general like the cytoplasmic membranes seen in all other cells of mammals, birds, amphibians, etc. Thus, these membranes have three distinct molecular strata. There is a central bimolecular layer of lipids, an outer unimolecular layer of protein and an inner monolayer of protein or possibly something else (carbohydrate). As indicated, the Schwann cell has been observed literally to wrap itself spirally around the axon (Fig. 100**A**).

Once this spiral wrapping has started, more than 100 spiral laminations may occur, to produce the extremely laminated myelin normally observed (Fig. 101). The cytoplasm of these pseudopodia-like extensions of the Schwann cell is apparently squeezed out almost completely as the 'wrap-around' process continues so that all the cytoplasmic organelles

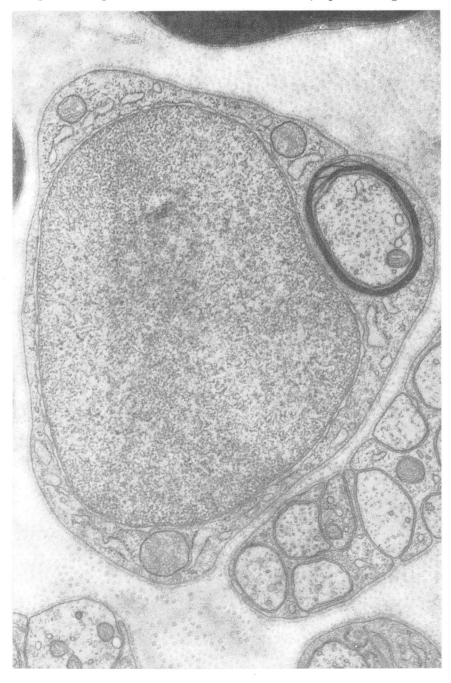

Fig. 102. Cross section, Guinea pig sciatic nerve. A small, myelinated axon lies within a Schwann cell which also contains mitochondria, endoplasmic reticulum, and the nucleus in this plane of section. The nerve fibers cut in cross section at the lower right of the field, represent 'unmyelinated' axons of the autonomic system with only a single layer of Schwann cell membrane wrapped around them. (× 36 000).

of the cell will in the final state be found near the nucleus or at the proximal-distal edges of the lamellar sheaths. This obviously serves to bring adjacent membranes of the Schwann cell processes in apposition with each other. Further, in the process of the spiral winding of lamellae, each lamella overlaps the preceding ones distally and proximally. The extent of this overlap may be observed at the nodes of Ranvier where adjacent Schwann cells meet (Fig. 103), or just fail to meet.

As observed electronmicroscopically, myelin appears as dense lines of about 25 Å repeated radially at a period of about 120 Å in fully myelinated fibers. Light zones appear between the dense lines and each light zone is bisected by an irregular (intraperiod) line which is not as dense as the dense lines. The major dense lines appear to be formed where the adjacent layers of the internal surface of mesaxon loops derived from the Schwann cell fuse together. The less dense intraperiod lines represent the line of fusion of the external surface of Schwann cell membranes,

Fig. 103. The node of Ranvier, as seen with the electron microscope. **M,** a myelin lamella. Note the overlap of each succeeding lamella at the node.

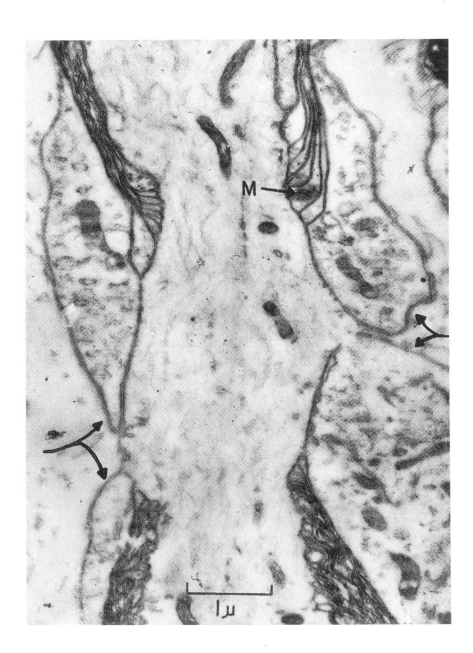

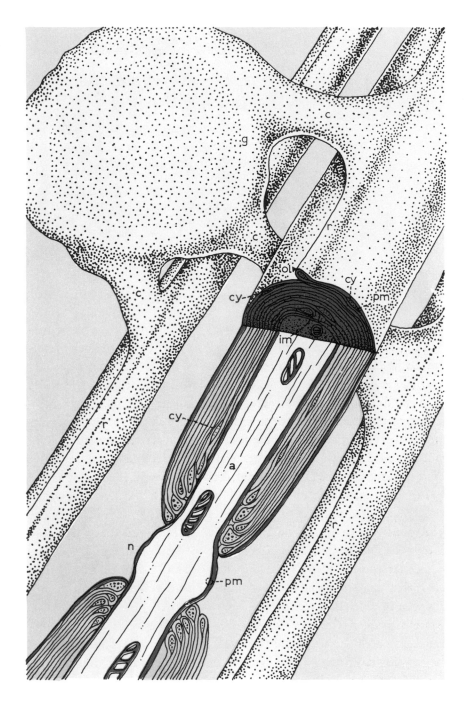

Fig. 104. Illustration indicating that a single oligodendroglial cell in the CNS may be involved in myelin formation for more than one axon.

g, oligodendroglial cell; **a,** axon; **c,** connection between glial cell body and myelin sheath; **cy,** cytoplasm; **pm,** plasma membrane; **n,** node of Ranvier; **ol,** loop of the plasma membrane; **im,** internal mesaxon; **r,** ridge.

when the cytoplasm is squeezed out of the spiral process which has become wrapped around the axon (Fig. 100, **B**). The light zone of the myelin sheath is usually considered to contain the lipid of myelin. However, according to Robertson, only a small portion of the central light zone contains lipid. The remainder appears to be a highly hydrated space between the two components of the bimolecular stratum of lipids[110, 111]. This space might presumably be available for ionic current flow. Thus, as finally constituted, the myelin consists of a multilamellar (Fig. 105, **B**) series of extensions of the Schwann cell cytomembrane wound helically around the axon. Since the Schwann cell cytoplasm has been virtually all squeezed out, this leaves primarily a series of cell mem-

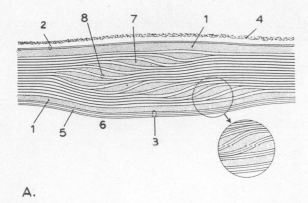

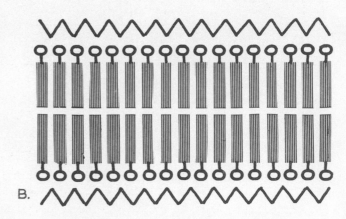

Fig. 105 A, Diagram of the ultra-structure of Schmidt-Lantermann clefts. **1,** Schwann cell cytoplasm; **2,** Schwann cell membrane; **3,** axon Schwann membrane; **4,** basement membrane; **5,** gap between axonal and Schwann membranes; **6,** axoplasm; **7,** interlamellar space; **8,** lamella.

Fig. 105 B. This figure illustrates the molecular structure of Schwann cell membranes. According to this conception the cell membrane consists of a single bi-molecular leaflet of lipid with the polar surfaces of the lipid molecules covered by mono-layers of non-lipid material. The open circles indicate the polar ends of the lipid molecules. The non-polar portions are indicated by small stripes. The non-lipid layers are indicated by the zigzag lines.

branes in apposition to each other with the electron-dense lines representing the protein of a cell membrane, and the light zones the lipid-aqueous interzone of a cell membrane.

Figs. 105 A, 106. Breaks in the myelin sheath other than at the nodes have been described by light microscopy. These are the Schmidt-Lantermann incisures, which were once thought to act as canals providing for entry or egress of materials between the axon and the extraneuronal fluid spaces. The existence of gaps in the myelin sheath has been confirmed by electron microscopy, which does not, however, reveal canals but rather areas where the lamellae of the sheath have become 'unstuck' and pulled partially apart, possibly, as suggested by Robertson[109], as a result of the histological processing. Since Robertson has observed that there may be considerable stretches of nerve fiber without clefts and that the number increases in fibers isolated in Ringers and other fluids, his view as to their being artifactual seems plausible despite reports of their having been seen in unfixed nerves by phase microscopy.

As indicated, not all peripheral nerves have been classified as myelinated. In particular are those fibers of the autonomic system termed postganglionic. They have long been considered unmyelinated. However, they, like other peripheral 'unmyelinated' nerves, exist in relation to Schwann cells, as do the 'myelinated' fibers. Viewed by electronmicroscopy, such fibers appear embedded within a depression of the Schwann cell, whose cell wall forms a single spiral lamina around the axon. Thus, the axon appears suspended within a fold of the Schwann-cell cytomembrane which projects into the cytoplasm of the Schwann cell as a mesaxon. One or more of such axons may be found in relation to a single Schwann cell (Fig. 102).

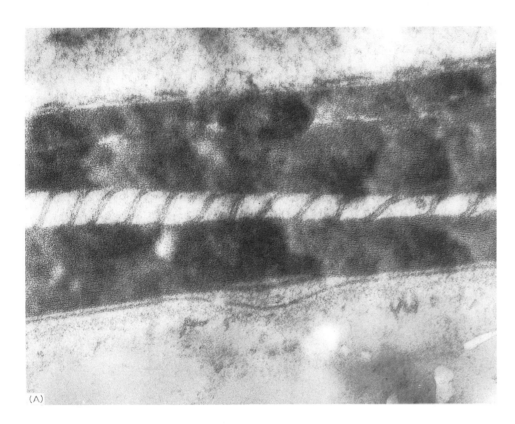

(A)

Fig. 106. Portion of longitudinal section of the Schmidt-Lantermann cleft traversed by myelin lamellae. **A,** × 67 000; **B,** × 100 000.

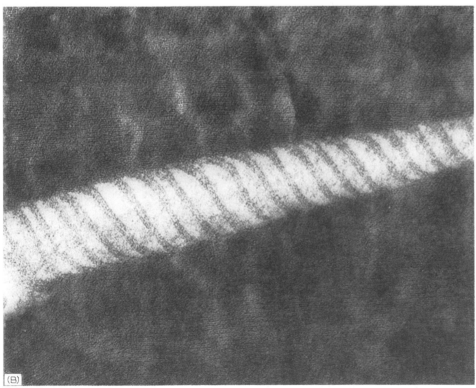

(B)

Fig. 107. These electron micrographs illustrate a direct connection between a glial cell and a forming myelin sheath. During the neonatal period of rapid myelin formation such connections are readily visible in spinal cord white matter; they have not yet been demonstrated in similar adult tissue. A process (**p**) of an oligodendrocyte (**oligo**) extends to the myelin sheath forming about axon a_1. This process is shown at another level in the inset. Here the plasma membrane of the process is seen to be directly continuous with the lamellae of the sheath. Thus, the sheath forms as a spiral extension of the oligodendrocytic plasmalemma, ending at the inner mesaxon (**arrow**). Connections between one oligodendrocyte and two myelin sheaths have been observed.

A portion of the oligodendrocyte nucleus (**n**) is visible. The extension to the sheath contains the usual cytoplasmic components found in the perikaryon. The myelin sheath about axon **a**, demonstrates the inner mesaxon (**arrow**) and outer loop (**ol**) typical of the sheath configuration. (Kitten spinal cord 5 days post partum, OsO_4 fixation, Epon embedment, lead citrate and uranyl acetate staining; × 26 000; inset × 34 500.)

7.12.2 Myelinization centrally

Fig. 107. The formation of myelin sheaths around the axons within the central nervous system is less clearly understood. Although nodes comparable to the nodes of Ranvier of peripheral nerves are not as frequently encountered centrally, they have been clearly shown by Peters[103] in the optic nerve (this is not a true nerve but a peripheral projection of the CNS itself), and in general throughout the CNS.

The myelin sheaths found in the CNS are also made up of multilamellar sheaths, apparently formed by processes derived from glial cells. Bunge *et al.*[18] believe that one glial cell is actually involved in the myelin sheaths of adjacent axonal fibers (Fig. 104, 107). Luse[90, 91] also suggests that myelin is formed centrally by processes from glial cells, particularly oligodendroglial. They observe that only a few lamellae surround an axon in early stages (mice and rats). Later, a large number of flattened glial processes surround the axon. Glial cytoplasm is entrapped within some of the membranes surrounding such axons, and the number of membranes within the sheath of a particular axon varies along the course of the fiber. Furthermore, it would appear that while the glial cell may provide processes for the sheaths of more than one adjacent axon, many glial cells are actually needed to form the complete multilamellar sheath of myelin found around the axon at any particular locus.

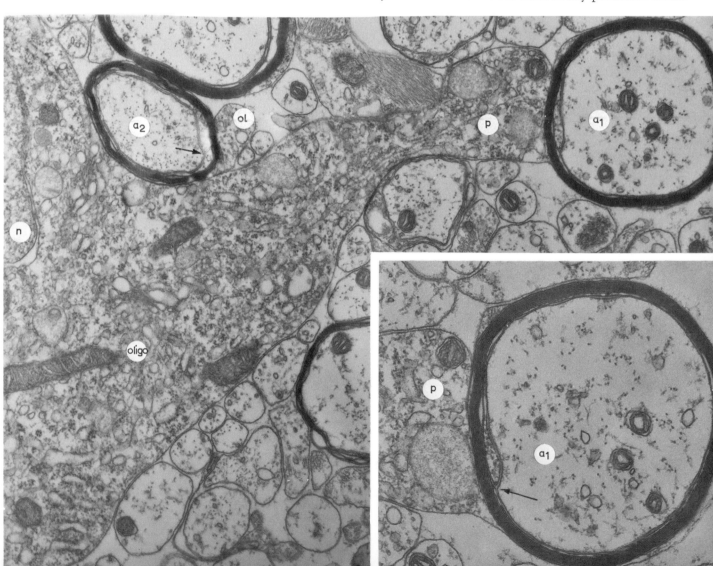

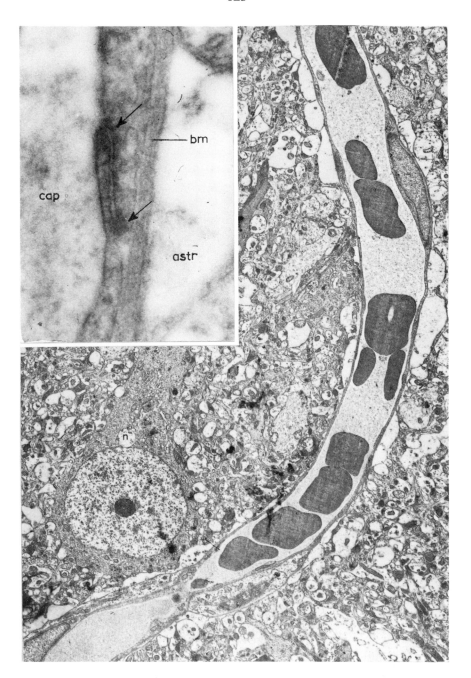

Fig. 108. Electron micrograph showing the relationship between capillaries, glia and nerve cells in rat cerebral cortex. The capillary endothelium as shown at a higher magnification in insert demonstrates the overlapping of endothelial cell margins which occurs in brain capillaries. **astr,** astrocyte foot processes; **bm** basement membrane; **cap,** capillary lumen; **n,** nucleus of a small nerve cell.

7.13 Neuron–glia relationships

Figs. 108, 109, 110. In the past, the neurons have been considered independently from the glial cells which surround and support them. At the same time, it was believed that there was a large extracellular space in the CNS which contained H_2O and electrolytes, etc. Thus, nutrients might leave the capillaries and pass into this 'space' and then enter the neurons[55]. Electron microscopy studies by many authors indicate that such a large space does not exist. The only 'free' spaces which do exist are the 100 to 200 Å wide spaces between the plasma membranes[24] which provide for an extracellular space of about 21% of the brain volume. All the area of the brain parenchyma is filled with nerve cells, their processes, glial cells and units of the vascular system. Astrocytes have

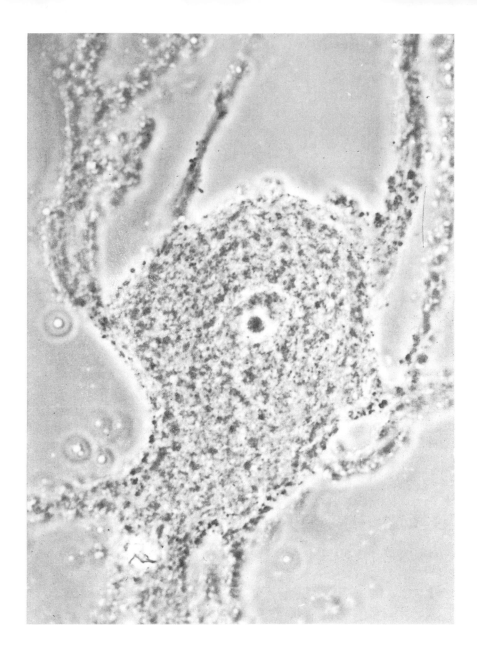

Fig. 109. Fresh, isolated nerve cell from the Deiters' nucleus, rabbit. Dissected out by hand, photographed in the phase contrast (× 320), in isotonic sucrose solution. Slightly stained by methylene blue to show the density of the synapses as small, dark knobs on the surface.

been observed to extend between capillaries and nerve cells and between capillaries and ependymal cells. Conceivably, such cellular units may serve to contain some of the water considered to exist in an extracellular space. Obviously, such fluid would now be intracellular, the astrocytes serving as a sort of extraneuronal space capable of containing the water, etc., usually considered as being extracellular[90, 91, 112, 135]. The facts that extracellular edema is not commonly produced and that various kinds of experimental edema occur within the glial cells[27] also suggest that the 'extracellular' water space of the CNS is partly within the glial cell. However, while most electron microscopists agree than an extracellular 'water space' in brain is limited to the 100–200 Å spaces between plasma membranes, Van Harreveld[135], on the basis of electron microscopy of quick frozen slices of cortex, feels that there may be spaces between cells which are much larger than 200 Å. Electron microscopy of the system further

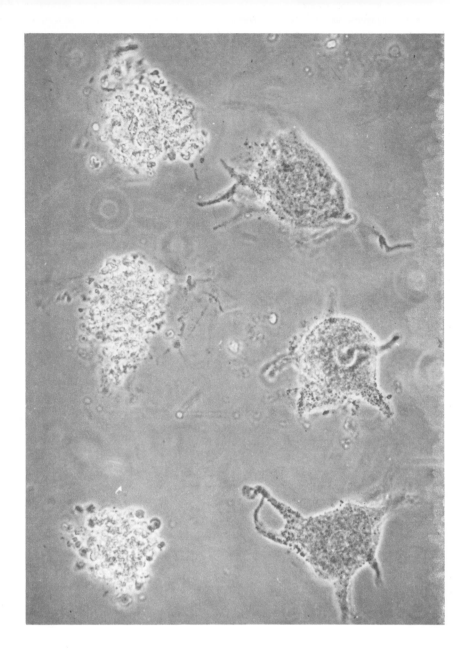

Fig. 110. Fresh Deiters' nerve cells and the glial cells originally closely surrounding each cell, dissected free, trimmed to the volume of their associated nerve cell, and arranged in a row at the left of the nerve cells. The clusters of glial cells slightly pressed against glass. (Phase contrast, × 24.)

demonstrates a close structural relationship between neurons and glia, indicating that neurons rarely contact blood vessels, but have glia interposed. Such glia may then also serve as a connecting link between the neuron and capillary for exchange of nutrients or wastes, supplementing exchanges occurring along the extracellular space. The use of such spaces would seem, however, to be limited by numerous 'tight' junctions between cells. Furthermore, the glial cell, as interposed between neurons and capillaries, may be capable of reacting as something more than a passive transfer cell[67].

Before discussing some of the demonstrated relationships other than structural which exist between neurons and glia, a few observations may be mentioned which pertain to the synthetic function of neurons.

Neurons have been shown to have tremendous capacity for producing RNA, the amount produced being related to the neuronal activity. It seems clear that nerve cells produce RNA and new protein in a manner similar to that of all other cells. Thus, there is a dependence on DNA which acts as a carrier of genetic material. Although neuronal divisions with accompanying duplication of DNA occur only rarely in most adult mammals[2, 4, 6], there is good evidence for a turnover of at least some of the purine and pyrimidine bases of nerve cell DNA[74]. A very high turnover of low molecular weight RNA has also been demonstrated.

In the formation of new nerve-cell protein, the same processes observed in other cells are apparently operational. Thus, amino acids become activated by an enzyme, the energy coming from ATP. These activated amino acids are then linked to a soluble acceptor or transfer RNA system to form an amino acyl-RNA. Each enzyme system concerned may be specific for 1 amino-acid derivative.

A more recent report[79], however, suggests that there may be some overlap in these systems. The soluble RNA acceptor system acts to transfer the activated amino acid to the template or messenger RNA. This messenger RNA presumably transmits the code message for the protein synthesis from the nuclear DNA to the ribosomal RNA. Thus, there are at least three classes of RNA. There is the ribosomal RNA which is intimately involved in protein synthesis. Then there is transfer RNA which has the unique property of binding enzymatically with amino acids, and lastly, there is messenger RNA whose role appears to be to transmit the message code regarding protein (enzyme or polypeptide) synthesis to the ribosomes. According to most available data, new protein seems to be synthesized in nerves as in other cells as a single complete protein instead of by addition of peptides and polypeptides to each other to produce the new protein. However, other evidence indicates that various amino acids in nerve cell protein have different half lives within the neural protein (different turnover rates) and may be replaced individually in the proteins. Thus, an activated amino acid may simply exchange for one already in a protein molecule. Whichever occurs, there is little doubt but that a dynamic state exists. It is interesting to note that nerve cells deprived of their normal stimuli during critical periods of formation fail to develop normally biochemically. Thus, retinal cells deprived of light in the newborn rabbit have only low amounts of RNA and protein, and they do not function properly.

Fig. 111. Some forms of glial-neuronal interrelationships have been known for some time. Thus, glial cells have been shown to react to brain (neuron) damage[128]. Perineuronal glial elements react when increased functional demands are made on the neurons they surround[77] as well as after nerve cell stimulation[79]. These observations and others have been considered as indicating that glial cells are involved in at least supporting nerve cell activity.

Other relationships between neurons and glia have been demonstrated by microchemical methods[69]. Some of these observations are as follows: (a) Glia have only 10% of the RNA of neurons on a dry weight basis. This may be due to a decreased synthesis, wider distribution of RNA in the large astrocyte cells with their many far flung pseudopodia-like processes, or possibly transference of RNA to the adjacent neurons; (b) stimulation of neurons for short periods leads to an increase in neuronal RNA, protein and respiratory enzyme activity and a concomitant decrease in these units in the surrounding glial structures. This suggests that there may be an exchange of material between glial and nerve cells. Prolonged stimulation decreases the RNA and protein of both neurons and glia; (c) in stimulated neurons, whose enzyme activity becomes raised, anaerobic glycolysis was depressed, whereas anaerobic glycolysis was significantly raised in the surrounding glial units. At the same time, the efficiency of the cytochrome oxidase system improved in the nerve cells. Since the efficiency of glucose utilization by the Krebs cycle (aerobic glycolysis) is 55% and only 3% during anaerobic glycolysis, it is apparent that the neurons are using most of the available energy when stimulated.

Glial ATP-ase has a higher activity than that of nerve cells. Furthermore, the pH maximum and ion requirements of glia and neurons differ, suggesting different biochemical requirements or states. Qualitative differences in the RNA bases in the glial and nerve cell units have been observed. Thus, there are higher guanine and lower cytosine values in nerve cell RNA and *vice versa* in the adjacent glial cells. Changes in the RNA of glia and neurons of one of the vestibular equilibratory nuclei have also been observed in rats learning to perform a complicated motor sequence involving balance.

When chemical agents which will enhance protein synthesis are administered, nerve cell RNA and protein increase, while the content in glial cells falls. The composition of the bases of RNA of nerve cells and adjacent glia also show inverse changes in such circumstances with respect to guanine and cytosine values.

Further experiments[58] suggest that the glial mass may be further subdivided into those units found predominantly around capillaries (contain more astrocytes than is found in the glial mass around neurons) and those predominantly around nerve cells. While the astrocyte would appear to have a relation to both capillaries and neurons, oligodendroglia, as satellites, appear to have more of a neuronal relationship. Thus, the glial cell mass around the neurons was about 90% oligodendroglia and 10% astrocytes. The capillary glia consisted of 70% oligodendroglia and 30% astrocytes. These observations are based on the relative position of the glial cell bodies as seen by light microscopy. The structural relationship, as revealed by electron microscopy, shows a rather extensive infiltration of astrocyte foot processes into the areas where oligodendroglial cell bodies predominate. These processes then appear to become

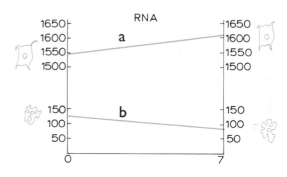

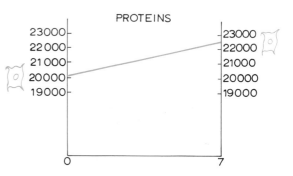

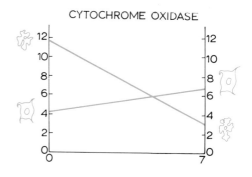

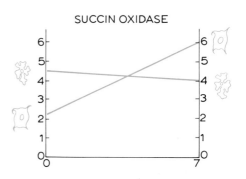

Fig. 111. Vestibular stimulation 25 min/day for 7 days. Schematic representation of the changes occurring concomitantly in the Deiters' nerve cells and in their (oligodendro-)glial cells on vestibular stimulation. RNA and proteins expressed as pg/cell. Enzyme activity expressed as $\mu l\ O_2 \times 10^{-4}/h/cell$. **a,** neurons; **b,** glia.

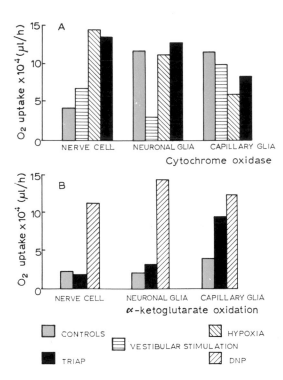

Fig. 112. **A**, summary of cytochrome oxidase assays; **B**, summary of α-ketoglutarate oxidation assays.

interposed between the oligodendroglia and nerve cells to a considerable degree. Hamberger's studies[58] on the effect of centrifugal rotation of rabbits on the oxidation of cytochrome c, succinate, α-ketoglutarate, and glutamate by the neuronal and capillary glia cell bodies of one of the vestibular nuclei indicate differences, induced by rotation, in the enzyme function in the two glial areas. Hamberger concluded that the reactions of neuronal glia favored a metabolic relation to the nerve cell, and the enzymatic properties of the glial mass adjacent to capillaries suggest that it may, in conjunction with the vascular endothelium, be involved in transport of material between blood and brain. How these two metabolic relationships in glia are actually related to nerve cell function is difficult to resolve since the astrocyte processes are so intimately associated with nerve cells. It may well be that astrocytes function in transport mechanisms and that oligodendroglia are more concerned with such synthetic mechanisms as involve an exchange of nucleic acid bases and proteins, etc., between glia and nerve cell units.

The various data and suggestions presented above are far from conclusive proof for a specific metabolic relationship between neurons and glia. However, the inference is strongly suggestive that an important metabolic interaction exists which may relieve the neurons of the necessity of being complete metabolic units in regard to total maintenance of their own structural units. The data which have accumulated on such metabolic interaction have to date been most suggestive in relation to protein and nucleic acid formation.

A similar situation appears to exist for the perikaryon of sensory ganglia. These cells have long been recognized as being surrounded by perisomatic satellite cells and an outer capsule of connective tissue elements. The extent to which the satellite elements envelop the sensory cell has only recently been ascertained. It appears that these cells form a complete, continuous sheath around the sensory cells, intertwining between the neurons and the capillaries. Thus, these 'peripheral glia' appear in the same relation to sensory ganglion cells as oligodendroglia and astrocytes do to the CNS neurons. Periaxonal satellites appear aminar and envelop segments of axon, building tubular sheaths. They may lie on the axon, with the various turns of the spiral course in contact with each other. This appears to be somewhat similar to the manner in which the Schwann cells form the myelin sheath. Indeed, Pannese[100] feels that the perisomatic and periaxonic satellites and the Schwann cell may not necessarily represent discretely different cell types, but differences in morphological arrangement induced by their location. This may perhaps be related to their common origin from the neural crest.

7.14 Pinocytosis in nervous tissue

The phenomenon of *pinocytosis* was first described by Lewis[86] in 1931. This term, which means literally 'drinking by cells', was used to describe a process whereby undulating cellular membranes were observed (in tissue culture) to entrap fluid within folds. This led to the formation of vacuoles which tended to migrate into the cytoplasm. Such activity has been observed in astrocytes[104] as well as in oligodendroglia and microglia[72] *in vitro*. The latter studies also demonstrated the uptake of protein by glia in tissue culture preparation. However, there was no evidence of such pinocytotic uptake of protein or fluid by dorsal root ganglion cells in the cultures. Furthermore, there is as yet no direct evidence for pinocytotic mechanisms in the living intact brain. Nevertheless, the data obtained by *in-vitro* techniques strongly suggest an active pinocytosis by the normal glial elements supporting the nerve cells. The possibility that transport of materials from the blood to the nerve cell through the glial cells involves pinocytosis of water and dissolved solutes as well as active biochemical transport mechanisms has attracted considerable attention. The observation that pinocytosis has been seen only in the glial cells serves to further support the concept that the glia are highly important in the maintenance of nerve cell metabolism.

7.15 Degeneration of neurons

Injury of nerve fibers peripherally is a common problem in medical practice today. A host of accidental situations ranging from industrial to automotive provide for a wide array of peripheral nerve injuries. Many histological changes occur in nerve fibers as a result of severe crushing or severence. From various studies (*cf.* Singer and Schadé[120, 121]), it appears that the velocity of degeneration depends somewhat on the size and degree of myelinization of the fibers, the large myelinated fibers degenerating faster than small ones[61].

Fig. 113. The spatial terminology for cell and fiber degeneration.

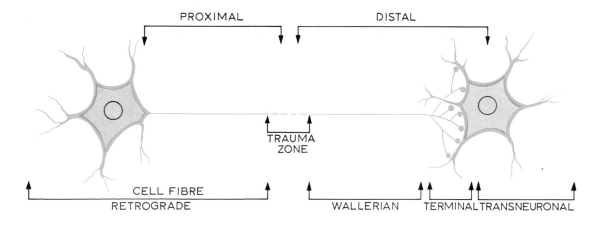

7.15.1 Distal changes (Wallerian degeneration)

Figs. 113, 114, 115. Following severence of a nerve fiber, the distal part undergoes complete degeneration. The part proximal to the section will show retrograde changes in the axon which extend centrally for two to three centimeters. Further degenerative changes in the axon will be minimal unless the section was too close to the cell body or if the cells were immature, as in a newborn mammal[83]. Such incompletely matured cells may not survive axonal sectioning. In the first 3 to 5 days after section, the peripheral segment will still respond to chemical or electrical stimulation. Despite this maintenance of some physiologic function, changes occur in the axon as early as 12 hours after injury which prophesy the ultimate degeneration. Within a short space the neurofibrils become hypertrophic[138], and the axon cylinders swell. Lee[84] observed an acute swelling of mitochondria and endoplasmic reticulum in the axon 19 hours after sectioning. The endoplasmic reticulum eventually disintegrates into fragments of uneven granular material[61]. Neurofibrils were observed to aggregate, and the number of mitochondria and dense bodies in the axon increased. The source of an increased number of mitochondria in the peripheral part of a sectioned nerve is difficult to explain other than as a local phenomenon. Since the axon starts to show anatomical signs of breaking up into fragments 2 days after sectioning, the presence of some response to stimulation up to 5 days after section raises the question as to possible Schwann cell participation in impulse propagation.

Within 12 to 19 hours after sectioning, a loosening of the myelin lamellae occurs. Such changes were more prominent in 24 hours. Furthermore, the myelin sheaths showed a complex folding with an increase in the number of Schmidt-Lantermann clefts proximal to the section. This appears to result from a splitting of the myelin sheath along the intermediate dense lines of the lamellar sheaths. This observation does not necessarily disagree with Robertson who felt that the clefts may be artifacts, since the physiologic states proximal and distal to the nerve section are not equivalent and the myelin sheath need not react the same way to the fixation process. That the underlying cause for the clefts may not be the same as in normal tissue is suggested by the fact that the clefts which occur in normal nerves arise as separations along the major dense rather than being associated with the intermediate dense lines. Changes in the external (surface) part of the Schwann cells begin later and proceed more slowly than do those in the myelin sheath derived from the Schwann cell membranes and axon (rat). The Schwann cell cytoplasm appears more abundant around degenerating fibers than around non-degenerating fibers. It is vacuolar and contains many granules about 100 Å in diameter. The cytoplasmic content of the Schwann cell increases during the first three to four days after nerve section and then decreases by the sixth to eighth day.

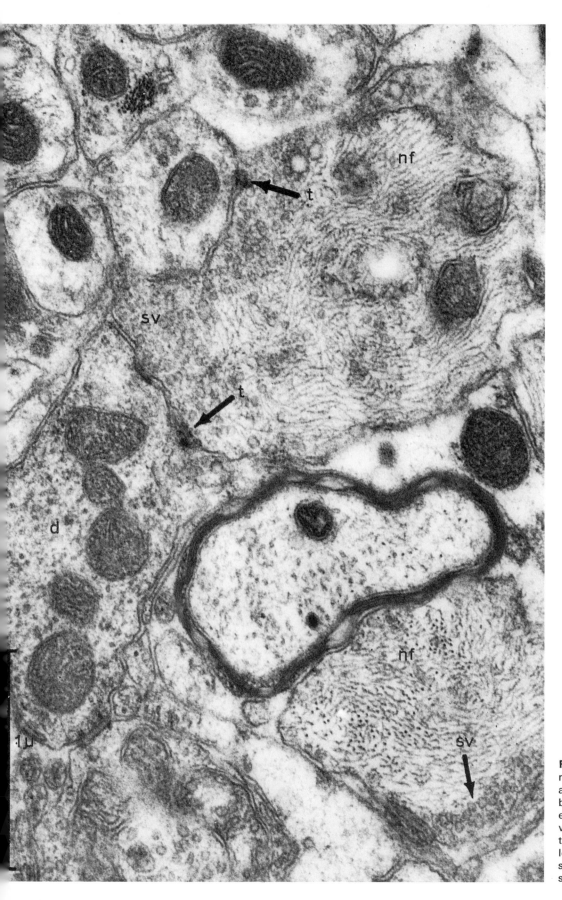

Fig. 114. Two degenerating axon terminals from the lateral geniculate nucleus of a monkey that had one eye removed 5 days before death. The terminals show an extensive network of neurofilaments (**nf**) which has displaced the synaptic vesicles towards one side of the terminal; in the left terminal the vesicles lie close to the synaptic thickenings (**t**); **d,** dendrite; **sv,** synaptic vesicles.

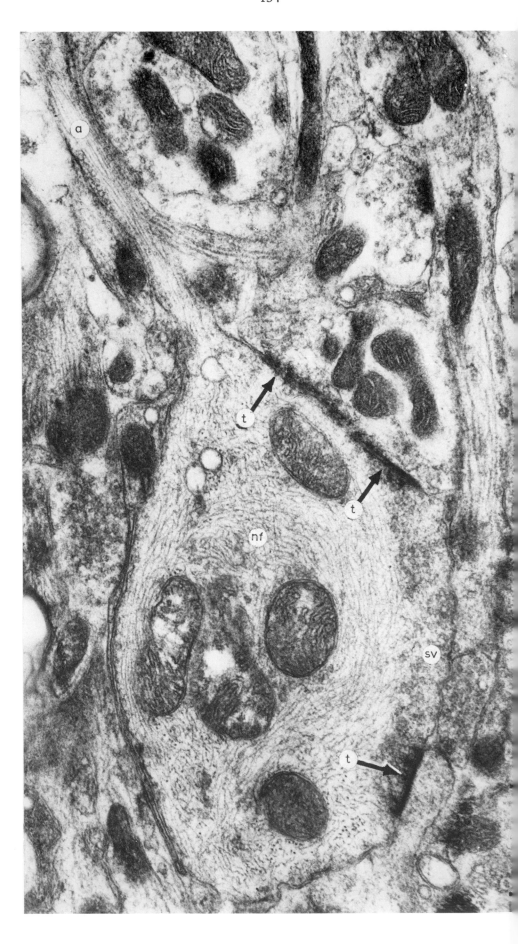

Fig. 115. A, degenerating terminal similar to those shown in **B**; 5 days survival. Note the axon (**a**) entering the top left part of the figure. **B,** degenerating terminal that shows a ring of neurofilaments similar to the neurofibrillar rings that can be seen with the light microscope. **nf,** neurofilaments; **sv,** synaptic vesicles; **t,** synaptic thickening.

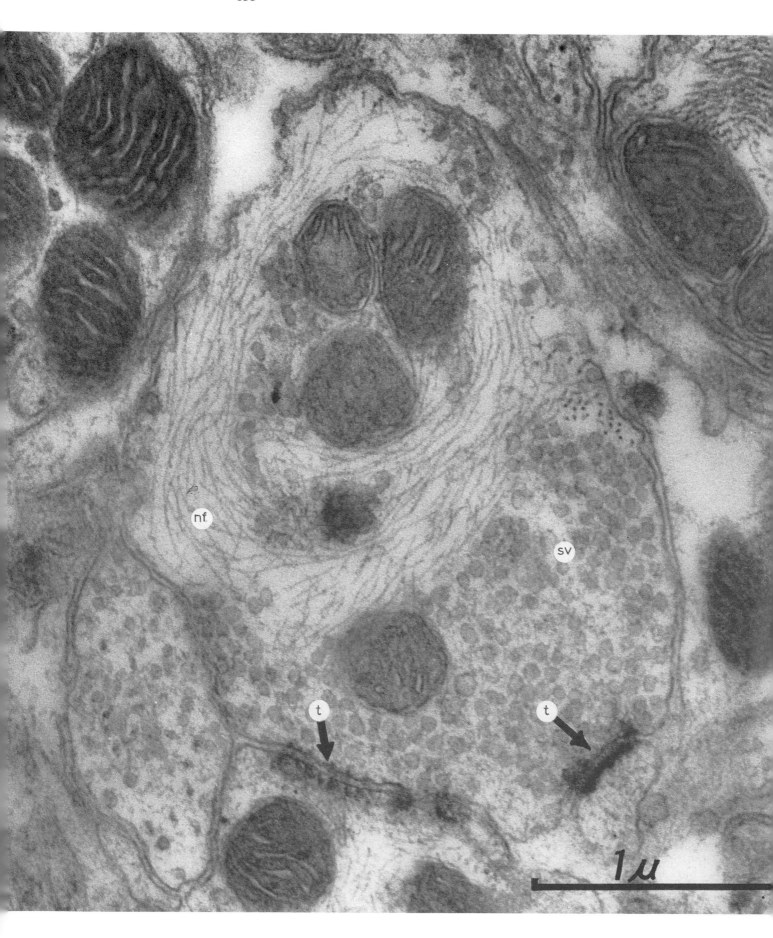

1μ

These sheath cells become very metachromatic following the axonal degeneration and have nuclei with intensely staining chromatin (metachromasia is the condition where cells do not stain true with a given dye). An increase in cytoplasmic organelles becomes apparent in Schwann cells of both myelinated and unmyelinated neurons within 2 days. They appear to start dividing mitotically around the fourth day, forming a syncytial nucleated band which comes to lie in the position previously occupied by the severed nerve fibers in their endoneural tubes. The collagen fibers of these tubes appear to be in part formed by Schwann cell. This syncytial cord apparently provides the 'contact guidance' pathway which the regenerating nerve fiber will follow and becomes continuous with a similar cord of proliferating Schwann cells arising from the proximal end of the cut nerve fiber.

The axoplasm contracts away from the myelin sheath in places and contains granular or filamentous material lying within clear matrices, sometimes associated with mitochondria, dense particles or vesicles. Between the seventh and twelfth day the axoplasmic organelles of mye-

Fig. 116. Cross section of Schwann cell in metachromatic leucodystrophy. Several myelin lamellae, occasionally separated by narrow zones of Schwann cell cytoplasm, are continuous with the external and internal mesaxons and form a simple spiral around the axon (× 38 000). (courtesy H. de F. Webster.)

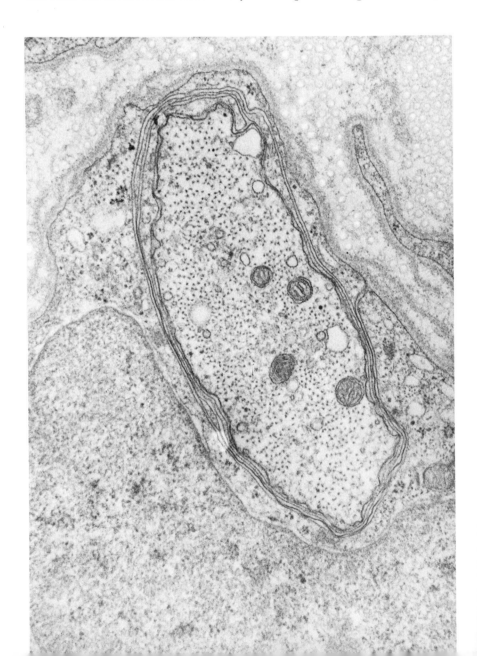

linated fibers gradually disappear leaving large or small spaces within the myelin sheath. In the rat, such axoplasmic organelles did not wholly disappear until after the 28th day, when some dense particles still remained. By the 35th day, no axonal remnants remained, only particles of free or phagocytised myelin[84]. While these axonal changes are occurring, the myelin as a whole undergoes further degenerative changes, becoming beaded, within the first 2 to 3 days, subsequently breaking up into fragments. This process is more or less complete within two weeks. The Schwann cells appear to become phagocytic when the myelin membranes they have formed break down. This phagocytosis extends through the 2nd and 3rd week after section. While being able to ingest the myelin, the presence of such proteolipid material within the Schwann cells as long as 3 months after nerve section suggests that they are very slow to digest such ingested myelin. The phagocytosis is apparently aided by connective tissue macrophages as well.

New nerve fibrils may be observed as small 0.5 μ axoplasmic protrusions from the proximal nerve trunk seven days after injury in crushed nerves, and fourteen days after injury in sectioned nerves. By eight weeks these fibrils are clearly definable as unmyelinated nerve fibers lying within Schwann cells. In a sense, they are undergoing the first phase of myelinization. Complete remyelinization of these fibers appears to follow their increase in size once having reached their 'target' structures and may not be complete even within one year. The preceding discussion attempts to interrelate the investigations of several workers whose observations are not all in agreement. Therefore, a conclusive statement on the changes occurring in the degenerating peripheral nerve is not yet available. The role of the Schwann cell is in particular challenged. Lee[84] observes that it has some phagocytic activity but does not undergo mitotic division. He does not mention a syncytial cord as described by Barton[10].

7.15.2 Retrograde degeneration

The degenerative changes in the proximal nerve fibers appear to be quite similar to those observed distally, but may be limited to a few centimeters, depending on the extent and nature of the injury. The axons become swollen with an increase in axoplasm and in the number of neurofibrils. Schwann cell cytoplasm increases, and there is at the site of injury a proliferation of Schwann cells which extend a syncytial cord toward that of the distal stump. The myelin sheath shows a beading and breakdown by light microscopy. Such a myelin sheath will then be ingested by phagocytic Schwann cells or tissue macrophages. By electronmicroscopy, the myelin just proximal to a cut, but not crushed nerve, shows an increase in what appears to be Schmidt-Lantermann clefts. Inasmuch as these clefts are not increased in number peripherally where Schwann cell changes are more extreme, it has been suggested that the presence of 'normal' Schwann cells is necessary for these extra intralaminar spaces to be formed.

7.15.3 Changes in the perikaryon after nerve root section

Sectioning of a nerve is accompanied almost immediately by intracellular changes which have frequently been interpreted as pertaining to the attempt by the cell to reconstitute its peripheral process. There is a dramatic increase in cell volume with a chromatolysis of the basophilic elements. A part of the chromatolysis may be related to an increased dispersion of basophilic material in the greatly swollen cell rather than to actual dissolution of the nucleic acids. The nucleus becomes eccentrically placed within the first four to six days. Studies on survival rate indicate that in cats with facial nerves sectioned at the stylomastoid foramen, most cells survive in animals 15 days or more in age. Thus, the chromatolysis and increase in nucleolar and nuclear size in such animals would appear to be normal physiologic responses directed toward synthesizing new axonal material. Studies by Hydén[65-67] and Rhodes and Ford[107] on the sectioned XIIth nerve indicate a marked increase in cell volume initially. Cell protein and RNA concentration both drop sharply, though RNA per cell drops only slightly. Thus, the chromatolysis of Nissl substance which occurs during the phase of cytoplasmic swelling is not simply

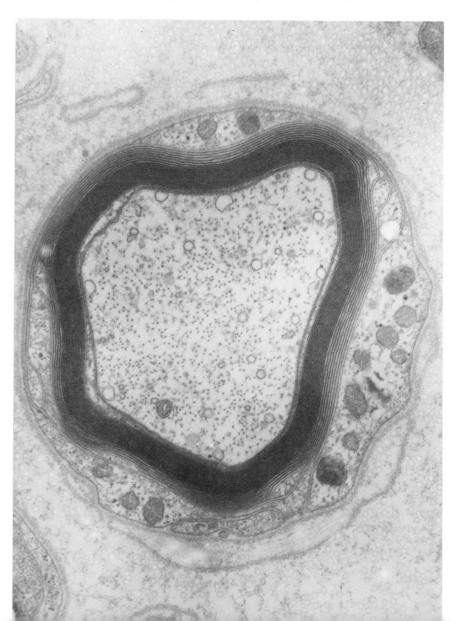

Fig. 117. Cross section, myelinated fiber in metachromatic leucodystrophy (× 29 000). A circumferential band of compact myelin lamellae adjacent to the axon shows an increase in overall density and a decrease in the period between dense lines to approximately 100 Å. The spacing of lamellae external to this band is slightly increased (130–140 Å) and two small inclusions are present in the Schwann cell cytoplasm.

indicative of a loss of RNA-P, but of a redistribution into an area of larger volume, possibly in a form not related to the endoplasmic reticulum. The RNA per cell then actually increases rapidly, reaching a peak about 40 days after nerve section. Protein concentration per cell appears to parallel the rapid increase in RNA per cell, which starts about 8 days after section for RNA and 1–2 days after section for total cell protein. Therefore, cellular efforts to provide for new axonal material, involving utilization of some RNA-P, formation of new RNA-P and new cellular protein appears to start almost at once in the perikaryon of the damaged neuron.

Early studies by Einarson[42] on fatigued nerve cells demonstrated that prolonged stimulation depletes Nissl substance. This has been confirmed biochemically by Hydén's group, who reported that RNA-P decreased in cells after prolonged stimulation. In subsequent regenerative phases, basophilic material (RNA and simple protein) appeared first around the nucleolus; it then migrated to the nuclear membrane through which it passed and finally appeared in the cytoplasm as a perinuclear halo which subsequently took the form of Nissl particles. Experiments with ^{14}C-lysine in regenerating facial nerves[106] indicate that ^{14}C-lysine has a similar perinuclear localization 14 days after sectioning the facial nerve. Inasmuch as the RNA of neurons and other cells appears related to general protein synthesis, the localization of a labeled amino acid in a position comparable to that previously described for new RNA suggests that the lysine is being incorporated into nerve protein in this location.

Maximal growth of the neuronal body becomes greatest about a month after a nerve crush injury. At this time, RNA, protein and lipids of the cell body could be more than twice that of normal cells. The return to normal levels occurs about 90 days after injury. The final maturation of the regenerating neurons appears related to whether or not contact is made with the peripheral 'target' by the regenerating neuron. The growth rate across the wound scar was estimated by Cajal to be about 0.25 mm/day. However, once the syncytial cord of neurilemmal Schwann cells is penetrated, the rate may be as fast as 4.84 mm/day, though rates between 3 and 4 mm seem more normal. The outgrowing fibers which appear in the proximal stump in about seven days in crushed myelinated fibers and fourteen days in nonmyelinated fibers are at first all more or less unmyelinated. They have, as previously indicated, only a single fold of Schwann cell membrane about them. The path taken by an outgrowing axon appears to be chosen largely by chance. Thus, motor fibers may well grow into the neurilemmal sheath of a sensory fiber, and *vice versa*. Therefore, the number of motor fibers growing back to a denervated muscle may be much less than was present prior to injury. However, functional loss is not proportional to the decrease in fibers reaching it, since neighboring uninjured neurons have been observed to give off collaterals which enter the syncytial cords of the old myelin-neurilemmal sheaths and provide for an innervation to the muscle. Part of the later recovery in poliomyelitis may depend on this phenomenon.

References

1 Agduhr, E. (1941) A contribution to the technique of determining the number of nerve cells per unit volume of tissue. *Anat. Rec.*, *80*, 191–202.

2 Altman, J. and Das, G. D. (1965) Postnatal origin of microneurons in the Rat Brain. *Nature*, *207*, 953–956.

3 Altman, J. and Das, G. D. (1966) Autoradiographic and histological studies of postnatal neurogenesis. I. A longitudinal investigation of the kinetics, migration and transformation of cells incorporating tritated thymidine in neonatal rats with especial reference to postnatal neurogenesis in some brain regions. *J. Comp. Neurol.*, *126*, 337–389.

4 Andrews, W. (1956) Structural alterations with aging in the nervous system. *J. Chron. Dis.*, *3*, 575–596.

5 Angevine, J. B. and Sidman, R. L. (1961) Autoradiographic study of cell migration during histogenesis of cerebral cortex in the mouse. *Nature (Lond.)*, *192*, 766–768.

6 Angevine, J. (1965) Time of origin of cells in the hippocampal region. An autoradiographic study in the mouse. *Exptl. Neurol. Suppl. 2*, 1–70.

7 Arey, L. B. (1965) *Development Anatomy. Textbook and Laboratory Manual of Embryology*. W. B. Saunders Co. Philadelphia, Penn.

8 Barr, M. L. and Bertram, E. G. (1951) The behavior of nuclear structures during depletion and restoration of Nissl material in motor neurons. *J. Anat.*, *85*, 171–181.

9 Barr, M. L., Bertram, L. F. and Lindsay, H. A. (1950) The morphology of the nerve cell nucleus according to sex. *Anat. Rec.*, *107*, 283.

10 Barton, A. A. (1962) An electron microscope study of degeneration and regeneration of nerve. *Brain*, *85*, 799–808.

11 Baxter, J. S. (1953) *Fraziers' Manual of Embryology. The Development of the Human Body*. Bailliere, Tindall and Cox, London.

12 Bodian, D. (1962) The generalized vertebrate neurone. *Science*, *137*, 323–326.

13 Bridgman, C. S. and Carmichael, L. (1935) An experimental study of the onset of behavior in the fetal guinea pig. *J. genet. Psychol.*, *47*, 247–267.

14 Brody, H. (1955) Organization of the cerebral cortex. III. A study of aging in the human cerebral cortex. *J. comp. Neurol.*, *102*, 511–556.

15 Bronte, G. (1949) Studies on lipids in the nervous system with special reference to quantitative chemical determination and topical distribution. *Acta physiol. Scand.*, *18*, Suppl. 63.

16 Brown, J. B. (1955) The development of the nucleus of the spinal tract of V in human fetuses of 14 to 21 weeks of menstrual age. *J. comp. Neurol.*, *106*, 383–424.

17 Brownson, R. H. (1956) Perineuronal satellite cells in the motor cortex of aging brains. *J. Neuropathol. exptl. Neurol.*, *15*, 190–195.

18 Bunge, M. B., Bunge, R. P. and Ris, H. (1961) Ultrastructural study of remyelination in an experimental lesion in adult cat spinal cord. *J. biophys. biochem. Cytol.*, *10*, 67–94.

19 Cajal, S. Ramon Y (1909–1911) *Histologie du système nerveux de l'Homme et de Vertébrés*, 2 Vol. Paris, Maloine.

20 Carmichael, L. (1934) An experimental study in the prenatal guinea pig of the origin and development of reflexes and patterns of behavior in relation to the stimulation of specific receptor areas during the period of active fetal life. *Genet. Psychol. Monogr.*, *16*, 337–491.

21 Clark, G. (1962) Area 3, a critical evaluation of cyto-architectonic studies. *J. comp. Anat.*, *119*, 21–24.

22 Dastur, D. K., Lane, M. H., Hansen, D. B., Kety, S. S., Butler, R. N., Perlin, S. and Sokoloff, L. (1963) Effects of aging on cerebral circulation and metabolism in man. *Human aging, a biological and behavioral study*. J. E. Birren, Editor. Public. Health Service Publication, No. 986. U.S. Gov. Printing Office.

23 David, G. B., Brown, A. W. and Mallion, K. B. (1961) On the identity of the "neurofibrils". "Nissl complex", "Golgi apparatus", and "Trophospongium" in the neurons of vertebrates. *Quart. J. micr. Sci.*, *102*, 481–493.

24 Dempsey, E. W. and Lüse, S. (1958) Fine structure of the neuropil in relation to neuroglia cells. *Biology of Neuroglia*. W. F. Windle (Ed.). Springfield, Thomas (pp. 99–108).

25 De Robertis, E. and Bennett, H. S. (1955) Some features of the submicroscopic morphology of synapses in frog and earth worm. *J. biophys. biochem. Cytol.*, *1*, 47–58.

26 De Robertis, E. and Gerschenfeld, H. M. (1961) Submicroscopic morphology and function of glial cells. *Intern. Rev. Neurobiol.*, *3*. C. C. Pfeiffer and J. R. Smythies (Eds.). New York–London, Academic Press (pp. 1–61).

27 De Robertis, E., Gerschenfeld, H. M. and Wald, F. (1960) Ultrastructure and function of glial cells. *Structure and function of the cerebral cortex*. D. B. Tower and J. P. Schadé (Eds.). Amsterdam–New York, Elsevier (pp. 69–80).

28 De Robertis, E. and Pellegrino de Iraldi, A. (1961) Plurivesicular secretory processes and nerve endings in the pineal gland of the rat. *J. biophys. biochem. Cytol.*, *10*, 361–372.

29 Detwiler, S. R. (1936) Growth response of spinal nerves to grafted brain tissue. *J. exptl. Zool.*, *74*, 477–495.

30 De Webster, H. F. (1964) Some ultrastructural features of segmental demyelination and myelin regeneration in peripheral nerve. Mechanisms of neural regeneration. *Progr. Brain Res.*, *13*. M. Singer and J. P. Schadé (Eds.). Amsterdam–London–New York, Elsevier (pp. 151–174).

31 Dobbing, J. (1963) The blood-brain barrier. Some recent developments. *Gray's Hosp. Rep.*, *112*, 267–286.

32 Dodgson, M. C. H. (1962) *The growing brain. An essay in developmental neurology*. Bristol, Wright and Sons.

33 Du Vigneaud, V., Ressler, C., Swan, J. M., Roberts, C. W., Katsoyannis, P. G. and Gordon, S. (1953) The synthesis of an octapeptide amide with the hormonal activity of oxytocin. *J. Amer. chem. Soc.*, *75*, 4879–4880.

34 Du Vigneaud, V., Gish, D. T., and Katsoyannis, P. G. (1954) A synthetic preparation processing biological properties associated with arginine vasopressin. *J. Amer. chem. Soc.*, *76*, 4751–4752.

35 Eayrs, J. T. (1955) The cerebral cortex of normal and hypothyroid rats. *Acta anat. (Basel)*, *25*, 160–183.

36 Eayrs, J. T. and Goodhead, B. (1959) Postnatal development of the cerebral cortex in the rat. *J. Anat. (London)*, *93*, 385–402.

37 Eayrs, J. T. and Lishman, W. G. (1955) The maturation of behavior in hypothyroidism and starvation. *J. Anat. (London)*, *85*, 350–358.

38 Edström, A. (1966) Amino acid incorporation in isolated mauthner nerve fiber components. *J. Neurochem.*, *13*, 315–321.

39 Edström, A. (1967) Inhibition of protein synthesis in mauthner nerve fibers components by Actinomycin, D., *J. Neurochem.*, *14*, 239–243.

40 Einarson, L. (1932) A method for progressive selective staining of Nissl and nuclear substance in nerve cells. *Amer. J. Pathol.*, *8*, 295–305.

41 Einarson, L. (1933) Notes on the morphology of the chromophilic material of nerve cells and its relation to nuclear substances. *Amer. J. Anat.*, *53*, 141–168.

42 Einarson, L. (1957) Cytological aspect of nucleic acid metabolism. *Metabolism of the nervous system*. D. Richter (Ed.). London, Pergamon Press (pp. 403–421).

43 Einarson, L., and Krogh, E. (1955) Variations in the basophilia of nerve cells associated with increased cell activity and functional stress. *J. Neurol., Neurosurg. Psychiat.*, *18*, 1.

44 Fernandez-Moran, H. (1950) Sheath and axon structures in the internode portion of vertebrates myelinated nerve fibers, an electron microscope study of rat and frog sciatic nerves. *Exptl. Cell Res.*, *1*, 309–337.

45 Flexner, L. B. (1955) Enzymatic and functional patterns of the developing mammalian brain. *Biochemistry of the Developing Nervous System*. H. Waelsch (Ed.). New York, Academic Press (pp. 281–300).

46 Flexner, L. B., Belknap, E. L., Jr. and Flexner, J. B. (1953) Biochemical and physiological differentiation during morphogenesis. XVI. Cytochrome oxidase, succinic dehydrogenase and succinoxidase in the developing cerebral cortex and liver of the fetal guinea pig. *J. cell. comp. Physiol.*, *42*, 151–162.

47 Flexner, L. B., Flexner, J. B. and Hellerman, L. (1956) Biochemical and physiological differentiation during morphogenesis. XX. *In vitro* observations on carbohydrate metabolism of the developing cerebral cortex of the fetal guinea pig. *J. cell. comp. Physiol.*, *47*, 469–482.

48 Flexner, L. B., Flexner, J. B. and Roberts, R. R. (1958) Biochemical and physiological differentiation during morphogenesis. XXII. Observations of amino acids and protein synthesis in the cerebral cortex and liver of the newborn mouse. *J. cell. comp. Physiol.*, *51*, 385–403.

49 Flexner, J. B., Greenblatt, C. L., Cooperbond, S. R. and Flexner, L. B. (1956) Biochemical and physiological differentiation during morphogenesis. XIX. Alkaline phosphatase and aldolase activity in the developing cerebral cortex and liver of the fetal guinea pig. *Amer. J. Anat.*, *98*, 129–138.

50 Folch-Pi, J. (1955) Composition of the brain in relation to maturation. *Biochemistry of the Developing Nervous System*. H. Waelsch (Ed.). New York, Academic Press (pp. 121–132).

51 Frankenhaeuser, B., and Hodgkin, A., (1956) The after-effects in impulses in the giant nerve fibers of Loligo. *J. Physiol.*, *131*, 341–376.

52 Gasser, H. S. (1955) Properties of dorsal root unmedullated fibers on two sides of the ganglion. *J. gen. Physiol.*, *38*, 709–728.

53 Gasser, H. S. (1956) Olfactory nerve fibers. *J. gen. Physiol.*, *39*, 473–496.

54 Geren, B. B. (1954) The formation from the Schwann cell surface of myelin in peripheral nerves of chick embryos. *Exp. Cell Res.*, *7*, 558–562.

55 Glees, P. (1961) *Experimental Neurology*. Oxford, Clarendon Press.

56 Gray, E. G. (1963) Electron microscopy of presynaptic organelles of the spinal cord. *J. Anat.*, *97*, 101–106.

57 Guillery, R. W. (1965) Some electron microscopical observations of degenerative changes in central nervous synapses. Degeneration patterns

in the nervous system. *Progr. Brain Res.*, *14*. M. Singer and J. P. Schadé (Eds.). Amsterdam–London–New York, Elsevier.

58 HAMBERGER, A. (1963) Difference between isolated neuronal and vascular glia with respect to respiratory activity. *Acta physiol. scand.*, *58*, *Suppl. 203*, 3–58.

59 HAMLYN, L. H. (1963) An electron microscope study of pyramidal neurones in the Ammon's horn of the rabbit. *J. Anat.*, *2*, 189–201.

60 HARRISON, R. G. (1910) The outgrowth of the nerve fibers as a mode of protoplasmic movement. *J. exptl. Neurol.*, *9*, 787–848.

61 HONJIN, R. and TAKAHASHI, A. (1962) Electron microscopy of nerve fibers. VI. On the myelin changes in the peripheral myelinated nerve fibers during Wallerian degeneration. *J. Electron Microscopy*, *11*, 139–156.

62 HOOKER, D. (1952) *The prenatal origin of behavior*. 18th Porter Lecture Series. Lawrence, University of Kansas Press.

63 HOOKER, D. (1954) Early behavior, with a preliminary note on double simultaneous fetal stimulation. *Research Publications of the Association for Research in Nervous and Mental Disease*, *33*, 98–113.

64 HUMPHREY, T. (1954) The trigeminal nerve in relation to early human fetal activity. *Research Publications of the Association for Research in Nervous and Mental Disease*, *33*, 127–154.

65 HYDÉN, H. (1943) Protein metabolism in the nerve cell during growth and function. *Acta physiol. scand.*, *6*, Suppl. 17.

66 HYDÉN, H. (1960) The neurone. *The cell, biochemistry, physiology, Vol. 4.* J. Brachet and A. E. Mirsky (Eds.). New York, Academic Press. (pp. 215–324).

67 HYDÉN, H. (1962) Cytophysiological aspects of the nucleic acids and proteins of nervous tissue. *Neurochemistry*. K. A. C. Elliot, I. H. Page and J. H. Quastel, Editors. Springfield, Thomas (pp. 331–375).

68 HYDÉN, H. and LINDSTRÖM, B. (1950) Microspectrographic studies on the yellow pigment in nerve cells. *Discussions Faraday Soc.*, *9*, 436–441.

69 HYDÉN, H. and PIGON, A. (1960) A cytoplasmical study of the functional relationship between oligodendroglial cells and nerve cells of Deiter's nucleus. *J. Neurochem.*, *6*, 57–72.

70 KAPLAN, H. and FORD, D. H. (1966) *The Brain Vascular System*, Elsevier, Amsterdam.

71 KETY, S. S. (1955) Changes in cerebral circulation and oxygen consumption which accompany maturation and aging. *Biochemistry of the Developing Nervous System*. H. Waelsch (Ed.). New York, Academic Press. (pp. 208–215).

72 KLATZO, I. and MIQUEL, J. (1960) Observations on pinocytosis in nervous tissue. *J. Neuropath. exptl. Neurol.*, *19*, 475–487.

73 KOENIG, H. (1958) Uptake of adenine-8-¹⁴C and Orotic-6-¹⁴C acid into nuclear DNA of non-dividing cells in the adult feline neuraxis. *J. biophys. biochem. Cytol.*, *4*, 664–666.

74 KOENIG, H. (1958) An autoradiographic study of nucleic acid and protein turnover in the mammalian neuraxis. *J. biophys. biochem. Cytoll*, *4*, 785–792.

75 KRIEG, W. J. S. (1953) *Functional neuroanatomy*. New York, McGraw-Hill.

76 KUHLENBECK, H. (1954) Some histologic age changes in the rat's brain and their relationship to comparable changes in the human brain. *Confin. neurol. (Basel)*, *14*, 329–342.

77 KULENKAMPFF, H. (1952) Das Verhalten der Neuroglia in den Vorderhörnern des Rückenmarks der Weissen Maus unter dem Reiz Physiologischer Tätigkeit. *Z. Anat. Entwickl.-Gesch.*, *116*, 304–312.

78 KUNTZ, A. and SULKIN, N. M. (1947) The neuroglia in the autonomic ganglia: cytologic structure and reactions to stimulation. *J. comp. Neurol.*, *86*, 467–477.

79 LAJTHA, A. (1962) The "Brain Barrier System". *Neurochemistry*. K. A. C. Elliott, I. H. Page and J. H. Quastel (Eds.). Springfield, Thomas (pp. 339–430).

80 LAJTHA, A. and FORD, D. H. (1968) The "Brain Barrier Systems", *Progr. Brain Res.*, *29*, Elsevier, Amsterdam.

81 LARSELL, O. (1937) The cerebellum: a review and interpretation. *Arch. Neurol. Phsychiat.*, *38*, 580–607.

82 LARSELL, O. (1947) The development of the cerebellum in man in relation to its comparative anatomy. *J. comp. Neurol.*, *87*, 85–129.

83 LAVELLE, A. and LAVELLE, F. (1958) Neuronal swelling and chromatolysis as influenced by the state of cell development. *Amer. J. Anat.*, *102*, 219–242.

84 LEE, J. C. (1963) Electron microscopy of Wallerian degeneration. *J. comp. Neurol.*, *120*, 65–79.

85 LEVEQUE, T. (1953) Changes in the neurosecretory cells of the rat hypothalamus following ingestion of sodium chloride. *Anat. Rec.*, *117*, 741–758.

86 LEWIS, W. H. (1931) Pinocytosis. *Bull. Johns Hopk. Hosp.*, *49*, 17–23.

87 LISS, L. (1960) Senile brain changes. Histopathology of the ganglion cells. *J. Neuropathol. exptl. Neurol.*, *19*, 559–571.

88 LORENTE DE NÓ, R. (1943) Studies on the structure of the cerebral cortex. Continuation of study of ammonic system. *J. Psychol. Neurol.*, *46*, 113–177.

89 LØVTRUP, S. and SVENNERHOLM, L. (1963) Chemical properties of brain mitochondria. *Exptl. Cell Res.*, *29*, 298–313.

90 LUSE, S. A. (1956) Formation of myelin in the central nervous system of mice and rats, as studied with the electron microscope. *J. biophys. biochem. Cytol.*, *2*, 777–784.

91 LUSE, S. A. (1956) Electron microscopic observations on the central nervous system. *J. biophys. biochem. Cytol.*, *2*, 531–542.

92 MALHATRA, S. K. (1959) What is the "Golgi" apparatus in its classical site within neurones of vertebrates. *Quart. J. Micr. Sci.*, *100*, 339–367.

93 MYERS, R. E. (1962) Transmission of visual information within and between the hemispheres. A behavioral study. *Interhemispheric Relations and Cerebral Dominance*. V. B. Mountcastle, Editor. Baltimore, Johns Hopkins Press (pp. 51–73).

94 NOBACK, C. R. and DEMAREST, R. J. (1967) *The Human Nervous System*. McGraw Hill, New York.

95 OLIVECRONA, H. (1957) Paraventricular nucleus and pituitary gland. gland. *Acta physiol. scand.*, *40*. Suppl. 136, 7–178.

96 OLSEN, S. and PETRI, C. (1963) Histochemical localization of acid phosphatase in the human cerebellar cortex. *Acta Neurol. Scand.*, *39*, 112–122.

97 OLSZEWSKI, J. (1947) Zur Morphologie und Entwicklung des Arbeitskerns unter besonderer Berücksichtigung des Nervenzellkerns. *Biol. Zbl.*, *66*, 265–304.

98 PALADE, G. E. (1953) An electron microscope study of the mitochondrial structure. *J. Histochem. Cytochem.*, *1*, 188–211.

99 PALAY, S. L. (1958) The morphology of synapses in the central nervous system. *Exptl. Cell Res.*, *5*, 275–293.

100 PANNESE, E. (1960) Observations on the morphology, submicroscopic structure and biological properties of satellite cells (S.C.) in sensory ganglia of mammals. *Z. Zellforsch.*, *52*, 567–597.

101 PAPPAS, G. D. and PURPURA, D. P. (1961) Fine structure of dendrites in the superficial neocortical neuropil. *Exptl. Neurol.*, *4*, 507–530.

102 PAPPAS, G. D. and PURPURA, D. P. (1964) Electron Microscopy of immature human and feline neocortex. Growth and Maturation of the Brain. *Progr. Brain Res.*, *4*. D. P. Purpura and J. P. Schadé (Eds.). Amsterdam–New York, Elsevier (pp. 176–186).

103 PETERS, A. (1960) The formation and structure of myelin sheaths in the central nervous system. *J. biophys. biochem. Cytol.*, *8*, 431–446.

104 POMERAT, C. M. (1952) Dynamic neuroglialogy. *Tex. Rep. Biol. Med.*, *10*, 885–913.

105 PURPURA, D. P. and SCHADÉ, J. P. (1964) Editors. Growth and maturation of the brain. *Progr. Brain Res.*, *4*. Amsterdam–London–New York, Elsevier.

106 PURPURA, D. P., SHOFER, R. J., HOUSEPIAN, E. M. and NOBACK, C. R. (1964) Comparative ontogenesis of structure-function relations in cerebral and cerebellar cortex. Growth and maturation of the Brain. *Progr. Brain Res.*, *4*. Amsterdam–London–New York, Elsevier (pp. 187–221).

107 RHODES, A., and FORD, D. H. (1963) Influence of the thyroid state on uptake of ¹⁴C-1-lysine by normal and regenerating neurones in the rat. *Anat. Rec.*, *145*, 346.

108 RITCHIE, J. M. and STRAUB, R. W. (1957) The hyperpolarization which follows activity in mammalian non-medullated fibers. *J. Physiol.*, *136*, 80–97.

109 ROBERTSON, J. D. (1958) The ultrastructure of Schmidt-Lantermann clefts and related shearing defects of the myelin sheath. *J. biophys. biochem. Cytol.*, *4*, 39–46.

110 ROBERTSON, J. D. (1959) The ultrastructure of cell membranes and their derivatives. *Biochem. Soc. Symp.*, *16*, 3–43.

111 ROBERTSON, J. D. (1960) The molecular structure and contact relationship of cell membranes. *Progr. Biophys.*, *10*, 343–418.

112 SCHADÉ, J. P. (1964) On the contribution of neuroglia to the function of the cerebral cortex. *Neurologic and electroencephalographic correlative studies in infancy*. P. Kellaway, Editor. New York, Grune and Stratton. In the press.

113 SCHADÉ, J. P. and BAXTER, C. F. (1960) Changes during growth in the volume and surface area of cortical neurons in the rabbit. *Exptl. Neurol.*, *2*, 158–178.

114 SCHADÉ, J. P., VAN BACKER, H. and COLON, E. (1964) Quantitative analysis of neuronal parameters in the maturing cerebral cortex. Growth and maturation of the brain. *Progr. Brain Res.*, *4*. D. P. Purpura and J. P. Schadé (Eds.). Amsterdam–London–New York, Elsevier (pp. 150–175).

115 SCHADÉ, J. P. and VAN GROENINGEN, W. B. (1961) Structural organization of the human cerebral cortex. I. Maturation of the middle frontal gyrus. *Acta Anat. (Basel)*, *47*, 74–111.

116 SCHARRER, E. and SCHARRER, B. (1954) Neurosekretion. *Handbuch der Mikroskopische Anatomie des Menschen. VI.* Möllendorff (Ed.). Heidelberg, Springer (pp. 953–1066).

117 SCHULTZ, R. L., MAYNARD, E. A. and PEASE, D. (1957) Electron microscopy of neurones and neuroglia of cerebral cortex and corpus callosum. *Amer. J. Anat.*, *100*, 369–407.

118 SHARIFF, G. A. (1953) Cell counts in the primate cerebral cortex. *J. comp. Neurol.*, *98*, 381–400.

119 SHERRINGTON, C. S. (1897) The central nervous system. Vol. 3. *A Textbook of Physiology*. M. Forster (Ed.). London, MacMillan.

120 SINGER, M. and SCHADÉ, J. P. (1964) (Eds.). Mechanisms of neural regeneration. *Progr. Brain Res.*, *13*. Amsterdam–New York, Elsevier.

121 SINGER, M. and SCHADÉ, J. P. (1965) (Eds.). Degeneration patterns in the nervous system. *Progr. Brain Res.*, *14*. Amsterdam–London–New York, Elsevier.

122 SJÖSTRAND, F. S. (1953) The lamellated structure of the nerve myelin sheath as revealed by high resolution electron microscopy. *Experientia (Basel)*, *9*, 68–69.

123 SJÖSTRAND, F. S. (1963) A comparison of plasma membrane, cytomembranes, and mitochondrial membrane elements with respect to ultrastructural features. *J. Ultrastruct. Res.* *9*, 561–580.

124 SMART, I. (1961) The subependymal layer of the mouse brain and its cell production as shown by radioautography after thymidine-³H injection. *J. exptl. Neurol.*, *116*, 325.

125 SPERRY, R. W. (1962) Some general aspects of interhemispheric integration. *Interhemispheric Relations and Cerebral Dominance*. V. B. Mountcastle, (Ed.). Baltimore, Johns Hopkins Press (pp. 43–49).

126 SPERRY, R. W. (1963) Evidence behind chemoaffinity theory of synaptic patterning. *Anat. Rec.*, *145*, 288.

127 SPERRY, R. W. (1964) The great cerebral commissure. *Scientific American*, *210*, 42–52.

128 SPIELMEYER, W. (1922) *Histopathologie des Nervensystems*. Berlin, Springer.

129 TEWARI, H. B. and BOURNE, G. H. (1962) Histochemical evidence of metabolic cycles in spinal ganglion cells of rat. *J. Histochem. Cytochem.*, *10*, 42–64.

130 TEWARI, H. B. and BOURNE, G. H. (1962) The histochemistry of the nucleus and nucleolus with reference to nucleic-cytoplasmic relations in the spinal ganglion neurone of the rat. *Acta Histochem.*, *13*, 323–350.

131 TORRES, F. (1963) Maturation of electrical activity of the brain. 42nd Ross Conference on Pediatric Research. *Recent advances in degenerative disease of the central nervous system in infants and children* (pp. 37–44).

132 UZMAN, B. G. and NOGUEIRA-GRAF, G. (1957) Electron microscopic studies of the formation of nodes of Ranvier in mouse sciatic nerves. *J. biophys. biochem. Cytol.*, *3*, 589–598.

133 VAN DER LOOS, H. (1963) Similarities and dissimiliarities in submicroscopical morpholgy of interneuronal contact sites of presumably different functional character. Topics in basic neurology, *Progr. Brain Res.*, *6*.

W. Bargmann and J. P. Schadé, Editors. Amsterdam–London–New York, Elsevier (pp. 43–58).

134 VAN DER LOOS, H. (1963) Fine structure of synapses in the cerebral cortex. *Z. Zellforsch.*, *60*, 815–825.

135 VAN HARREVELD, A. and SCHADÉ, J. P. (1960) On the distribution and movement of water and electrolytes in the cerebral cortex. *Structure and Function of the Cerebral Cortex*. D. B. Tower and J. P. Schadé, (Eds.). Amsterdam, Elsevier (pp. 239–256).

136 VERNADAKES, A. and WOODBURY, D. M. (1962) Electrolyte and amino acid changes in rat brain during maturation. *Amer. J. Physiol.*, *203*, 748–752.

137 VESALIUS, A. (1555) *De Humani corporis fabrica*, libri septem. Basileae, J. Oporinus.

138 VIAL, J. D. (1958) The early changes in the axoplasm in Wallerian degeneration. *J. biophys. biochem. Cytol.*, *4*, 551–556.

139 VRAA-JENSEN, G. (1956) On the correlation between the function and structure of nerve cells. *Acta psychiat. scand.*, *Suppl. 109*, 9–88.

140 WARWICK, R. (1951) A study of retrograde degeneration on the oculomotor nucleus of the rhesus monkey. *Brain*, *73*, 532–543.

141 WARWICK, R. (1955) The so-called nucleus of convergence. *Brain*, *78*, 92–114.

142 WARWICK, R. and MITCHELL, G. A. G. (1956) The phrenic nucleus of the macaque. *J. comp. Neurol.*, *105*, 553–586.

143 WEISS, P. and HISCOE, H. B. (1948) Experiments on the mechanism of nerve growth. *J. exptl. Zool.*, *107*, 315–396.

144 WHITTAKER, V. P. and GRAY, E. G. (1962) The synapse: Biology and Morphology. *Brit. med. Bull.*, *18*, 223–228.

145 WILLIER, B. H., WEISS, P. A. and HAMBURGER, V. (1955) *Analysis of development*. Philadelphia, Saunders.

146 WINDLE, W. F. (1950) Reflexes of mammalian embryos and fetuses. *Genetic Neurology*. Report of the International Congress on the Development, Growth, and Regeneration of the Nervous System. P. Weiss (Ed.). Chicago, University of Chicago Press (p.p. 214–222).

147 WINZLER, R. J., MOLDAVE, K., RAFELSON, M. E., JR., and PEARSON, H. E. (1952) Conversion of glucose to amino acids by brain and liver of the newborn mouse. *J. biol. Chem.*, *199*, 485–492.

148 WISCHNITZER, S. (1960) The ultrastructure of the nucleus and nucleocytoplasmic relations. *Int. Rev. Cytol.*, *19*, 137–162.

149 WORTHINGTON, W. C., JR. and CATHCART, R. S. (1963) Ependymal cilia: Distribution and activity in the adult human brain. *Science*, *139*, 221.

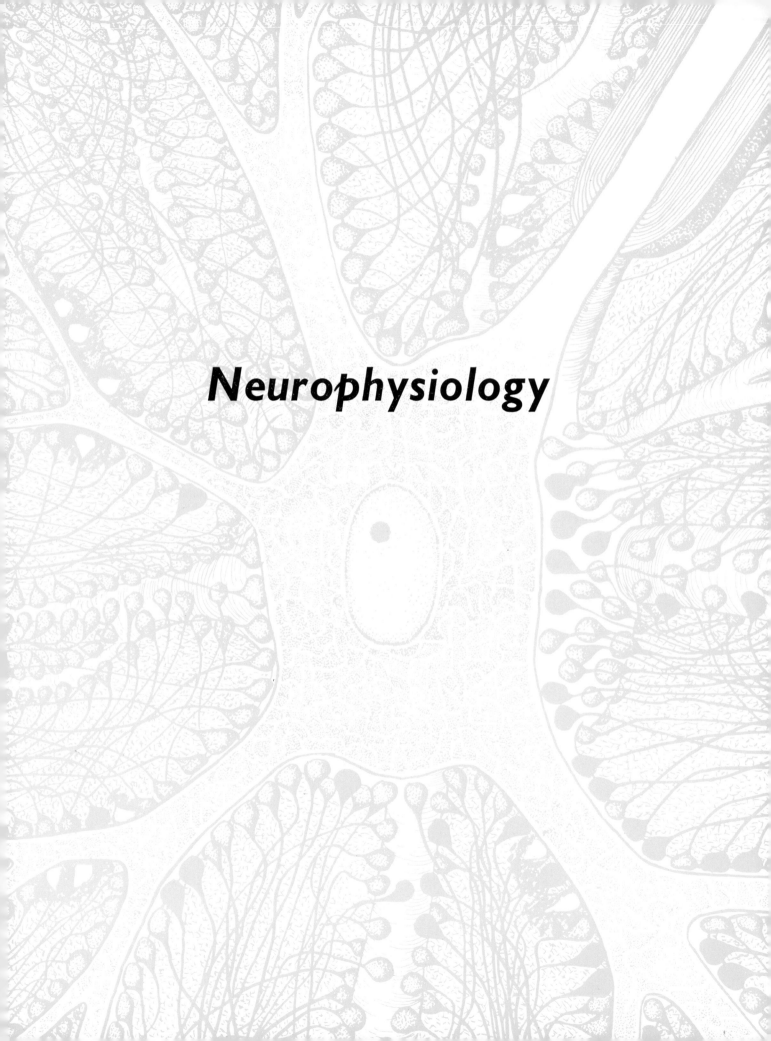

Neurophysiology

Survey of Contents

8. Historical development

8.1 Introduction

Neurophysiology is the branch of the neurological sciences which is particularly concerned with the study of function and the processing of information in nervous tissue. In general terms this simply means that the neurophysiologist is interested in how a single nerve cell, or the complete brain works. In his attempt to discover or to understand nerve and brain mechanisms the neurophysiologist makes special use of the great advances in electrical stimulation and recording. Most of the methods of investigation adopted recently by physiologists have been directed towards studying the electrical characteristics and activity of nervous tissue with the aid of modern electronic equipment. Although the function of the neuron also expresses itself in many other ways (*e.g.* heat production, metabolic changes, morphological changes, excitation or inhibition of other tissues, etc.), the electrical properties give the best information about the transport and processing of information in the nervous system. Although neurophysiology studies nervous events within the framework of physiology, many other fields of science, such as physics, mathematics, computer sciences, physical chemistry and biochemistry contribute to its understanding and techniques. One can say that neurophysiology actually stretches from the biophysics of the single nerve cell itself to the physiological interpretation of diseases of the nervous system.

Fig. 118. Earliest experiments in neuromuscular physiology by Swammerdam (18th century). Fig. V is an experiment to show the change in shape of a muscle when stimulated by pinching its nerve. Fig. VI illustrates the pulling together of the pins holding the tendons when the muscle contracts.

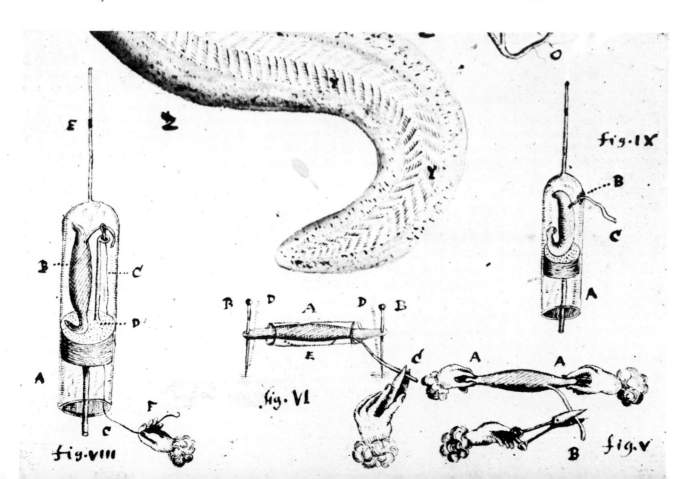

Major efforts are being concentrated upon the investigation of the electrical activities of parts of neurons, of whole neurons and of neuronal aggregates, such as nuclei, or even of bigger structures such as the hippocampus, cerebellum, cortical areas, etc. It can be safely predicted that with the improvement of techniques neurophysiologists may unravel within the coming decades many of the basic mechanisms underlying processes such as memory and consciousness.

The major phases in the historical development of neurophysiology closely parallel the development of electrical and electronic instrumentation (*cf.* Brazier[10, 12]). Early workers in this field watched the deflection of a galvanometer needle when studying a nervous event. Later, by placing electrodes upon the brain or attaching them to the surface of the skull, investigators studied the electrical wave patterns of the brain by means of primitive amplifiers and called them 'electro-encephalograms' (from the Greek word $\varepsilon\gamma\kappa\varepsilon\varphi\alpha\lambda o\varsigma$ = brain and $\gamma\varrho\alpha\varphi\varepsilon\iota\nu$ = to write). Nowadays million-dollar electronic computers are used to analyse the electrical patterns occurring within very small brain areas and even within single neurons.

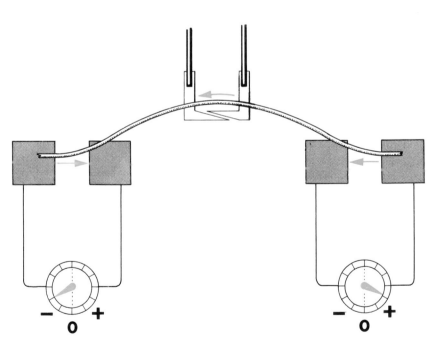

Fig. 119. Schematic diagram showing one of the arrangements used by Du Bois-Reymond (1849) for demonstration of electrical signs of the process which propagates along the nerve.

8.2 Galvani and Du Bois-Reymond

In the course of time neurophysiology was gradually brought to its present understanding of the electrical aspects of the nervous event. The great pioneers of this science came from famous universities in Italy, Germany, England, Poland and Russia, but the search is now being pressed forward in scientific laboratories in almost every country in the world. In 1786 Luigi Galvani, professor of Anatomy at the University of Bologna, accidentally discovered that a frog's leg touching an iron railing propagated an electrical current. In a general statement appearing in his

'Commentary' in 1791 he wrote that in some fashion nervous tissue and electricity were related. Great advances were made in 1848 with the work of the German E. Du Bois-Reymond who, with the aid of a galvanometer and a pair of electrodes (one attached to the horizontal surface of a peripheral nerve and the other to the cut end of that same nerve), demonstrated that there was a flow of electricity whenever the nerve propagated an impulse. The galvanometer indicated that this flow was from a positive level of electrical potential to a negative level, and he called this shift a 'negative variation'. In 1875, the famous English school of neurophysiologists began with Richard Caton, who later became Professor of Physiology at University College of Liverpool (the same position many years later occupied by Sherrington).

Caton became interested in Du Bois-Reymond's technique and he was the first one to apply it to the brain[20, 21]. From investigations of the brain of rabbit and monkey he reported: 'In every brain hitherto examined the galvanometer has indicated the existence of electric currents... Feeble currents of varying direction pass through the multiplier when the electrodes are placed on two points of the external surface of the skull. The electric current of the grey matter appeared to have a relation to its function.'

He thus discovered, perhaps unknowingly, the principle of the electroencephalogram. Lacking any knowledge of Caton's work, a young man by the name of Adolf Beck, working under the great Polish physiologist Cybulski at the University of Krakow, arrived in 1888 at many of Caton's same conclusions. He also recorded the electroencephalogram and localized various functional areas of the brain.

Cybulski himself studied many of the characteristics of the brain waves, making the further clarification that 'spontaneous waves' are 8 to 10 cycles per second in the dog, and 15 to 20 in the monkey, and that these frequencies increase to 18 to 22 per second upon peripheral stimulation. In addition, his concept that the electrical nature of a nervous event resulted from chemical differences across the membrane foreshadowed the modern concept.

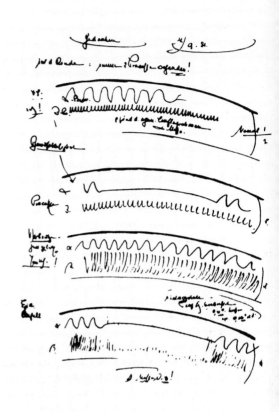

Fig. 120. A page from the note-book of Dr. Hans Berger, a German psychiatrist, the first to record electroencephalographic potentials from man, and the founder of clinical electroencephalography.

8.3 19th Century neurophysiology

During the 19th century, concepts of nervous functioning and its electrical concomitants were characterized by a more or less clear separation into two lines of research:

(a) the study of propagated impulses or 'action potentials' in peripheral nerves, and

(b) the so-called spontaneous brain waves and related phenomena in the central nervous system, *i.e.*, the electroencephalogram.

The research subsumed under (a) is concerned with the mode of operation of the basic components of nervous tissue, whereas (b) is related to the functioning of neuronal assemblies within the central

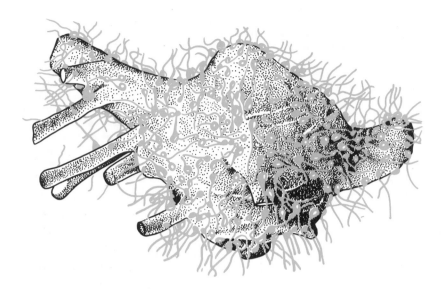

Fig. 121. A, photograph of a reconstructed model of a motoneuron with the initial portions of the dendrites; the synaptic end knobs are shown in green.

nervous system. The major part of the following chapters will be concerned with the analysis of electrical events in single neurons and the transfer of information from one cell to another cell. As will be shown, the mode of operation of these basic units constitutes the fundamental feature in the functioning of the nervous system as a whole. At the end of this book we will deal with some aspects of integrative mechanisms and neuronal circuits.

At the end of the last century a number of important neurohistologists (Forel, His, Ramón y Cajal) laid the foundation for the 'neuron theory', *viz.* that the nerve cells are the functional units of the nervous system. The most important implication of the neuron theory was the assumption that neurons must enter into functional contact with one another by *contiguity*, and not by cellular *continuity*. This latter idea was defended by such reputable histologists as Gerlach and Golgi, who formulated their observations as the 'reticular theory'.

Two neurophysiologists, Adrian and Sherrington, have made significant contributions to the understanding of the function of the individual neuron and the transmission of information from one cell to another. They were jointly awarded the Nobel Prize in 1932 'for their discoveries regarding the functions of the neuron'. Adrian[1] worked on various problems connected with the conduction of the action potential, and had established as early as 1912 the 'all-or-nothing' nature of this phenomenon. Sherrington studied the interactions among different neurons and introduced an extremely useful preparation: the electrophysiological investigation of the reflex arc. A stimulus (in general evoked at a receptor unit) is produced in an afferent fiber, which conducts impulses into the spinal cord (or brain stem), whereupon other neurons are excited. These cells ultimately evoke impulses in efferent nerve fibers which result in the activation of muscle fibers or other effector organs. Special conditions are associated with the transfer of a stimulus from one neuron to another.

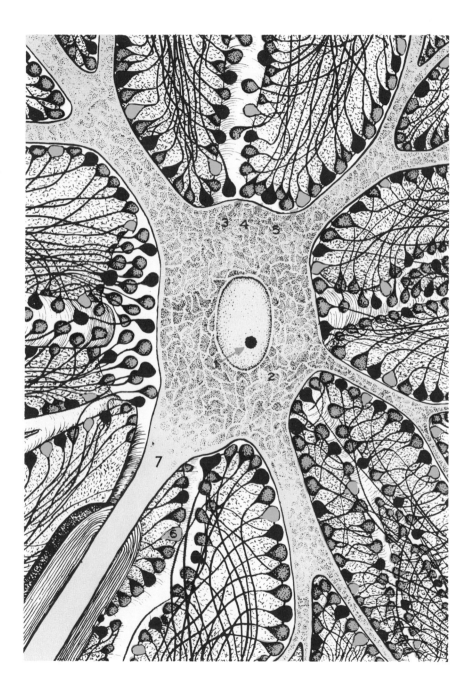

Fig. 121. B, model of a motoneuron, used in the following paragraphs to explain electrical events.
1, nucleus; **2,** Nissl body; **3,** inactive synapse; **4,** excitatory synapse; **5, 6,** inhibitory synapse; **7,** axon hillock.

8.4 Birth of synaptology

Sherrington proposed in 1897 the term 'synapse' (from the Greek $\sigma\upsilon\nu\alpha\pi\tau\omega$ = to clasp) for the regions of close juxtaposition between two neurons. Reflexes are of fundamental importance and the study of the electrical aspects of the reflex arc has given so many clues in recent years that almost all electrical events in the nervous system can be explained by properly analysing and interpreting what happens in the various parts of the reflex arc[137, 138].

We will follow a stimulus through the reflex arc and see what type of events occur. Fig. 122 shows a conceptual model of a reflex arc consisting of the following elements: a receptor in the muscle, an afferent fiber to the spinal cord, an efferent fiber from the spinal cord to the muscle (the effector), and the effector itself. In the spinal cord a direct connection between afferent and efferent fibers can be made (monosynaptic reflex) or one or more interneurons may be interposed between the two (polysynaptic reflex). An excitation of some kind is evoked in the receptor by the form of energy (pressure, touch, heat, etc.) to which it is attuned.

Receptors are generally specialized to respond only to a single type of stimulus, but there are a few exceptions to this rule. The receptors act as biological transducers, which convert 'receptor energy' into the electrical energy of the nerve impulse. This impulse is conducted as the action potential along the axon of the afferent neuron. Transmission takes place in the spinal cord so that the information from the excited afferent cell is passed on to the motoneurons, either directly or indirectly *via* one or more interneurons. After effective integration of all impinging signals, action potentials are set up and conducted along the axon of the motoneuron. This impulse ends by exciting the muscle across the neuromuscular junction. In following a stimulus through a reflex arc, we encounter various junctions or places where the electrical activity of one cell influences or modulates the electrical activity of a succeeding cell. Between receptor and neuron, between neurons, and between neuron and effector, in all these places we find junctional transmission of information. In general only the junctions between neurons are called synapses, although there is no real reason why we could not call the other junctions synapses too. As we will see, an analogous type of electrical events occurs at all synapses, and it is basically different process than the conduction of an action potential along an axon.

8.5 The reflex arc

Most of the fundamental modes of operation of the nervous system seem to be present in the reflex arc and we can distinguish the following types of activity:

(1) Response to energy by the receptor and its conversion into excitation of the afferent cell,

(2) Conduction of action potentials along the axons of afferent, efferent fibers and interneurons,

(3) Transfer of activity from one neuron to another,

(4) Excitation of the effector by the efferent fiber.

The mechanisms underlying (1), (3) and (4) have many features in common since they all concern the transferring of information from one cell to another. Furthermore since each cell is an independent unit enclosed within a membrane, communication takes place across junctions. This basic set of phenomena may well be the most important of the functional responses that are to be found in the nervous system.

Fig. 122. It is by means of electrical recording and stimulation that the activities of neurons, receptors and effectors can be most intimately followed. The changes in electrical potential monitor nerve activity in an accurate and quantitative way. Even the expression 'a nerve at rest' actually refers to a steady electrical activity.

Neurons conduct and generate electrical potentials, despite the fact that they consist for the most part of a very unsuitable material, namely water. The neuronal membrane separates two aqueous solutions of low resistance while the specific resistance of the membrane itself, for neurons in the mammalian spinal cord, is of the order of 1000 ohms/cm². The specific capacitance is about 2–5 μfarads/cm². Two groups of investigators have added considerably in recent years to our knowledge of the function of individual neurons. Hodgkin and Huxley[88-91], working with single axons, formulated the ionic theory of the nerve impulse in the axon. The experimental investigation of synaptic transmission was revolutionized in 1951 by Sir John Eccles and his coworkers[33-35] who developed techniques for recording electrically from the interior of neurons within the spinal cord. It is now possible to penetrate neurons in the central nervous system with microelectrodes (small glass capillaries of 0.5 μ or less, filled with a conducting salt solution or with some metal) and thereby to record the electrical events from normally functioning cells. Eccles, Hodgkin and Huxley were awarded the Nobel Prize for medicine and physiology in 1963, for their brilliant research concerning the microphysiology of neurons.

Since we will deal in the following chapters with the analysis of electrical properties and electrical events in neurons we must first discuss some basic facts about the electrical parameters and ionic composition of neurons.

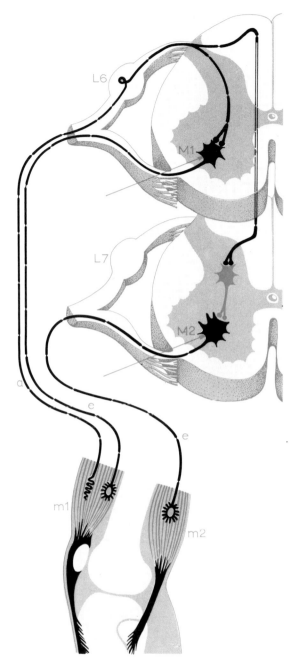

Fig. 122. Diagram showing the pathways of a stimulus from a receptor (an annulospiral ending) in the quadriceps muscle (**m 1**) at the **L 6** and **L 7** segmental levels of the spinal cord. One branch of the afferent neuron (**a**) monosynaptically excites a quadriceps motoneuron (**M 1**), the other branch descends to **L 7** and excites an interneuron, which in turn inhibits a motoneuron (**M 2**) of the antagonistic muscle, biceps semitendinosus (**m 2**). The **arrows** indicate the placement of the recording electrodes.

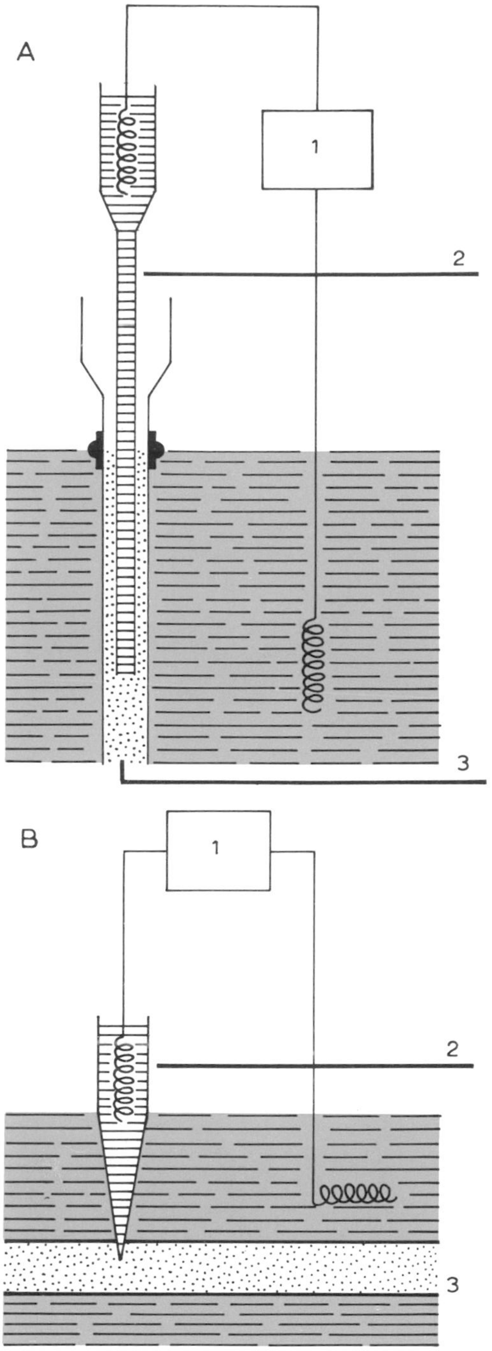

9. Electrical parameters and ionic composition of neurons

9.1 Neuronal potentials

Fig. 123. Pushing a microelectrode through the membrane of a neuron at rest, causes a sudden shift of potential of about -70 mV, as recorded on the oscilloscope. This is the 'resting potential'. The giant axons of squid and cuttle fish have usually been used for this type of investigation, since they have a diameter up to 1000 μ, which makes them easily penetrable by microelectrodes[83, 87, 101]. The cell bodies of large neurons in the central nervous system are also suitable objects.

The resting potential is mainly a consequence of the fact that the aqueous solutions inside and outside the neuronal membrane have a different ionic composition. Three ions are of particular importance: sodium, chloride and potassium. Sodium and chloride are present in much higher concentration in the extracellular fluid while potassium is much more concentrated inside the neuron. The resting potential created across this semipermeable membrane follows nearly all the conditions given by the Nernst equation for electrolytes.

The Nernst equation in simplified form can be expressed in the following manner for *e.g.* potassium ions:

$$E_k = 60 \log_{10} \frac{(K_0)}{(K_1)}$$

where E_k = the equilibrium potential for potassium ions: K_0 and K_1 = the concentrations of potassium ions outside and inside the neuron respectively. The condition for equilibrium for potassium ions is that the electrochemical potential for potassium ions is zero. We now have to ask the question: 'What is the electrochemical potential for a particular ion?' It is the sum of the electrical and the concentration energy differences across the membrane. Since ions are positively and negatively charged, a difference in these charges builds up a difference of potential. A difference in concentration of an ion across a membrane also builds up a potential across it, since there is a tendency for the more concentrated solute to move to regions where it is more dilute. The condition of equilibrium is, in other words, that the electrical forces just balance out the concentration forces. Focusing our attention more upon the membrane itself we could also say that the equilibrium potential for a given ion is equal to that potential across the membrane which causes the

Fig. 123. A and B, recording techniques with microelectrodes in giant axons. **1,** recording apparatus; **2,** microelectrode; **3,** nerve fiber.

flux (rate of flow) of that ion to be equal in both directions. From the values for the intra- and extracellular ion concentration, the equilibrium potential for potassium, sodium and chloride can be calculated using the Nernst equations.

9.2 Electrolytes in nerve tissue

9.2.1 Chloride ions

This ionic species is the only one which is in electrochemical equilibrium with the resting potential. Since chloride ions have a negative charge, the electrical field across the neuronal membrane drives chloride ions out of the neuron and maintains a low internal concentration. The distribution of the ions is therefore controlled by the membrane potential. The ions diffuse freely through the membrane and do not control the membrane potential at rest.

Equilibrium potentials

$$E_{Cl} \ (mV) = 60 \log_{10} \frac{Cl_i}{Cl_o} = ca. -70 \, mV$$

$$E_{K} \ (mV) = 60 \log_{10} \frac{K_o}{K_i} = ca. -90 \, mV$$

$$E_{Na} \ (mV) = 60 \log_{10} \frac{Na_o}{Na_i} = ca. +60 \, mV$$

Fig. 124. Development of transmembrane voltage by an ion-concentration gradient. The membrane shown (bar in the middle of the figure) has some, but not all, properties of a real cell membrane. This hypothetical membrane is pierced by pores of such size that K⁺ and Cl⁻ ions can move through them easily, Na⁺ ions with difficulty, and A⁻ (organic anions) not at all. Sizes of symbols in left- and right-hand columns indicate relative concentrations of ions in fluids bathing the membrane. Dashed arrows and circles show paths taken by K⁺, A⁻, Na⁺ and Cl⁻-ions as a K⁺ or Cl⁻ travels through a pore. Penetration of the pore by a K⁺ or Cl⁻ follows a collision between the K⁺ or Cl⁻ and water molecules (not shown), giving the K⁺ or Cl⁻ the necessary kinetic energy and proper direction. An A⁻ or Na⁺ is unable to cross the membrane and is left behind when a K⁺ or Cl⁻, respectively, diffuses through a pore. Because K⁺ is more concentrated on left than on right, more K⁺ diffuses from left to right than from right to left, and conversely for Cl⁻. Therefore, the right-hand border of the membrane becomes positively charged (K⁺, Na⁺) and the left-hand negatively charged (Cl⁻, A⁻). Fluids away from the membrane are electrically neutral because of attraction between + and − charges. Charges separated by membrane stay near it because of their attraction.

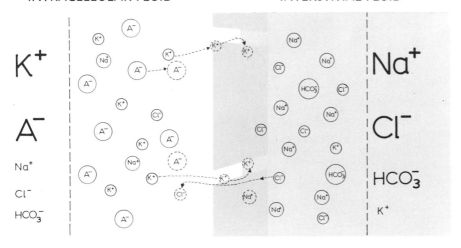

INTRACELLULAR FLUID   INTERSTITIAL FLUID

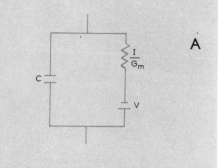

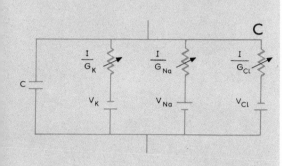

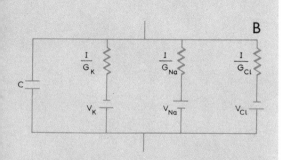

Fig. 125. A, simplest electrical circuit which simulates electrical properties of a neuron; **B,** electrical circuit with separation of batteries and membrane conducting channels related to potassium, sodium and chloride; **C,** electrical circuit illustrating the active ionic pathways.

9.2.2 Potassium ions

The equilibrium potential for potassium ions is slightly higher than the membrane potential. The distribution of this ionic species is thus controlled for the most part by the membrane potential and the ions diffuse relatively freely through the neuronal membrane. The remainder of the potassium ions concentrated inside the cell (which accounts for the difference between the resting potential and the equilibrium potential for potassium ions) must therefore be actively transported against an electrochemical gradient of about 20 mV. Since the membrane and equilibrium potential do not differ very greatly from each other there is relatively little energy needed to transport the required amount of potassium ions across the membrane. An active (metabolic) mechanism is postulated for this transport: the 'potassium pump' *(vide infra)*.

9.2.3 Sodium ions

The calculated equilibrium potential is in this case very much different from the level of the resting potential. The behavior of the sodium ions is determined almost exclusively by the way in which the resting potential is generated and maintained by the cell. The equilibrium potential is so much different that the electrochemical potential is in the order of 100 mV. There are two forces which act to drive sodium ions into the neuron; namely the concentration gradient and the membrane potential. Again a transport mechanism must be postulated: the 'sodium pump' causing the sodium ions to move outward. The neuronal membrane at rest, however, is considerably less permeable to sodium ions than to potassium and chloride ions. Both the sodium and the potassium pumps are linked very closely and are, at least in their qualitative aspects, mirror images of each other.

9.3 Membrane potential

Fig. 125. Since we are speaking primarily of the electrical properties of neurons we will end this section with a representation of the neuron in terms of an equivalent circuit. In an electrical circuit diagram a zigzag line represents an ideal resistance and $\frac{1}{T}$ an ideal capacitor, a straight line represents an ideal conductor. Diagram **A** shows the approximate equivalent electrical circuit of the resting membrane of a standard motoneuron.

The neuronal membrane has a high electrical capacity, as would be expected for a membrane this thin (50–70 Å), and a high electrical resistance corresponding to the low ionic permeability. The membrane potential is represented by a battery of 70 mV. In **B** and **C** the potassium, sodium and chloride channels are introduced into the diagram. We will now turn to the changes in these parameters which occur during the propagation of the action potential.

Fig. 126. The generation of the membrane potential at rest by the sodium-potassium pump is nicely illustrated by the diagram of Eccles. The scheme illustrates the active and passive transport of sodium and potassium. Active transport implies that the process requires a continuous supply of energy, which is supplied by the metabolic machinery of the neuron. Passive transport implies the diffusion of a substance down its electrochemical gradient. The ionic flux channels numbered 1 to 4 are indicated by columns of varying thickness and size. The slopes in the flux channel between the interior and exterior sides of the neuronal membrane represent the electrochemical gradients for potassium and sodium. At the resting potential of -70 mV the electrochemical gradient for potassium ions corresponds to a potential which is 20 mV more positive (drawn upward) than the equilibrium potential. The electrochemical gradient for sodium ions corresponds to a potential which is 130 mV more negative (drawn downward) than the equilibrium potential. Since the magnitude of the fluxes is indicated by the width of the channel, the outward diffusional flux of sodium ions is not shown because it is negligible. The exact molecular mechanism of the sodium-potassium exchange is still unknown, but it seems likely, however, that many enzymes play a significant role.

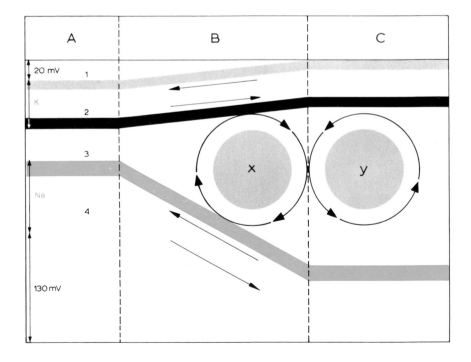

Fig. 126. Diagrammatic representation of K$^+$ and Na$^+$ fluxes through the neuronal membrane in the resting state.
A, extraneuronal space; **B**, neuronal membrane; **C**, intraneuronal space; **X**, K-Na-pump; **Y**, metabolic drive of pump; **1** and **4**, diffusion fluxes; **2** and **3**, pump fluxes.

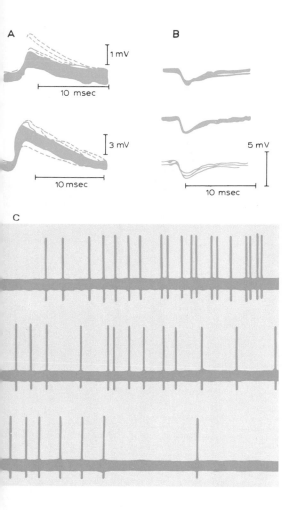

Fig. 127. Various types of electrical potential in the nervous system. **A,** excitatory synaptic potentials; **B,** inhibitory synaptic potentials; **C,** action potentials.

10. Action potential

10.1 Excitability and conductivity

The maintenance of a resting potential across the membrane is one of the most characteristic properties not only of neurons but of all living cells. Cell membranes all have the ability to separate ions, but nerve and muscle cells, in addition, possess two highly distinctive properties: excitability and conductivity.

Excitability: A stimulus (change in the environment) brings about transient changes in the properties of the membrane (changes in ionic permeability and membrane potential).

Conductivity: The changes evoked by the stimulus are not confined to the vicinity of the stimulus but, once initiated, propagate rapidly to adjacent regions of the membrane.

These properties can be easily demonstrated in experiments on single axons. When a brief electrical current is caused to flow outward across the membrane of an axon, a series of changes occurs in it which result in the breakdown of the barrier against the flow of sodium ions. These rush inward due to the large gradients causing the action potential. The sudden change in electrical state is also called a spike potential because of its very brief duration.

Not all electrical stimuli will generate action potentials. The stimulus must be large enough to decrease the membrane potential to a certain critical level, called the threshold. All stimuli equal to or greater than this threshold value, however, evoke an action potential of a constant magnitude. Since the axon thus responds either with a full-size action potential or with none at all, this characteristic has been called: all-or-nothing. Once the action potential has been elicited it travels along the membrane of the axon independent of further stimulation. This is a second and equally important feature of the action potential: the axon contains within itself the energy required for propagating the action potential; the stimulus acts only to trigger the axon into activity. In short action potentials show the following characteristics[96, 104]:

(1) *Threshold*: the cell fires at a specific level of depolarization;

(2) *Propagation*: internal current causes depolarization of other membrane areas when one area of an elongated cell undergoes an action potential; only under unusual circumstances is the action potential generation limited to a small area;

(3) *All-or-nothing* phenomenon;

(4) *Refractory period.*

10.2 Cable properties of axon

Fig. 128. The membrane of a neuron has a high electrical resistance (ranging from 500 to 10,000 ohm/cm² , depending on the species and on the neuron size) and a high electrical capacity (ranging from 1 to 5 μF/cm²). It separates two highly conductive solutions, the internal and external fluid spaces of the axon[39].

In general it is customary to discuss excitation and propagation in terms of the *cable* properties of the axon[109, 110]. However, the electrical properties of an axon are very poor when compared, for instance, with a cable of copper wire. The membrane of the axon is at least 1,000,000 times leakier to electrical current while the resistance of the interior of the axon is more than 10,000,000 times greater.

In stimulating an axon electrically by using two electrodes (see Fig. 128**A**), most of the current flows from the anode to the cathode *via* the fluid external to the axon, because of its low resistance. Some of the current in the vicinity of the anode, however, flows inwards across the membrane through the axoplasm of the axon, and out again across the membrane in the vicinity of the cathode. As is shown in Fig. 128**B** the current density is greatest immediately under the anode and cathode. Current flow along the exterior or interior of the axon has apparently no effect, but the flow across the membrane has a very pronounced effect upon the membrane potential. Current flowing outward across the membrane (at the cathode) causes a drop in its potential. This change in the potential level of the membrane is called: 'depolarization', although it might be better to speak of *hypo*polarization. Current flowing inward across the membrane (at the anode), on the other hand, causes an increase of the membrane potential. This is called 'hyperpolarization'. We will encounter this phenomenon in discussing inhibitory mechanisms of the neuron. If the current density through the membrane is sufficient to reduce the membrane potential to its threshold value, the action potential is triggered. The threshold value lies at about −50 mV, which means that in order to evoke an action potential, the outward current through the membrane should be sufficiently dense to decrease the membrane potential by 20 mV. In the following paragraphs we will see how such a cathodal current is normally elicited across an excitable membrane. This can occur at the junction between receptor cell and afferent fiber, at the junctions between neurons (excitatory synapses) and at the neuromuscular junction (the site of contact between an efferent nerve fiber and a muscle fiber).

Fig. 128. A, current distribution in a nerve fiber during passage of constant current from outside; **B,** density of membrane current against distance along nerve. **1,** cathode; **2,** anode; **3,** outside; **4,** membrane; **5,** inside.

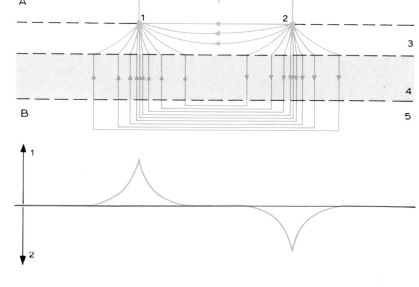

10.3 Ionic permeability changes

Fig. 129. Experiments of Hodgkin and Huxley[84-95] on the giant axon of squid have elucidated many of the basic phenomena regarding the transmission of impulses in nerve fibers. The action potential lasts for about 1 msec (**A**). At the peak of the spike the membrane potential does not merely fall to zero, but actually is reversed in sign. The charge on the inside of the membrane becomes positive with respect to the exterior space by 30 to 40 mV for a short period of time (**B**). The explanation for this is that the permeability of the membrane to sodium ions increases suddenly at the critical depolarization level and, consequently, a rapid inward flux of sodium ions occurs. This inward flux carries a large enough amount of positive charge into the cell to reverse the sign of the membrane potential. This reversal of the net charge in the interior of an active region of the axon corresponds with the measured exterior wave of negativity. At the peak of the spike the membrane potential approaches the equilibrium for sodium ions. The change in sodium permeability lasts for only a fraction of a msec, and is followed by a period of relatively high potassium permeability. This allows a rapid outward movement of potassium ions so that the membrane is recharged and the membrane potential restored almost to normal. Subsequently the sodium ions which had entered, are pumped out slowly, so that the membrane does not ultimately run down.

Fig. 129**B** shows the inward movement of sodium ions during the rising phase of the action potential and the outward movement of potassium ions during its falling phase. **C** illustrates the changes in membrane conductance for sodium and for potassium ions. The time course of the potassium conductance change is slightly different from that for sodium so that the initial level of the membrane potential is not immediately restored. A small hyperpolarization of 10–15 mV is observed, due to the residual efflux of potassium ions. Despite the poor cable properties of the axon, the action potential can travel at a relatively high speed (up to about 120 m per sec in large myelinated fibers) for an indefinite distance without change in size. This remarkable performance is explained by the fact that only very small parts of the axon membrane need to be discharged to the threshold value in order to initiate the action potential. The most important feature is the generation of the explosive increase in sodium permeability when the critical depolarization value is reached. The propagation of the impulse can occur because the outward current across the membrane adjacent to the active region is of sufficient magnitude to trigger the change in sodium conductance. The flow of inward and outward current is shown in part **D** of Fig. 129.

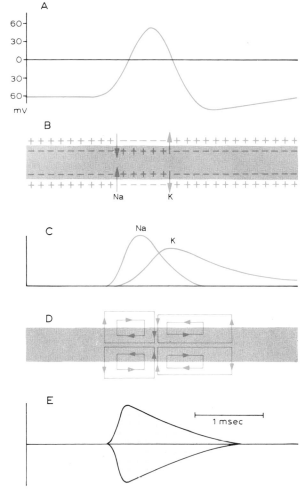

Fig. 129. Summary of the events occurring during propagation of an impulse along a squid giant axon. **A,** action potential; **B,** polarity of potential difference across the membrane; **C,** changes in sodium and potassium permeabilities; **D,** local circuit current flows; **E,** variation in total membrane conductance.

10.4 Positive and negative feedback

Fig. 130. The conductance for potassium ions is many times greater in the membrane at rest than that for sodium ions: $g_K \gg g_{Na}$. At the peak of the action potential, g_{Na} has become larger than g_K and the membrane potential then approaches the equilibrium potential for sodium ions. Some fractions of a msec later g_K is again larger than both g_{Na} and its initial value. During the hyperpolarization, which immediately follows the action potential, the membrane potential approaches the equilibrium potential for potassium ions. The whole process is self contained and it shows the significant role of sodium ions in the propagation of the action potential. The regenerative character of the action potential is illustrated by the fact that the altered potential across the membrane in turn causes electrical currents in the exterior and interior of the axon. The excitation of the membrane is a good example of positive feedback. A small decrease in resting potential produces an increase in sodium conductance. The latter results in a further depolarization, which in turn produces a further increase in sodium conductance. Any positive feedback below threshold is counterbalanced by a negative feedback to restore the resting potential. The positive feedback becomes manifest at threshold, and then the system explodes into an all-or-nothing action potential. The change in potassium conductance is an example of negative feedback. In summarizing: the potential change is due to a large increase of permeability to sodium ions which are distributed far from electrochemical equilibrium. The energy dissipated during an action potential stems ultimately from metabolism *via* the ionic (sodium-potassium) pump which sets up the non-equilibrium ion distributions. Although transmembrane ionic flux (mainly sodium ions inward) is involved in the potential change, altering the charge on the membrane capacity, the action potential does not depend on any major change in concentration of the ions on either side of the membrane. The ionic pump will actually restore the situation which existed as before firing of the action potential.

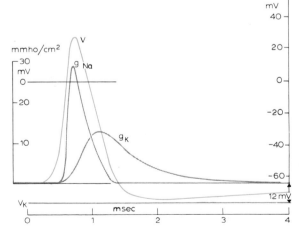

Fig. 130. Theoretical action potential (V) and membrane conductance changes g_{Na} and g_K obtained by solving the equations derived by Hodgkin and Huxley for the giant axon of squid at 18.5°C.

10.5 Strength–duration relationships

Fig. 131. The 'all-or-nothing' law does not imply that the action potential always has the same amplitude. This is illustrated in **A** where action potentials in a nerve are recorded at decreasing temperatures, from 37.7° to 24°C. The amplitude decreases markedly and the propagation is slower, which is indicated by the distance between the stimulus artifact and the peak of the action potential. For any given set of parameters the axon responds maximally to any stimulus of threshold intensity.

Although sufficient in magnitude, a current, usually generated by a stimulator as a square wave, must also have a minimal duration in order to decrease the membrane potential to the threshold value. The threshold strength for a longlasting stimulus is thus less than that required for a stimulus of shorter duration. A strength–duration curve can be determined which expresses the relationship between the strength of a stimulus and the duration which it must have in order for the membrane to be adequately depolarized. This curve also indicates the minimum strength which an applied current could have ('rheobase') and still excite the membrane, *i.e.* if it were applied infinitely long.

One may measure the excitability of a tissue by determining the time during which a current of twice the rheobase value must flow in order to excite the tissue. This is called the *chronaxy*, or excitation time. It is interesting to note that the shape of the strength–duration curve is about the same for all excitable tissues, only the time and the current scales varying from one case to another.

The action potential lasts usually for about 1–3 msec. One can now pose the question of what is the shortest time interval which must elapse before a second action potential could travel along the nerve fiber. For a brief period following an action potential it is impossible to elicit a second one. This interval is called the absolute refractory period and results from the still elevated potassium permeability, which prevents the membrane from becoming depolarized. Following this, another action potential can be elicited, but only if the stimulus strength is increased above the threshold for the first one. This results from the gradual return in potassium permeability to its resting value and is called the relative refractory period. The threshold gradually returns, during this period, to its original value.

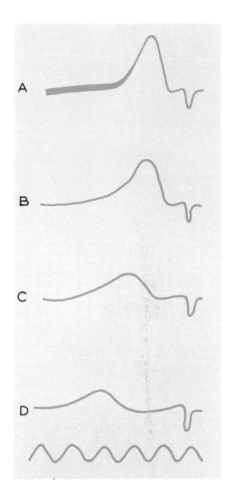

Fig. 131. **A-D** the effect of temperature on the monosynaptic action potential in a single fiber of the cat's nerve. Temperature: **A,** 37.7°C; **B,** 33.0°C; **C,** 27.2°C; **D,** 24.0°C. The downward deflection on the right of each record indicates the moment of stimulation. Time signal: 2000 c/sec. (time is measured from right to left).

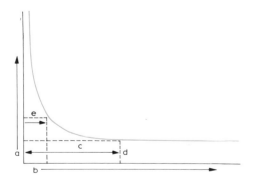

Fig. 131. E, the strength-duration curve; **a,** strength; **b,** duration; **c,** utilization time; **d,** rheobase; **e,** chronaxy.

10.6 Saltatory conduction

Fig. 132. The discussions in the preceding paragraphs on excitability and conduction were based mainly upon analyses of the mechanisms operating in unmyelinated nerves. Most peripheral nerves in vertebrates, however, have a thick covering of myelin, consisting of a lipid–protein sheath around the axon. This myelin sheath is a very effective insulator of the membrane from electrical currents. It is not a continuous coating but it is interrupted by the nodes of Ranvier at intervals of up to 1.5 to 2 mm along the length of the axon. The myelin sheath is absent at the nodes. The width of the node of Ranvier is from 0.5 to 2.5 μ. There is an approximately constant ratio between the diameter of the axon and the distance between two of its nodes of the order of 1 to 100. Fibers may be classified as either myelinated or unmyelinated depending on the thickness of the myelin sheath. It is customary, to call axons unmyelinated if no myelin can be detected under the light microscope. This covering of the major portion of the axon by an insulating material has important implications for the propagation of the action potential[139, 141, 142].

TABLE 3

BIOPHYSICAL CHARACTERISTICS OF MYELINATED NERVE FIBERS*

(Approximate values)

Axoplasm
  resistance 15 mΩ/mm
Myelin sheath
  resistance   300 mΩ/mm
  capacitance   1.5 pF/mm
Node of Ranvier
  membrane resistance   40 mΩ
  membrane capacitance   1.5 pF
internal K$^+$ concentration 120   mM
external K$^+$ concentration   2.5 mM
internal Na$^+$ concentration 13.5 mM
external Na$^+$ concentration 115   mM
K$^+$ permeability constant   1.2 $\times$ 10^3 cm/sec
Na$^+$ permeability constant   8 $\times$ 10^3 cm/sec
non-specific permeability constant 0.54 $\times$ 10^3 cm/sec

* Conductive part of the neuron.

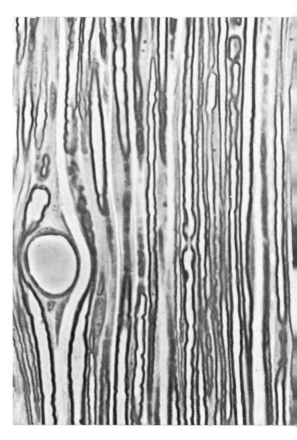

Fig. 132. Longitudinal section of a rat peripheral nerve, to show the presence of nodes of Ranvier.

Fig. 133. Experiments of Tasaki[141], Stämpfli and co-workers[139] have demonstrated that the myelin sheath has a high resistance to direct current (Table 3). Tasaki determined the threshold of a single myelinated fiber by moving a small electrode along its length. The threshold was found to be lowest when the electrode was placed directly over the node and highest when the electrode was midway between the nodes. The myelinated nerve fiber also has a cable structure so that when one node is excited, local currents flow towards it from adjacent nodes (see Fig. 133**B**). The axon membrane is in effective electrical contact with the low resistance interior and exterior of the fiber only at the nodes so that these currents reduce the charge, and thus the membrane potential, only or mainly at the nodes. The nodes of Ranvier are depolarized in this way to their threshold value whereupon an action potential is elicited. Consequently, the impulse 'jumps' from node to node and this phenomenon is therefore called *saltatory conduction* (from Latin *saltare* = to jump).

Saltatory conduction enables the conduction speed to be considerably increased since only the nodes of the axon need to be depolarized in order for the impulse to be propagated. The conduction speed may be as much as 20 to 25 times greater in myelinated nerve fibers than in unmyelinated ones of the same size. This provides a considerable economy of space in the vertebrate nervous system where large numbers of fibers conducting over long distances are found.

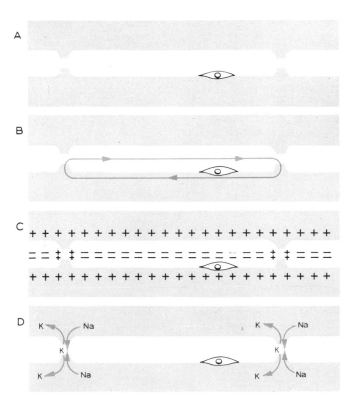

Fig. 133. Some of the events occurring during propagation of an action potential in a myelinated nerve fiber. **A,** diagram of the axon with myelin sheath and two nodes of Ranvier; **B,** circuit current flow through nodes; **C,** polarity of potential differences across the membrane during propagation of action potentials in both nodes; **D,** scheme of ion movements.

10.7 Compound action potential

Fig. 134. A completely different pattern from those hitherto described is seen when the electrical activity produced by stimulation of a nerve trunk is recorded. The action potential has a polymodal character, consisting of several components, and is thus called a compound action potential. The occurrence of several peaks indicates that impulses are travelling in the nerve trunk at different velocities. Careful analysis of the compound action potential has demonstrated two important features of potentials in nerve: (a) the conduction velocity is proportional to the diameter of the nerve fiber and (b) the thicker nerve fibers have a lower threshold than the thinner ones. The first characteristic can be demonstrated by the following experimental test. Fig. 134**C** shows the analysis of the various components of the compound action potential recorded in the sciatic nerve of a frog at different distances from the point of stimulation. If the distance between the stimulating and recording electrodes is known and also the time interval between the stimulus and the arrival of the impulse at the recording electrodes, the conduction velocity can easily be calculated. In the first two traces the two elevations are seen to become gradually separated with successively longer conduction distances. In the third and the fourth lead the two peaks are clearly separated. The peaks become increasingly separated from each other as the conduction length increases because they reflect the activity of groups of fibers having different conduction rates. A clear picture can be obtained of the relationship between fiber diameter and conduction velocity by cutting part of the nerve trunk and isolating single nerve fibers for study.

The axons have been classified into three types: A (subdivided into α, β, γ), B, and C. Table 4 lists a number of characteristics of the various fibers.

The second characteristic can be demonstrated in the same preparation. By increasing successively the strength of the electrical stimulus to al nerve trunk, the different components appear in the record. The potentia

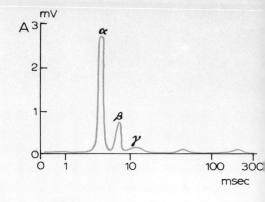

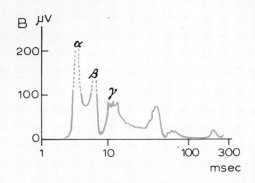

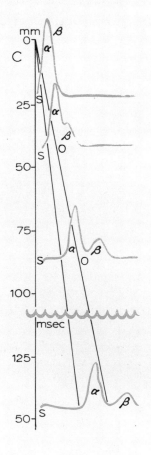

Fig. 134. **A** and **B,** compound action potential led off from the sciatic nerve of frog. **B** is at ten times the magnification of **A. C,** demonstration of the constant velocity of propagation of the α and β waves in the action potential of the sciatic nerve of a frog. The distance from the site of stimulation to the recording electrode is indicated on the vertical line. The starting points of the oscillograph trace show the distances at which the records were taken.

labeled α appears first in the record followed by β. The α potential, as shown in the previous experiment, represents the electrical activity in the fastest conducting axons, showing that conduction velocity and electrical threshold are inversely related to each other.

TABLE 4

CHARACTERISTICS OF THE MAJOR TYPES OF MAMMALIAN NERVE FIBERS

	A (motor and fast sensory)	B (autonomic preganglionic axons)	C (autonomic postganglionic axons)
Diameters of fibers (μ)	20 to 1	< 3	1.35 (unmyelinated)
Conduction velocity (m/sec)	100 to < 5	14 to < 3	< 2
Spike duration (msec)	0.4 to 0.5	1.2	2.0
Negative after-potential			
Amount (% of spike)	3 to 5	None	3 to 5
Duration (msec)	12 to 20	—	50 to 80
Positive after-potential			
Amount (% of spike)	0.2	1.5 to 4.0	1.5
Duration (msec)	40 to 60	100 to 300	300 to > 1000
Absolute refractory period (msec)	0.4α 0.6δ, cat 1.0δ, rabbit	1.2	2.0

11. Excitatory synaptic action

11.1 What is an EPSP?

Fig. 135. One of the simplest kinds of synaptic mechanisms is the mono-synaptic action generated in a mononeuron by stimulating the afferent fibers from a muscle receptor: the annulo-spiral ending of a muscle spindle (group Ia fibers)[15, 20, 23, 27]. The figures illustrate the electrical events recorded in a biceps-semitendinosus motoneuron by afferent volleys of progressively increasing size, elicited in the nerve to the biceps-semitendinosus muscle. Since the potentials are directed upward, it indicates a diminution of the electrical charge on the cell membrane *i.e.* a depolarization. The main feature of the potential is a rapid rise to the summit and a slower, approximately exponential, decay. By increasing the afferent stimulus this potential becomes progressively larger. The inset lines at the left of the main records show the moment of the stimulus, recorded close to the entry of the afferent fibers dorsally into the spinal cord. The depolarizing potentials of the postsynaptic membrane are produced by excitatory synapses and are therefore called: 'excitatory postsynaptic potentials' or 'EPSPs'[34, 35, 40].

The EPSPs become larger in **A** to **C** as the number of activated synapses increases. A few excitatory synapses may be active even in the resting state. There is at present no exact information regarding the distribution of different terminals on the surface of the motoneurons. The terminals of the Ia afferents of the same muscle as that innervated by the motoneuron shown may well be terminating on a specific part of the receptive pole.

The increase of the EPSP is very considerable: the records were taken at an amplification that decreases from **A** to **C** as the response increases (all records were made by superposition of a great number of faint traces). The EPSP begins about 0.5 msec after the stimulus in the Ia afferents has reached the spinal cord. The time between the arrival of the impulse at the presynaptic terminals and the beginning of the post-synaptic depolarization is called *synaptic delay* or *latency*.

A clear summation of EPSPs is seen by the increase in amplitude when the afferent impulse is made stronger. This is seen not only when EPSPs are produced in a motoneuron by a monosynaptic input from its own muscle, but also when the motoneuron is excited by monosynaptic impulses from several Ia afferent systems at the same time.

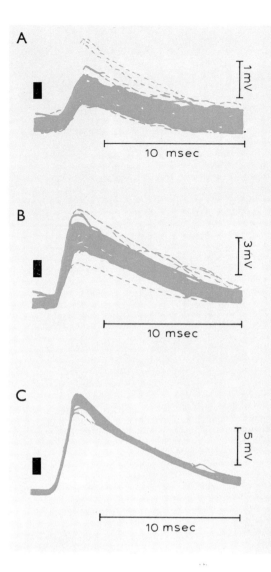

Fig. 135. EPSPs obtained in a biceps-semitendinosus motoneuron with afferent volleys of different size.

Fig. 136. Records of EPSPs recorded in a peroneus longus motoneuron in response to maximum stimulation of the Ia afferent nerve fibers from m. peroneus brevis (**J**), extensor digitorum longus (**K**) and peroneus longus (**L**). The cumulative effect of stimulating all three nerves is given in **M** as an example of spatial summation.

11.2 Parameters of the EPSP

Comparison of the records of the action potentials with those of the EPSPs of motoneurons makes it clear that the production of the EPSP is based upon a different mechanism from that which gives rise to the action potential. An important difference is that the EPSP is a *graded response*: which means that its amplitude varies with the intensity of the applied stimulation. The amplitude of the EPSP never exceeds 20 mV, while the size of the action potential may be five times as high.

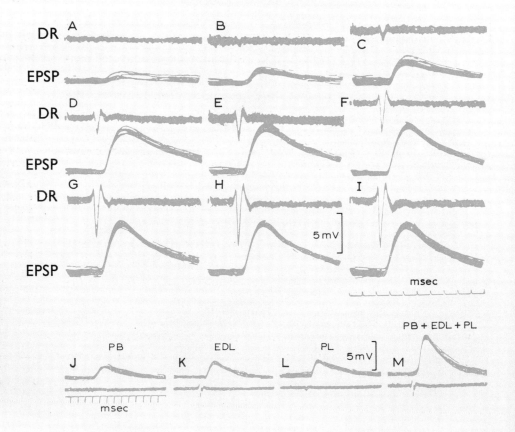

Fig. 136. Monosynaptic EPSPs recorded intracellularly in motoneurons of the lumbar region of cat spinal cord, each record being formed by the superposition of about 25 faint traces. In **A–I** the EPSP is generated in a medial gastrocnemius motoneuron by an afferent volley from the medial gastrocnemius nerve of progressively increasing size, as indicated by the spike potentials in the upper records from the dorsal roots (**DR**). The EPSP attained its maximum in **F**, where the volley was probably maximum for group Ia. In **J–M**, EPSPs are similarly recorded in a peroneus longus motoneuron in response to maximum group Ia volleys from the nerves to peroneus brevis (**PB**) extensor digitorum longus (**EDL**) and peroneus longus (**PL**), and by all three volleys together, as indicated by the symbols.

In analysing synaptic potentials usually four parameters are considered[96]:

(1) *synaptic delay*: the time interval between the stimulus and the onset of the synaptic potential,

(2) *rise time*: the time interval between the onset of the potential and the attainment of its peak amplitude,

(3) *decay time*: the time interval between the peak amplitude and the decay to some selected point. Generally the value for half decay time and time decay to l/e – the time constant – is given,

(4) *amplitude*: the vertical distance between the base line and the peak or top of the potential.

The synaptic delay is made up of the interval between the depolarization of the presynaptic ending and the release of neurotransmitter together with the time needed for the neurotransmitter to diffuse across the synaptic cleft and its reaction with the postsynaptic membrane.

After the synaptic delay the EPSP rises to a summit in about 1–1.5 msec and thereafter decays with a time constant of 4–5 msec. This decay is approximately exponential. The time constant remains the same even if the amplitude of the EPSP increases considerably due to stronger afferent stimuli.

The same order of magnitude for the parameters of the EPSPs have been found in a number of vertebrates as shown in Table 5.

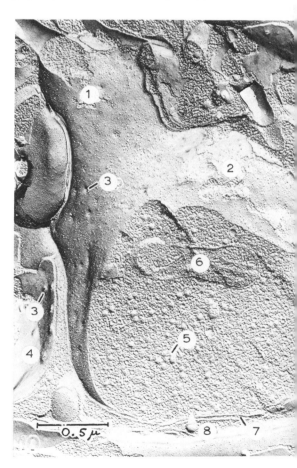

Fig. 137. Freeze-etched preparation of presynaptic nerve terminal. Cat subfornical organ; **1,** preterminal axon. Note the external surface (**2**) covered with scattered granules giving a rough appearance. Micropinocytosis (**3**) at the left side; **4,** inner surface of neuronal plasmalemma. The cut surface of the bouton contains spherical profiles of synaptic vesicles (**5**) and mitochondrion (**6**); **7,** synaptic cleft; **8,** postsynaptic element. Primary magnification × 20 000. (Photograph by Akert and coworkers, 1969.)

TABLE 5

VALUES FOR SOME PARAMETERS OF THE EPSP IN MOTONEURONS[24, 25, 101, 135]

Type motoneuron	Synaptic delay (msec)	Rise time (msec)	Decay time (constant) (msec)
mammal	0.3	1.0-1.5	3.5-6.0
frog	1.0-1.2	2.5-3.0	6.5-10
toad	1.5	2.1	8.0

In the transfer of signals in the synapse a series of events occurs namely, the presynaptic action potential, the release of the neurotransmitter and a number of postsynaptic electrical changes. Since adequate electrophysiological studies of presynaptic function is extremely difficult, this discussion on excitatory synaptic action will focus on the neurotransmitter mechanisms and the postsynaptic events.

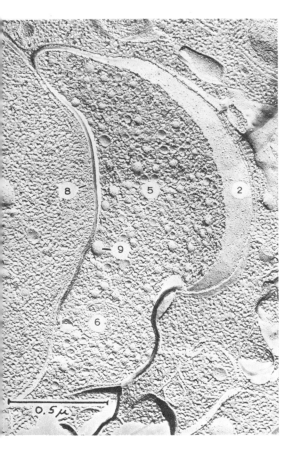

Fig. 138. Freeze-etched presynaptic nerve terminal in the cat subfornical organ. It contains numerous convex and concave profiles of synaptic vesicles (**5**) and one mitochondrion (**6**). The larger profiles represent dense-cored vesicles (**9**). At the left is presumably a synaptic contact, blurred by an uncoated (white) zone. The outer surface (**2**) of the plasmalemma is visible at the right. **8**, synaptic cleft. Primary magnification × 20 000. (Photograph by Akert and coworkers, 1969.)

11.3 Relationship of presynaptic action potentials to EPSP

The action potential travels in all-or-nothing manner into the presynaptic fiber, which ends in an expanded terminal called the synaptic knob. This knob is in intimate contact with a portion of the postsynaptic neuron; often called the subsynaptic membrane. The separation between the presynaptic membrane and the postsynaptic membrane (the synaptic cleft) is a remarkably uniform space of about 200 Å. This synaptic cleft is continuous with the extracellular space.

The action potential travelling into the terminals of the presynaptic fiber on its way to the synaptic area traverses a region of progressively thinning myelin. The myelin sheath peals off, layer by layer at the terminals, just as it does at the nodes of Ranvier. The terminal then expands into the synaptic knob, which, probably in the great majority of the synapses, is formed by unmyelinated axonal membranes.

The chemical theory of synaptic transmission requires that upon stimulation the presynaptic element releases an appropriate amount of neurotransmitter in the synaptic cleft, which subsequently acts upon the postsynaptic element.

Current concepts of the changes occurring at a synaptic ending are the following: The presynaptic impulses cause the following sequence of events in the synaptic area.

Firstly, depolarization of the presynaptic terminal occurs, the exact degree of the depolarization being unknown. Local circuit currents are thus caused to flow in the presynaptic membrane. These events make the presynaptic membrane 'ready' for the activation and release of the contents of the vesicles present in the synaptic ending. They probably also mobilize these vesicles and move them to the synaptic area. Secondly, specific chemical substances (neurotransmitters), which are liberated from the presynaptic membrane, diffuse into the synaptic cleft. Thirdly, a reaction of the neurotransmitter with the postsynaptic membrane occurs. The ionic permeability of the postsynaptic membrane is altered which initiates specific ionic movements across this membrane. Finally, the ionic movements cause small electrical currents to flow inward immediately under the synapse, across the subsynaptic membrane and outward again across adjacent portions of the postsynaptic membrane. These currents are responsible for the changes in polarization level, which in the case of excitatory synaptic action leads to the occurrence of the EPSPs. The transmitter substance is generally rapidly inactivated under normal circumstances by a specific enzyme (as is the case with acetylcholine), so that the subsynaptic membrane quickly returns to its resting state.

11.4 Neurotransmitter mechanisms

As can be seen in the electronmicrographs of synapses, one of the most prominent features is the presence in the presynaptic terminal of small, uniform vesicles close to the synaptic membrane. Structural and functional studies come into very close contact here thanks to the clear picture given by electronmicroscopy of one of the main structures that is required for the explanation of chemical transmission at synapses[31, 32, 39, 71]. Sufficient evidence has accumulated to support the assumption that these vesicles contain the transmitter substance. Experiments on the release of acetylcholine, the transmitter substance at neuromuscular junctions, show that the release has a quantal character[61, 102-113]. The impulse arriving in the presynaptic terminal is of an all-or-nothing nature, with a fixed amplitude. Therefore, it is not difficult to imagine, under normal circumstances, that a constant amount of neurotransmitter will be always released from the presynaptic membrane by each impulse. The amount of neurotransmitter generating a postsynaptic potential is in proportion to the amplitude of the potential, provided there is no alteration of the postsynaptic membrane. The EPSPs represent then a summation of unitary activities: a spatial summation of individual synaptic events. The neurotransmitter is released in multimolecular packets, whose release occurs also spontaneously, but at a very low rate. The small spontaneous potentials are called miniature potentials and can be recorded at a neuromuscular synapse (mEPP) or at a neuronal synapse (mPSP). The miniature potentials represent the basic coin of transmitter release. The rate of release is markedly increased for a brief period of time by an action potential in the presynaptic element.

A beautiful series of experiments by MacIntosh and coworkers[121, 122, 123] has elucidated most of the mechanism in the manufacture and release of *acetylcholine*, still the most firmly established of the few transmitter substances. The results of their experiments on the superior cervical ganglion of the cat supply a future for other transmitter substances and other synaptic systems within the central nervous system. In general the manufacture and release of transmitter substances at synapses in the central nervous system are extremely difficult to approach experimentally because of the great complexity of the interlacing fiber structures. The method of direct assay is limited to a few preparations such as the sympathetic ganglion and the phrenic nerve. Methods of indirect assay are relatively easy to use, and depend largely on the analysis of postsynaptic potentials.

MacIntosh has made very accurate measurements of the acetylcholine (ACh) content and output of this ganglion. In order to unravel the

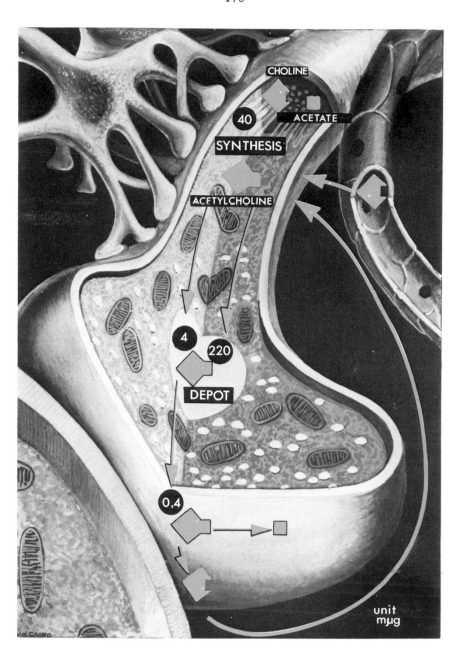

Fig. 139. Conceptual model of a synapse Some data on the synthesis, storage and release of acetylcholine are presented. The data reflect the mechanism of a cholinergic synapse at rest.
Upper left, neuroglial element; **upper right,** blood vessel; **middle,** presynaptic element; **lower left,** postsynaptic element.

metabolism of ACh, use was made of hemicholinium-3, a drug which inhibits the synthesis of ACh, and of anticholinesterases such as eserine and tetraethylpyrophosphate (TEPP) which inhibit the action of acetylcholinesterase (AChE).

Figs. 139, 140. Conceptual models of a synapse based on data of MacIntosh. The ganglia were perfused with oxygenated physiological solutions to which choline and glucose were added, substances necessary for the synthesis of ACh. The content and the output of the ganglia was then studied both under resting conditions and after prolonged activation.

The ACh is contained in a number of compartments, the main compartment being localized inside the synaptic vesicles. Two other compartments, together containing only about 20% of the total ACh, were

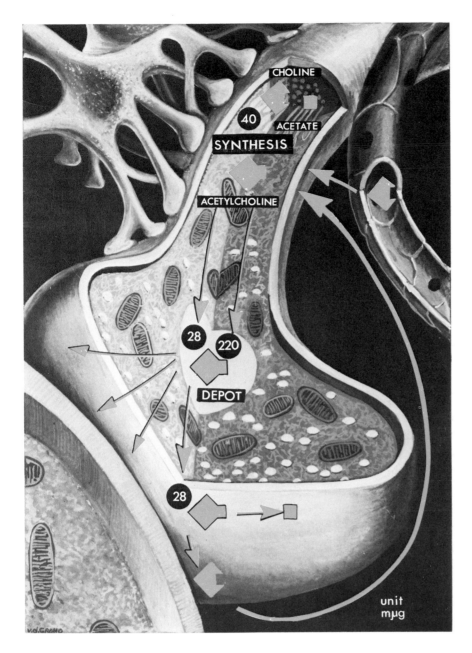

Fig. 140. Conceptual model of a synapse. The data reflect the mechanism of a cholinergic synapse at maximal activity.

localized outside the synaptic vesicles. Presynaptic stimuli showed at least two changes in the ACh metabolism:

(a) The rate of liberation of ACh from the presynaptic membrane into the synaptic clefts was considerably increased and reached a level as high as 28 ng/min. The level was then maintained indefinitely when cholinesterase activity was inhibited.

(b) The rate of synthesis of ACh increases to a level of about 28 ng/min.

Ca ions were also needed for the liberation of ACh during activity. The manufacture of the ACh is assumed to occur within the synaptic vesicles, which also contain the large depot of ACh. ACh was continuously produced in the resting state at a rate of about 4 ng/min. About 90% of this production diffuses into the surplus ACh compartment and about 10% is released into the synaptic cleft. The latter may act upon the postsynaptic membrane to give rise to miniature EPSPs. These are so small as to be hardly detectable, but may be a source of the synaptic noise. When hemicholinium-3 is added to the perfusion fluid, the output of ACh soon ceases because the synthesis of ACh is blocked and only the depot ACh can be used. The depot ACh is never depleted under normal circumstances even after long stimulation.

The synaptic vesicles probably contain a very high concentration of ACh. When a presynaptic impulse causes the vesicles to release part of their ACh (probably not the entire content) into the synaptic cleft, increased synthesis of ACh starts immediately in the vesicles. The neurotransmitter is believed to be contained in various stores, a main presynaptic store, a mobilization store and an immediately available store. The latter is rather small and an action potential releases only a fraction of its contents. It has been calculated that the mobilization store is about 100 times larger than the immediately available store. Experiments have shown that on the average some 250,000 quanta of neurotransmitter are present in a presynaptic ending of a motor phrenic nerve, of which 100–300 are released by an action potential.

Ultracentrifugation techniques combined with electronmicroscopy have recently shown that the fraction which is rich in ACh also contains a very large number of particles which could be recognized as presynaptic terminals containing vesicles and mitochondria. The presence of mitochondria in the synaptic area is very important, as they are the small 'power-houses' which provide the energy needed for all the activity which occurs. The number of vesicles in an average presynaptic terminal in the central nervous system may amount to 10,000–15,000. This should provide enough transmitter substances for a very large number of impulses. It seems reasonable at present to suppose that the synaptic delay in chemical transmission of synapses is caused mainly by the liberation of the transmitter substance and its attachment to the postsynaptic membrane.

Since we are now informed to some extent about the potentials registered by a microelectrode in the cell body of the motoneuron upon monosynaptically evoked excitatory action, we will channel the discussion into two divergent directions:

(a) What is the mechanism by which EPSPs evoke the discharge of an impulse (the action potential) along the axon of the motoneuron?

(b) What are the means by which presynaptic nerve impulses cause the depolarization of the postsynaptic membrane, thus evoking an EPSP?

11.5 Neurotransmitter–receptor complex

The action of the neurotransmitter is mediated as the result of the combination of the substance with a specific receptor. The receptor is part of the postsynaptic membrane and is a chemically defined area of large molecules which combine with a neurotransmitter by virtue of their chemically complimentary nature. Only a few specific neurotransmitters have thus far been identified in the central nervous system: acetylcholine, dopamine, adrenaline, noradrenaline, serotonin and γ-aminobutyric acid. Many rather stringent criteria must be satisfied before a substance may be classified as a synaptic neurotransmitter[39, 80, 96]. To name a few (Fig. **141**).

(1) The presynaptic terminals must contain both the substance in question, and in sufficient quantities, and the enzyme responsible for its synthesis.

(2) Stimulation of the presynaptic elements must release the substance from the terminals.

(3) When the substance is applied to the postsynaptic membrane the action must resemble synaptic activity.

A neuron is chemosensitive means not only that it has receptors which interact with a neurotransmitter, but also that some sort of functional action takes place. To determine the distribution of receptors of the postsynaptic membrane, the method of choice is the localized application of the substance and the measurement of the response-activity. The best technique is the iontophoretic application of substances with the aid of micropipettes and the simultaneous intracellular recording of electrical events.

Termination of the action of the neurotransmitter may be effected by two mechanisms:

(1) Enzymatic destruction of the substance. This phenomenon is well proven only at synapses where acetylcholine is the neurotransmitter. Acetylcholinesterase – a hydrolytic enzyme – which splits acetylcholine to choline and acetic acid is present in high concentrations in the postsynaptic membrane.

(2) Active uptake of the neurotransmitter into the presynaptic endings. The neurotransmitter action may be terminated by active uptake – as has been shown for noradrenaline. The mechanism is made up of two systems; a system which transports the neurotransmitter into the presynaptic ending and a system which transports the neurotransmitter into the synaptic vesicles. Both mechanisms can be disturbed by drug action.

There are but a few data on the chemical nature of the receptor. Acetylcholine is a cation at physiological pH. It seems likely that its receptor is anionic.

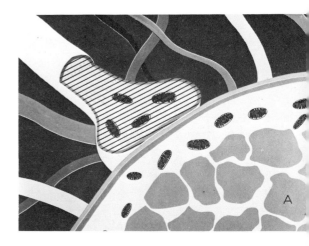

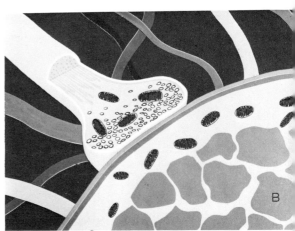

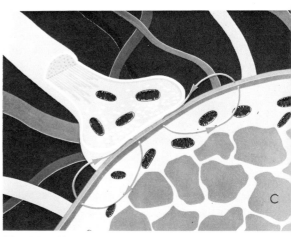

Fig. 141. Models of a synapse showing excitatory synaptic action. **A,** arrival of an all-or-nothing spike potential at the presynaptic terminal; **B,** mobilization of synaptic vesicles; **C,** generation of excitatory postsynaptic potentials.

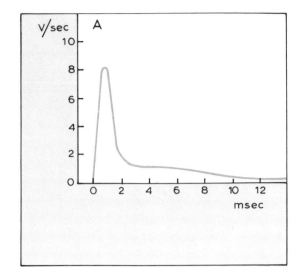

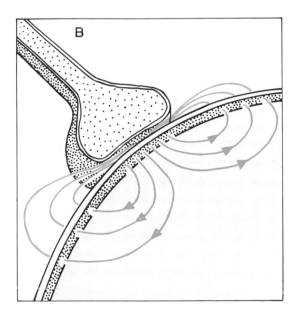

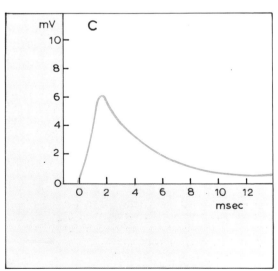

11.6 Excitatory ionic mechanisms

Fig. 142. The neurotransmitter-receptor complex initiates a change in conductance of the postsynaptic membrane, particularly for those ions which are present in abundance; *viz.* sodium, potassium and chloride. The increase in conductance of sodium and potassium in that order is much greater than that of chloride, which is presumably excluded by fixed negative charges in the membrane. In the case of sodium and potassium this conductance change is for ions with equilibrium potentials removed from the membrane potential, the resultant ion movement changes the membrane potential towards a new level characteristic of the combined ion species. The structural basis of the permeability changes may be the appearance of very small channels or pores in the postsynaptic membrane upon reaction with the neurotransmitter. The membrane would then for a very short period of time assume a sieve-like character, permitting ionic flow particularly of the cations sodium and potassium across it at a rate thousands of times faster than normally.

The equilibrium potentials for sodium and potassium are about + 60 mV and − 90 mV respectively, so that the zero level for the EPSP would be readily explicable if the permeability for sodium were about 50% more than that for potassium.

The intense ionic movements across the postsynaptic membrane will, as in the axon, cause electric currents to be generated. These will flow inward immediately under the synapse while there will be an outward current flow at the adjacent portions of the postsynaptic membrane. The outflow then depolarizes these regions of the membrane, giving rise to the EPSP. The current which produces the EPSP is not switched off suddenly, but a small residual current continues to flow. This is probably due to the fact that some transmitter substance continues to be released, which delays the repolarization of the membrane during the declining phase of the EPSP. The direct measurement of the subsynaptic current has encountered great difficulties, but Araki and Terzuolo[4] obtained records of the current by clamping the membrane potential at the resting level. The current flow required for this clamping during exc.tatory synaptic action is then a good record of the subsynaptic current flow.

Although we have talked only about the excitatory synaptic events upon stimulation of the IA afferents to the motoneurons in the spinal cord, there is now sufficient evidence that the phenomena described are also to be found in many other types of neurons and along different stimulation pathways.

Fig. 142. A, time course of the subsynaptic current required to generate the EPSP; **B,** generation of small electrical currents which flow inward under the synapse and outward across the adjacent portion of the postsynaptic membrane; **C,** mean of several monosynaptic EPSPs.

11.7 Conversion of EPSPs into action potentials

Fig. 143. As we have seen on page 165, a stronger afferent stimulus will evoke a greater EPSP. The figures on this page are drawn at a scale about five times as large as the other figures, which illustrate the electrical events for stimuli that are made stronger and stronger. When the depolarization of the postsynaptic membrane reaches a critical level the discharge of an action potential is evoked. The action potential always arises at the same level of depolarization. In the first picture (**A**) a regular EPSP is still seen. In **B**, **C** and **D** we see the generation of an action potential at the threshold of depolarization. In contrast to the EPSP we do not see any increase in the size of the action potential (as we would expect from its all-or-nothing character). The increasing stimulus strength causes it, however, to be generated with a progressively decreasing latency.

The phenomenon that excitatory synaptic action is due to the production of EPSPs, which in turn generate an action potential by causing a depolarization of the membrane to a critical level has been shown to exist in a wide variety of nerve cells in the central nervous system of both vertebrates and invertebrates. The action potential can also be produced in the motoneurons by conditioning procedures. Thus a depolarizing current is made to flow through a microelectrode. The action potential which is generated by a synaptic volley, occurs earlier the larger the intensity of the depolarizing current. The required degree of depolarization is, however, always the same for a particular neuron, say 15 mV. In the latter case this value is made up of the conditioning depolarization plus the superimposed EPSPs. One can finally also superimpose EPSPs upon preceding EPSPs until the critical depolarization level is reached *i.e. temporal summation.* These are examples of the ways in which subliminal EPSPs can be made to generate an action potential.

Since the individual EPSPs are very small in amplitude, it can be assumed that the activation of a single excitatory synapse in the mammalian central nervous system is not enough to discharge a neuron. Several excitatory synapses on the cell body and dendrites must be activated (at about the same time) for a neuron to be discharged.

We must now ask the question: what is the exact localization of the origin of the action potential; *i.e.* the 'generator site' of the spike?

At a short distance from the axon hillock the axon becomes covered with a thick layer of myelin. This first, rather 'naked' portion is called the initial segment (IS). The symbol 'SD' is commonly used in neurophysiological literature for the soma and dendrites. In order to locate the generator site of the action potential the axon of the motoneuron has been stimulated, so that the impulse travels then *antidromically* ('against the road') up to the cell body.

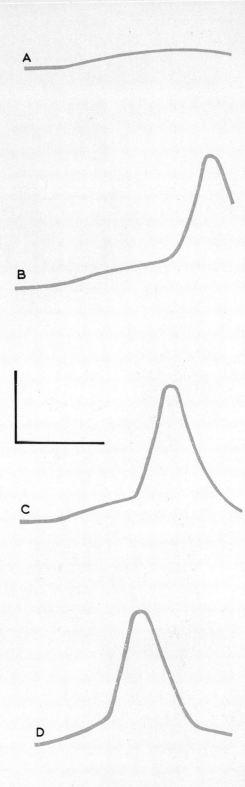

Fig. 143. Intracellularly recorded potentials of a gastrocnemius motoneuron evoked by a monosynaptic activation that was progressively increased from **A** to **D**. Calibration: 1 msec; 50 mV.

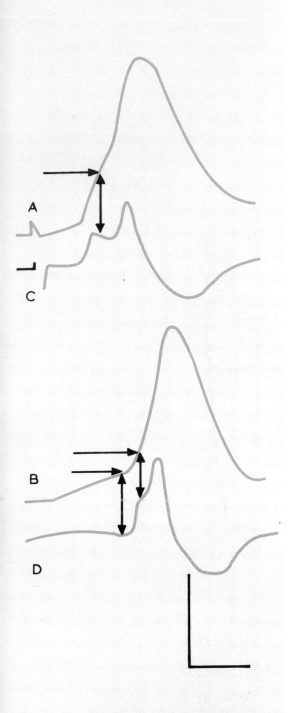

Fig. 144. Tracings of intracellularly recorded action potentials evoked by antidromic (**A**) and monosynaptic (**B**) stimulation of a motoneuron respectively. **C** and **D** show the electrically differentiated records. Calibration: 0.5 msec; 60 mV.

Fig. 144. A shows the intracellularly recorded action potential evoked by antidromic stimulation and **B** the spike potential evoked by monosynaptic stimulation. The two other drawings show the electrically differentiated records.

The analysis of the small inflections on the rising phase of the two action potentials in **A** and **B**, which is particularly evident when the recordings are examined after electrical differentiation (**C** and **D**), is much used for locating the generator-site of the action potential. It has been shown by Eccles and coworkers that the initial small spike in **C** and **D** is generated by an impulse in the initial segment and was therefore called the IS spike. The larger spike, which occurs later invades the soma-dendritic membrane and was therefore called the SD spike. Even in synaptically evoked action potentials it is possible, particularly in the electrically differentiated record, to distinguish between an IS and a SD spike.

The perpendicular lines indicate the origin of the IS and SD spikes while the horizontal lines indicate the respective threshold depolarizations. With all types of stimulation (synaptic, antidromic or direct electrical), it was found that the first response was the IS spike. Comprehensive investigations from various laboratories have led to the conclusion that the threshold for depolarization of the initial segment is always less than half that of the soma. Average values of about 10 mV for the IS spike and of about 27 mV for the SD spike were found in motoneurons. It was therefore postulated that the EPSPs are effective by electronic spread of the depolarizations to the initial segment rather than by generating a propagated impulse in the soma and dendrites of the motoneuron.

The early activation (due to its low threshold) of the initial segment adds very effectively to the depolarization of the somadendritic membrane so that the threshold of this membrane is then reached and the SD spike generated. Both the soma and dendrites are less readily excitable electrically than axons and the impulse propagation is usually very slow: below 1 meter/sec. The action potentials start to travel along the medullated axon about 0.05 msec after the initiation of the IS spike. The figures therefore indicate two components of the spike potential both with an all-or-nothing character generated in different regions of the motoneuron. The action potential in the myelinated axon of the neuron is probably generated in the first node of Ranvier. Pyramidal cells in the neocortex and the hippocampus also show the same composition of the action potential as do the motoneurons in the spinal cord. The lower threshold of the initial segment may have a very important functional meaning: it will act as a better integrator of the diversified excitatory and inhibitory actions over the somadendritic membrane than would be the case if spike potentials could be generated over the whole somadendritic membrane. The initial segment is then the special portion of the motoneuron where excitatory and inhibitory synaptic actions meet. The further action of the neuron is believed to be determined, as in a small computer by algebraic summation of the separate effects.

To sum up excitatory synaptic action, exemplified by a monosynaptic chemically transmitting synapse is brought about by the following sequence of events:

(1) the arrival of all-or-nothing action potentials in the presynaptic terminals (Fig. 141 **A**);

(2) the mobilization of synaptic vesicles which move to the presynaptic membrane and there release quanta of excitatory transmitter substance into the synaptic cleft (Fig. 141 **B**);

(3) the action of excitatory transmitter substance upon the subsynaptic membrane producing changes in the ionic permeability of the membrane, particularly to sodium and potassium; the transmitter is rapidly broken down by an enzyme (Fig. 141 **C**);

(4) the generation of small electrical currents which flow inward under the synapse and outward across the adjacent portions of the postsynaptic membrane (Fig. 142 **B**);

(5) the occurrence of local and graded potentials across the post-synaptic membrane: EPSPs (Fig. 142 **A**);

(6) the algebraic summation of the separate EPSPs by the initial segment of the axons;

(7) the summated EPSPs cause a critical level of depolarization to be reached and an IS spike is generated. This in turn evokes an action potential which is propagated along the axon in an all-or-nothing manner (Fig. 144 **B**).

Excitatory synaptic transmission thus shows the following sequence: all-or-nothing action potential – graded EPSPs – all-or-nothing action potential. In other words we start with a cable-like transmission in the presynaptic fiber, which is completely broken down in the synapse, and converted into a graded response. A reconversion takes place at the initial segment of the postsynaptic neuron and an action potential is further propagated along the axon. It is evident that the transfer of information from one excited neuron to another across the synapse involves a basically different process than the propagation of an action potential along an axon.

Erratum: Small arrow in lower right hand part of Fig. 145 C and pointing to axon hillock should be disregarded.

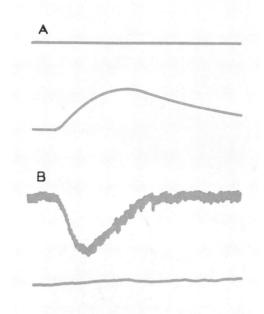

Fig. 145. A, B, voltage clamp method of Araki and Terzuolo to determine the excitatory synaptic current flow. Lower trace in A shows monosynaptic EPSP. Under voltage clamp conditions at the resting membrane potential the same monosynaptic excitation evokes the currents shown in **B**.

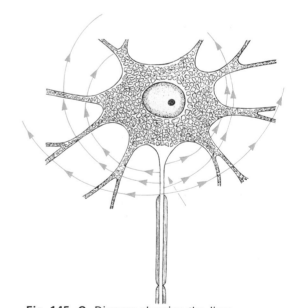

Fig. 145. C, Diagram showing the lines of current flow that occur when a synaptically induced depolarization of the somadendritic membrane electrotonically spreads to the initial segment.

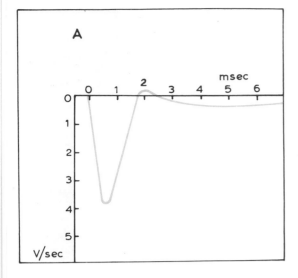

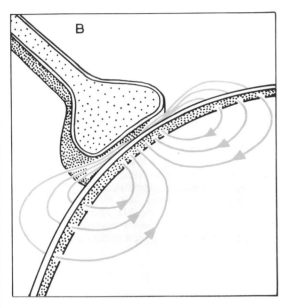

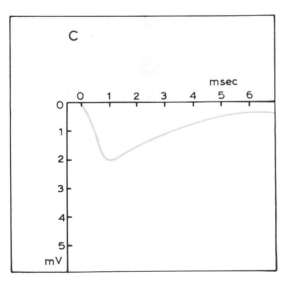

Fig. 150. A, time course of the sub-synaptic current required to generate the IPSP; B, generation of small electrical currents which flow outward under the synapse and inward across the adjacent portion of the postsynaptic membrane; C, mean of several monosynaptic IPSPs.

subsynaptic membrane of a rather uniform size, such that only ions with a radius of less than 5 Å in the hydrated state can pass. Chloride and to a lesser degree potassium are the only anions present in significant concentration. The pores must be small enough furthermore, to exclude the movement of sodium ions, which would otherwise cause a depolarization and the possible generation of an action potential. The fundamental difference, with respect to the permeability of postsynaptic membranes, between excitatory and inhibitory synapses is then that sodium permeability is high in the former and very low in the latter. The potassium ions play a role in both of them. The equilibrium potential for chloride is about -70 mV whereas the equilibrium potential for the IPSP is about -80 mV. Potassium ions make up most of this difference. The investigation of all the other ions was carried out only to elucidate the ionic mechanisms underlying inhibitory action, since only potassium, chloride and sodium are actually present in significant concentrations as free-moving ions.

Fig. 150. The conductance changes in the postsynaptic membrane cause currents to be generated (*i.e.* intense ionic movements), which are outwardly directed across the subsynaptic membrane and inwardly across adjacent portions of the membrane. This current causes the hyperpolarization of the membrane, seen as the IPSP. The lines of current are therefore drawn in the opposite direction as was done for the excitatory synapse. Knowing the shape of the IPSP and the time constant of the membrane, the time course of the 'IPSP-generating-current' can be calculated. The figures are not exact mirror-images of the EPSPs and the 'EPSP-generating-current' and a few differences are particularly noteworthy. The time constant of the IPSP is only slightly longer than that of the neuronal membrane. The declining phase of the time course of the current falls immediately to zero, indicating that there is no residual action of the transmitter substance. This conclusion can be drawn because the time course of the current is at once an indicator of the release of inhibitory transmitter substance and of the time course of the membrane permeability changes.

Since the current falls almost to zero right after the summit of the IPSP, it seems likely that the declining phase of the IPSP is due simply to the passive recovery of the membrane potential.

Araki and Terzuolo[4] were able to measure the postsynaptic inhibitory current directly by means of the voltage-clamping technique. Their recordings (Fig. 154**A**, **B**, and **C**) demonstrate the electrical events recorded by two microelectrodes located 10 μ apart inside a biceps-semitendinosus motoneuron. In **A**, two IPSPs recorded upon stimulation of the IA afferents from the quadriceps muscle are shown. In **B**, the lower beam has been switched so as to record the membrane current. In **C**, the membrane potential was clamped, at its resting level during the activation of an inhibitory synapse. The resulting current is recorded on the lower beam and is almost a mirror image of the one seen during the activation of an excitatory synapse.

12.5 Recurrent inhibition

Many neurophysiologists, and particularly Sherrington[137, 138], have been fascinated by the problem of inhibition in the central nervous system. To illustrate how close Sherrington[138] was in 1932 to our present-day concept of postsynaptic inhibition, we can quote the following passage from his Nobel oration (which had as its title, *Inhibition as a coordinative factor*):

'the inhibitory stabilization of the membrane might be pictured as a heightening of the 'resting' polarization, somewhat on the lines of an electrotonus'.

Fig. 151. Another great physiologist, Renshaw, has also contributed a great deal to our knowledge of inhibition. Recurrent or antidromic inhibition is named after him 'Renshaw inhibition' and the interneurons which perform this type of inhibition are called 'Renshaw cells'.

In 1941 Renshaw[133] gave a description of the inhibition of the activity of motoneurons upon antidromic stimulation of the axons of these cells. In subsequent years the anatomical basis for this inhibition was found and is diagrammed in Fig. 151a.

Collateral branches of the axons make synaptic contact with small interneurons lying in the area where the axons of the motoneurons leave the ventral horn of the spinal cord. The axons of these cells (Renshaw cells) in turn make synaptic contact with the motoneurons. A characteristic feature of this type of inhibition is that an antidromic volley elicits a prolonged effect. Fig. 151b shows the reaction to a single volley in the Renshaw cell. A long-lasting burst of action potentials occurs, the frequency of which is much higher in the beginning than at the end. Renshaw cells have, furthermore, the same properties as inhibitory interneurons, *viz.* action potentials invading their presynaptic terminals evoke IPSPs in the motoneurons. The IPSP produced in the motoneuron has the same features in both case. Fig. 151b, c, d, shows a portion of an IPSP upon which a ripple is seen which is a reflection of the burst of action potentials in the Renshaw cells. The function of this recurrent pathway is a clear example of a negative feedback, in that the Renshaw inhibition opposes the discharge of the motoneuron in direct proportion to the firing frequency of the latter. This negative feedback is not restricted to the motoneuron which is discharging at the time; many other motoneurons are affected supplying both the same muscle and other muscles in the same region.

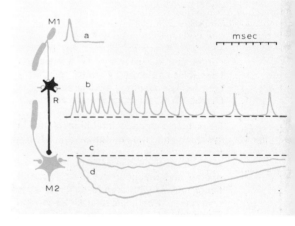

Fig. 151. Scheme of the pathway for Renshaw inhibition.
Diagram illustrating the postulated sequence of events from an impulse in a motoneuron (**M1**) to the inhibition of the motoneuron (**M2**).
a, impulse in the collaterals of the motoneuron axon; **b,** impulse evoked in the Renshaw cells by the cumulative effect of many synapses; **c,** the IPSP generated in the motoneuron by the firing of the Renshaw cells; **d,** the cumulative IPSP evoked in the motoneuron that is repeatedly bombarded by many Renshaw cells.

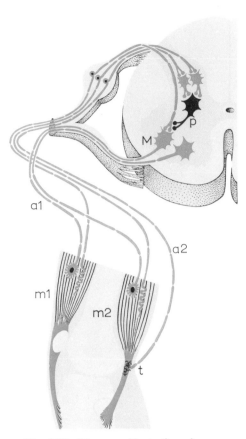

Fig. 152. Diagram illustrating how a contracting extensor muscle excites the knee joint and strongly stretches a flexor muscle. The resulting discharges up the IA and IB fibers from the flexor muscle excite an interneuronal pathway that leads to presynaptic inhibition of the Ia synapses on the motoneurons of the extensor muscle.

m1, extensor muscle plus annulo-spinal ending and myoneuronal endplate; **m2**, flexor muscle with annulo-spinal ending, myoneuronal endplate and Golgi tendon organ (**t**); **M**, motoneurons to flexor and extensor muscle; **p** = interneuron exerting presynaptic inhibition; **a1**, inhibited motoneuron; **a2**, sensory neuron activating interneuronal inhibitory pathway.

12.6 Disinhibition

From studies on many types of neurons in the vertebrate nervous system it may be concluded that synapses can be grouped into two general categories:

(1) excitatory synapses, which generate depolarizing potentials across the postsynaptic membrane, and

(2) inhibitory synapses, which generate hyperpolarizing potentials.

However, membrane potential changes are also seen when a sustained bombardment of synaptic activity is removed from a given neuron. Removal of excitatory synaptic activity or inhibitory synaptic activity have both been demonstrated in various parts of the central nervous system. The phenomena are called disfacilitation and disinhibition respectively[96].

Disfacilitation is easily demonstrated in spinal motoneurons innervating extensor muscles, when the cerebellum exerts a specific inhibitory effect. A sustained hyperpolarization of the membrane is seen, caused by the removal of a background depolarization. The maximum value of this phenomenon is the resting membrane potential of the neuron. This hyperpolarization is thus always less than the one produced by inhibitory synaptic activity.

Disinhibition is produced in a similar manner. An increase in the amplitude of the EPSP can be observed under certain conditions in spinal motoneurons when the effect of some inhibitory synapses is removed. The inhibitory background activity of certain interneurons mediated by the collateral activation of Renshaw cells has been shown to be effected by this mechanism.

Although it seems likely that both disfacilitation and disinhibition play a role in the functioning of the nervous system, it is presently not clear to what extend.

Excitatory and inhibitory synaptic potentials have a number of characteristics in common (Figs. 145, 154):

(1) they are graded phenomena and the amplitude of the potentials is related to the number of presynaptic fibers activated at a given time;

(2) they have a specific time course, which is characterized by a relatively fast rise and slow decay;

(3) the potentials in the postsynaptic membrane are generated by specific ionic mechanisms, which are secondary between a neurotransmitter and the receptor of the postsynaptic membrane;

(4) the synaptic potentials are electrotonically conducted along the receptive surface of the neuron.

12.7 Presynaptic inhibition

Fig. 153. The famous neurophysiologist John C. Eccles and his collaborators have in the last decade accumulated a wealth of experimental evidence that a second, quite different type of inhibition exists in the central nervous system, namely, presynaptic inhibition[39, 41, 54, 55, 56].

It was noted by several investigators that stimuli in the IA afferent fibers could diminish the size of the monosynaptic EPSP without affecting electrical parameters such as the membrane potential, the ionic permeability of the postsynaptic membrane, etc. Therefore it was concluded that the decrease in size of the EPSP must be due to changes in the excitatory action of the IA presynaptic impulses[39, 64, 65].

We will now briefly discuss some of the experimental evidence that has led to the hypothesis that depolarization of the presynaptic fibers is responsible for the observed diminution of the EPSP. Although presynaptic inhibition has since been shown to exist in many systems, the IA afferents, which make monosynaptic contact with the motoneuron, will be chosen for description of this phenomenon.

The following discussion will cover in sequence three aspects of presynaptic inhibition: (1) the depression of the monosynaptic excitatory

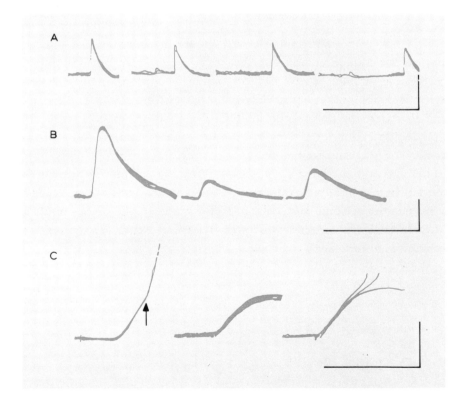

Fig. 153. A, depression of monosynaptic EPSPs by presynaptic inhibition. The EPSP in a plantaris motoneuron is seen to be depressed by 4 group I conditioning volleys in the nerve to the knee flexors, posterior biceps and semitendinosus. Calibration: 50 msec, 5 mV. **B,** control EPSP (1st record) of another experiment is seen to be greatly depressed both at 5 (2nd record) and 83 (3rd record) msec after conditioning techniques of 22 group I volleys. Calibration: 10 msec, 5 mV. **C,** presynaptic inhibition of monosynaptically generated reflex discharges. In the first record the superimposed control EPSPs are seen always to generate a discharge of the impulse at the arrow, whereas conditioning presynaptic inhibition (2nd and 3rd records) causes impulse generation to fall or be delayed. Calibration: 2 msec, 5 mV.

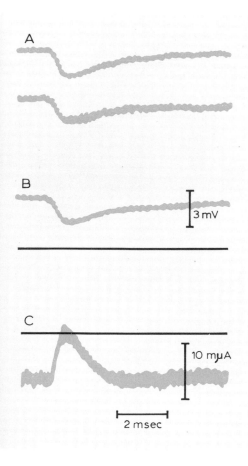

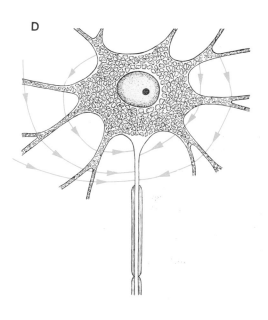

action (EPSP), (2) the depolarization of the presynaptic fiber, and (3) some pharmacological aspects of possible transmitter substances.

Figs. 153**A** and **B** illustrate the most direct evidence of presynaptic inhibition. In **A** impulses from the flexor muscle (post. biceps-semitendinosus) depress the monosynaptic EPSP of the plantar motoneuron relative to the control response. **B** illustrates the same phenomenon: stimuli arising from the same flexors diminish greatly in size the monosynaptic EPSP of the gastrocnemius motoneuron. The diminution of the EPSP may prevent it from generating an action potential at the axon hillock or at least delay its generation. Intracellular recordings from groups of IA primary fibers have shown the expected depolarization. The time course of this presynaptic depolarization was found to be in very good agreement with that of the depression of the EPSP. The latent period is about 4 msec, a summit at about 20 msec, and a total duration of at least 200 msec.

Although the transmitter substances mediating presynaptic and postsynaptic inhibitory action in the spinal cord have not been identified, there is much experimental evidence suggesting that a distinctive pharmacological mechanism is involved in each of these processes. As previously indicated, postsynaptic inhibitory action is depressed by a number of convulsant drugs, such as strychnine, thebaine and brucein. The action of these drugs is assumed to result from a competitive binding of the receptor sites for the postsynaptic inhibitory transmitter substance.

The most important result was the finding that picrotoxin depressed presynaptic inhibition but was ineffective on postsynaptic inhibition. Strychnine, which depresses postsynaptic inhibition, increased presynaptic inhibition. A number of barbiturates such as nembutal prolonged and increased the presynaptic inhibition of monosynaptic reflexes. All presynaptic inhibitory actions possess the same pharmacological properties. The pharmacological investigations reveal fundamental differences in the pre- and postsynaptic inhibition. Presynaptic inhibitory action is exerted by chemically transmitting synapses which act by depolarizing the excitatory synaptic terminals. In this way the amplitude of impulses in these terminals and the consequent release of excitatory transmitter substance are decreased.

Fig. 154. Membrane current during an IPSP. **A**, IPSP in a biceps-semitendinosus motoneuron by an afferent volley in the quadriceps nerve, recorded by both micro-electrodes; **B**, lower beam switched to record the membrane current; **C**, membrane potential clamped at its resting level during the IPSP (upper beam). The current is recorded in the lower beam; **D**, diagram showing the lines of current flow that occur when a synaptically induced hyperpolarization of the soma dendritic membrane electronically spreads to the initial segment.

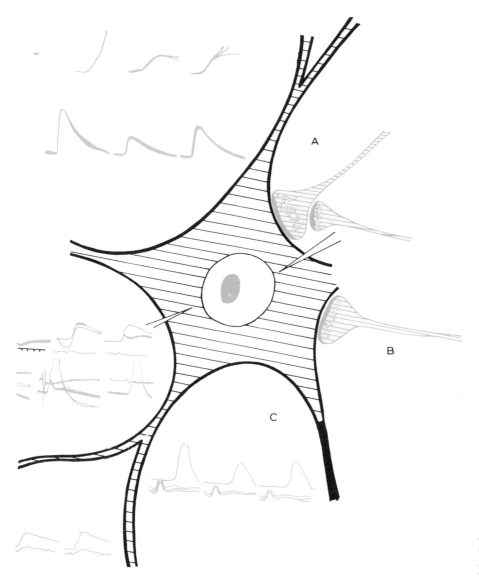

Fig. 155. Summary of electrical events accompanying pre- and postsynaptic inhibitory action in the motoneuron. **A,** presynaptic fibers; **B,** postsynaptic fiber; **C,** axon hillock.

Fig. 155. Summary of specimen records of the various types of responses associated with synaptic action. In the middle left quadrant is an intracellular electrode with records of IPSPs (downward deflections) and EPSPs (upward deflections), and their interactions. Two examples of spike inhibition are shown in the lower row. In the upper right hand part is shown a presynaptic inhibitory terminal on an excitatory fiber. The latter is seen to be depolarized, as shown by intracellular recording. This phenomenon is clearly shown by the differences in both intracellular and extracellular recordings following 2, and 4 volleys (lower left). In the upper left quadrant the effects of presynaptic depolarization upon excitatory synaptic action are recorded intracellularly. The upper row indicates how the presynaptic inhibitory action depresses the EPSP, so that it often fails to generate a spike. In the lower quadrant is seen the diminution of the reflex spike discharge in the ventral roots.

13. Electrical events in other synaptic functions

13.1 In receptor cells

One of the most significant factors in the survival of an organism is its ability to respond to stimuli from the external environment and to regulate its own internal environment. Sense organs are specialized to perform this function. The essential elements of all sense organs are receptor cells, which respond to physical and chemical disturbances and transmit information about them to the central nervous system. The transmission of pain stimuli is an exception to this rule.

Each type of receptor is in general attuned to a narrow range of stimulus energies: *e.g.* photoreceptors of the retina to 'light', thermo-

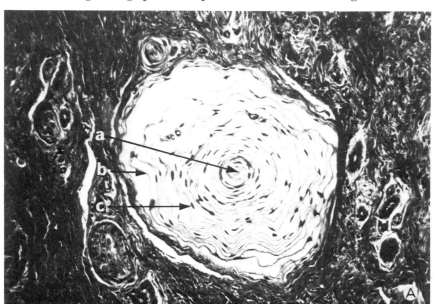

Fig. 156. A, histological section of a corpuscle of Vater Pacini; **a,** central core; **b,** lamella; **c,** nucleus of lamella.

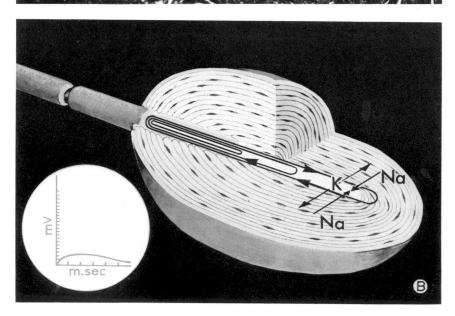

Fig. 156. B, schematic representation of the electrical events accompanying the generation of the receptor potential. The inset at the left shows the receptor potential. The movement of ions accompanying the receptor potential is indicated.

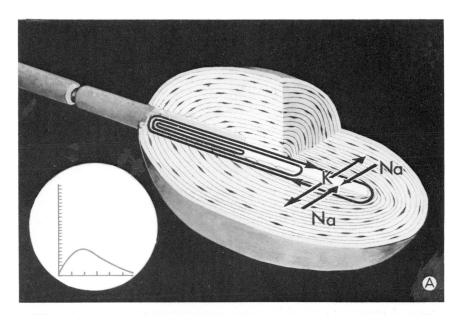

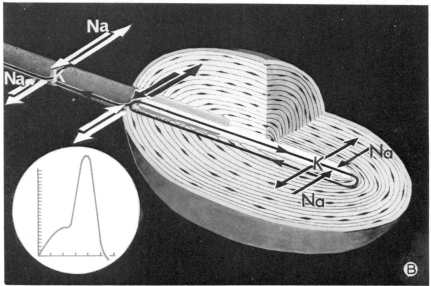

Fig. 157. (continuation of Fig. 156 **B**). **A**, a stronger stimulus produces a stronger generator potential. An increase in ionic movements and generator currents is shown; **B**, summated receptor potentials reach a critical level of depolarization and an action potential is generated (see inset).

receptors in the skin respond to 'heat' and 'cold', etc.

Receptor cells may be divided into two main categories:

(A) *Exteroceptors*–to gain information about external environment;

(B) *Interoceptors*–to gain information about internal environment.

Among the exteroceptors one can distinguish:

(A1) *Photoreceptors*, receivers of light, located in the retina.

(A2) *Chemoreceptors*, receivers of taste stimuli, located in the tongue, and receivers of smell stimuli, located in the nasal epithelium.

(A3) *Mechanoreceptors*, receivers of sound stimuli, located in the cochlea, and receptors for pain and touch (Meissner's and Pacinian corpuscles Fig. 156**A**) in the skin.

(A4) *Thermoreceptors*, cells in the skin, responding to heat and to cold (sense organs of Krause and Ruffini).

The interoceptors may be divided into the following groups:

(B1) *Chemoreceptors*, cells located in the walls of carotid arteries and

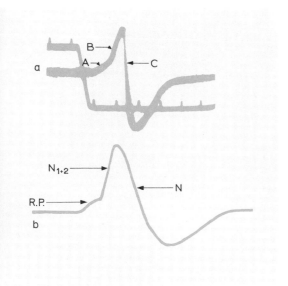

Fig. 158. a, potential recorded from a Pacinian corpuscle. Top beam (left) signals time course and amplitude of stimulus and time in msec. **A, B** and **C** show the three places of response; **b,** diagram of recorded potential similar to that in **A**; **R.P.**, receptor potential; **N1+2** and **N,** phases of all-or-nothing activity.

the aorta to respond to blood oxygen tension; in the respiratory center of the brain stem to respond to blood CO_2 tension, etc.

(B2) *Mechanoreceptors* of the labyrinth (semicircular canals, utricle, saccule) for recording of movement and position: stretchreceptors of muscle, etc.

(B3) *Osmoreceptors* of the hypothalamus and probably other brain areas to record blood osmotic pressure.

13.2 Receptor cells as transducers

The terminals of afferent nerve fibers are scattered over the whole surface of the body. The stimuli are received either by free nerve endings or by specialized sensory endings. All of the special sense cells in the skin consist of a connective tissue cushion in which is embedded the unmyelinated terminal of a larger myelinated nerve fiber. The receptors and afferent connections should be considered not only as groups of receptors excited by particular external events but as organs capable of presenting a detailed report of patterns of stimuli received from the environment. The receptor cells in the skin (and underlying tissue) can give a great deal of information about the nature of the object in contact with it. Even the slightest contact with an object will produce patterns of impulses in a great variety of afferent fibers. Unfortunately, little is known about the relationship of the histological structure of the sense cells and the discharge patterns. Only the Pacinian corpuscle has been studied in isolation and this sense cell will therefore be taken as an example for the discussion of the electrical events associated with the reception of stimuli from the external environment.

Figs. 156, 157, 158. All receptor cells have a common function in that they are transducers, *i.e.* they convert one form of energy into another. The sense organs in the skin convert mechanical and thermal energy into the electrical energy of the nerve potentials. In general, receptor cells do not themselves fire off action potentials, but they show graded potential changes which generate action potentials in the afferent nerve fiber with which they are connected.

Two potentials are usually defined in order to describe the sequence of electrical events of the transducer function of the receptor cell.

(1) The *receptor potential* is the graded response of a receptor to a stimulus: the first electrical potential to arise in the causal sequence.

(2) The *generator potential* is the potential which triggers the impulse in the axon: the last electrical potential before the all-or-none coding.

The potentials are inseparable from the associated membrane current (the 'generator current'), which triggers the action potentials. Only if specialized receptor cells are present (*viz.* rods and cones) can one distinguish separate receptor and generator potentials. In the case of the Pacinian corpuscle, where no special receptor cells are present, the two potentials are synonymous.

13.3 Receptor and generator potentials

Under the microscope the Pacinian corpuscle looks like an onion (Fig. 156, **A**). It is from 500 to 1000μ long and from 300 to 700 μ thick, and consists of many concentric lamellae or layers. The oval area in the center contains the corpuscle core, which encloses the unmyelinated part of the afferent nerve fiber. The first node of Ranvier is also located within the corpuscle. Many mitochondria are present in the central area, indicating the production of large amounts of energy.

By stimulating the corpuscle with a piezoelectric crystal, Loewenstein[119, 120] detected characteristic generator and action potentials in the afferent axon. To locate the transducer site in the corpuscle he and his coworkers peeled off the various layers of the corpuscle and stimulated the preparation at various phases of the dissection. Even a preparation with only the inner core intact showed characteristic potentials.

The generator potential has the same features as the excitatory post-synaptic potentials *viz.* a weak stimulus produces a weak generator potential while stronger stimuli produce proportionally stronger generator potentials. The potentials indicate a graded depolarization of the resting membrane potential. When the threshold is reached, an all-or-nothing action potential is triggered. Even partial destruction of the core sheath did not prevent the triggering of an action potential. Loewenstein then used a degeneration technique to produce an 'ending-less' core by severing the nerve fiber and allowing the nerve ending to degenerate. This preparation failed to produce a generator potential, indicating that the nerve ending itself was the transducer site. The generator potential does not travel along the axon but triggers at the first node of Ranvier an action potential. If the first node of Ranvier was blocked, no action potential could be induced in the nerve fiber.

The ionic mechanism of the receptor potential is also similar to that for the EPSP, *viz.* the deformation of the lamellae in the case of the Pacinian corpuscle causes an increased conductance for sodium and potassium ions.

In short the following sequence of events occurs:

(1) small electrical currents are generated (generator currents), which flow from the unmyelinated portion of the axon to the nodes of Ranvier;

(2) local, graded potentials (receptor potentials) occur across the neuronal membrane;

(3) the separate receptor potentials are algebraically summated by the first node of Ranvier;

(4) the summated receptor potentials cause a critical level of depolarization to be reached and an action potential is generated, which is then propagated along the axon in an all-or-nothing manner. The receptor potentials thus show all the characteristics established for the EPSP.

13.4 In neuromuscular transmission

Fig. 159. Upon excitation of the motoneuron action potentials are discharged along the efferent axons to the muscle. Transmission occurs at the neuromuscular junction. The fine terminal branches of the efferent axon reach the muscle fibers through the connective tissue which surrounds the various muscle bundles. The presynaptic ending is made up of the club-like endings of the axon terminals. They contain mitochondria and synaptic vesicles. The postsynaptic membrane consists of the motor endplates, which have a very specialized form (Fig. 159**A**).

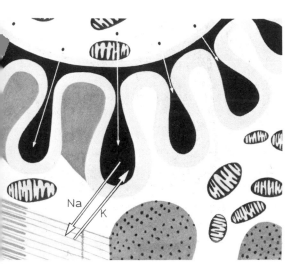

Fig. 159. A, Schematic diagram of junction between efferent fiber and muscle fiber; **a,** presynaptic terminal; **b,** cross section through presynaptic terminal containing mitochondria and synaptic vesicles; **c,** folds in the postsynaptic membrane; **d,** mitochondria; **e,** myofibrils; **B,** schematic picture of the various structures in the neuromuscular synapse.

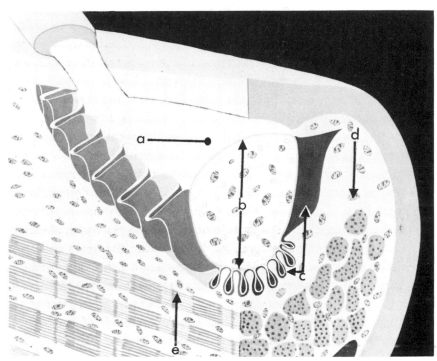

A schematic picture of the various structures in the neuromuscular synapse is given in Fig. 159**B**. The postsynaptic membrane has an extraordinary large contact surface because of its invaginated structure. The synaptic cleft measures from 200 to 600 Å.

Upon reaching the neuromuscular synapse the action potentials cause the same sequence of events as that occurring at the excitatory synapse. The synaptic vesicles are mobilized, move to the presynaptic membrane, and release there large quantities of the transmitter substance into the synaptic cleft. For striated muscle the transmitter substance has been shown to be acetylcholine. The action of acetylcholine upon the postsynaptic membrane produces changes in the ionic permeability of the membrane, particularly to sodium and potassium. The small electrical currents which then flow inward under the neuromuscular synapse and outward across the adjacent portions of the membrane are of the same nature as discussed in the case of the excitatory synapse. The transient depolarizations occurring in the motor endplates are called endplate potentials (EPPs). If sufficient to reach the firing level this depolarization will evoke a propagated muscle action potential. The EPP is a summated response, showing decremental conduction along the membrane.

Fig. 160. Five EPPs recorded intracellularly from a single curarized muscle fiber of a frog. The series of records (a–e) were taken at intervals of 1 mm along the muscle fiber; (a) shows the response at the neuro-muscular synapse. The decrease in amplitude exemplifies the decremental conduction. There is also a continuous occurrence of miniature EPPs of about 0.5 mV each and about 20 msec. They are produced by the spontaneous, random release of small amounts of acetylcholine in the absence of action potentials.

13.5 Muscle membrane receptors

Many attempts have been made to determine the distribution of receptors on the membrane of the muscle fiber. As mentioned before, the method of choice is now the electrophoretic application of substances combined with intracellular recording. In the study of the localization of receptor sites, acetylcholine is injected from the tip of a fine glass micropipette by a voltage pulse, and the depolarizing response is recorded by a second microelectrode inserted in the muscle fiber. The rat diaphragm phrenic nerve preparation is often used for the study of electrical events *in vitro*. The relative density of the receptors can be estimated by calculating the ratios of the depolarization by the acetylcholine to the applying current strength at different points along the muscle fiber. In doing so, the acetylcholine receptors are found in greatest density in the synaptic region, but also occur outside the neuromuscular junction on the surrounding muscle membrane.

The electrophoretic method can also be used to measure the alteration in distribution of receptor-sites under pathological conditions. In this way it has been possible to show changes in receptor density upon denervation, renervation and in the course of some myopathies. The sensitivity of the muscle membrane appeared to be closely related to the number of receptors.

The studies of Katz and Miledi[106–113] have shown that the chemosensitive area of the muscle membrane depends on the state of innervation. A muscle deprived of its motor innervation or poisoned with botulinum toxin has receptors uniformly distributed over the membrane. Upon reinnervation the receptor area of the membrane shrinks to a small focus.

It is generally assumed that receptors are located on the outside of the membrane. This can be proved by applying agents on the outside and inside of the membrane and analyzing the differences in response pattern. Intracellularly applied acetylcholine does not show a specific neurotransmitter effect.

As already noted before, it seems likely that receptors are anionic in nature. Such receptor sites would have some affinity for inorganic cations.

Fig. 160. Five endplate potentials (EPPs) recorded intracellularly from a single curarized muscle fiber of a frog.

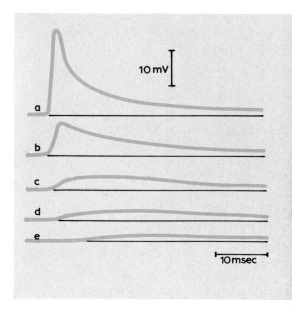

It has been reported that calcium and magnesium reduce the affinity of the receptors of the muscle membrane for tubocurarine.

In the past decade the study of the electrical events in the neuro-muscular synapse has elucidated many mechanisms responsible for the transfer of information between neurons and muscles. The significance of this research has been recognized by the awarding of the Nobel prize 1970 to B. Katz, one of the pioneers in this field.

14. Integrative mechanisms: Neuronal circuits

14.1 Introduction

The basic functional mechanisms discussed in the previous chapters represent perhaps all the types of membrane responses which are involved in the entire complicated machinery of the brain. We should then recognize that action potentials and synaptic potentials are the modes of electrical functioning of neurons, and that there exists an essential similarity of transducer-, excitatory synaptic, and motor end-plate activity. These latter phenomena process the same characteristics: graded summation and decremental spreading, and all have the effect of lowering the resting membrane potential. Inhibitory synaptic action opposes excitatory action.

We are still far from a clear understanding of the transfer and processing of information in the nervous system. The firing pattern of a given neuron may show a bewildering variability from moment to moment. Even more intriguing are the integrated mechanisms which depend on the functional integrity of neuronal networks.

Since we have gained some knowledge about the basic functional properties of neurons we will now move to the discussion of some integrative mechanisms. The description in this chapter will deal with aspects of neuron circuitry in four regions of the central nervous system:

(a) the *spinal cord*: the seat of integration of reflexes; (b) the *cerebellum*: the neuronal computer for all information regarding movements; (c) the *thalamus*: the major sensory relay station, and (d) the *cerebral cortex*: the grey mantle of the forebrain where the perception of sensory stimuli takes place and where also the commands for movements originate.

In the next chapter we will move to a more macroscopic level, and a description will be given of the major pathways.

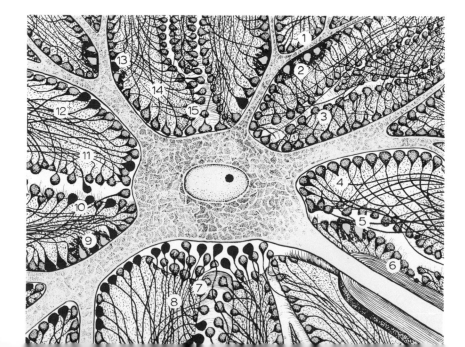

Fig. 161. Diagram of segmental afferent inputs, converging on a typical motoneuron, supplying the extensor muscle. Black knobs indicate excitatory, green inhibitory and mixed ones inactive synapses. **1-5,** Contralateral inputs; **6,** antidromic inhibition by Renshaw interneurons; **7-15,** ipsilateral inputs; **7-12,** multisynaptic reflex loop; **13-15** monosynaptic reflex loop.
1, secondary sensory ending of muscle spindle; **2,** touch and pressure from skin; **3,** free nerve endings; **4,** primary sensory ending of muscle spindle; **5,** Golgi tendon organ; **6,** antidromic inhibition by Renshaw interneurons; **7,** Golgi tendon organ (het. antagonistic); **8,** Golgi tendon organ (het. synergistic); **9,** Golgi tendon organ (homon); **10,** free nerve endings; **11,** touch and pressure; **12,** secondary sensory endings of muscle spindle; **13,** primary sensory ending (het. antagonistic); **14,** primary sensory ending (het. synergistic); **15,** primary sensory ending (homon).

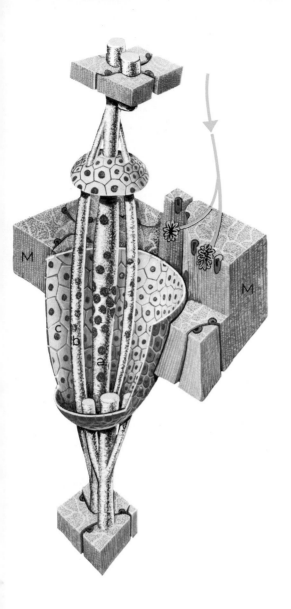

Fig. 162. Model of a typical muscle spindle. At the upper right is indicated the motor supply of the extrafusal fibers by endings of the α-neuron.
M, extrafusal fibers; **a,** nuclear bag fiber (s1); **b,** nuclear chain fiber (s2); **c,** capsule.

14.1.1 The spinal cord. Organization of the final common pathway

The α-motoneuron is an integrating unit that sends action potentials along its efferent axon to the muscle. Upon reaching the neuromuscular synapse the action potentials cause a sequence of events that occur also at the excitatory synapse. At the transmitting end of the motoneuron only excitatory phenomena take place, but at the receiving end of the neuron– the receptive pole– both excitatory and inhibitory synaptic processes influence the polarisation state of the membrane. The integrated actions of motoneurons by synaptic inputs of spinal and supraspinal origin are of a complex origin. From quantitative histological data an estimate has been gained of the synaptic input of a motoneuron of an average size and an average dendritic tree. Taking into account that the percent of membrane covered by synaptic endings ranges from about 50% for the soma and the dendrites originating from the soma to about 30% for dendrites of a diameter of 1–2 μ one arrives at an average number of synapses for a human motoneuron of 25,000 to 35,000. These synapses are non-randomly distributed, which is of primary structural and functional significance, since the location of a given input within the receptive pole of the neuron determines its contribution to the integrative processes of motoneurons. Thus it has been shown that the synapses belonging to the proprioceptive input from the periphery together with the synapses belonging to the reticular descending tracts are located on the dendrites at some distance from the soma. On the other hand, the direct inhibitory input of supraspinal origin is confined to the soma. A number of important facts concerning the structure and function of the integrative properties of the final common pathway have thus emerged from recent investigations.

(1) The receptive or integrative part of the membrane of motoneurons is influenced by excitatory and inhibitory synaptic inputs, mediated through neurotransmitters. The neurotransmitter may belong to various classes of chemical substances: cholinergic, catecholaminergic, indolaminergic, etc.

(2) The input to a motoneuron shows a bewildering complexity, the arrangement of excitatory and inhibitory synaptic endings is generally nonrandom, many thousands of synapses may function at the same time.

(3) Each motoneuron is thus subjected to a multitude of influences, originating at spinal and supraspinal levels; the balance of the excitatory and inhibitory influences at the same time determines the membrane polarization and hence the excitability of the motoneuron. The final common path thus integrates in a simple way (adding and subtracting) the messages which impinge upon it.

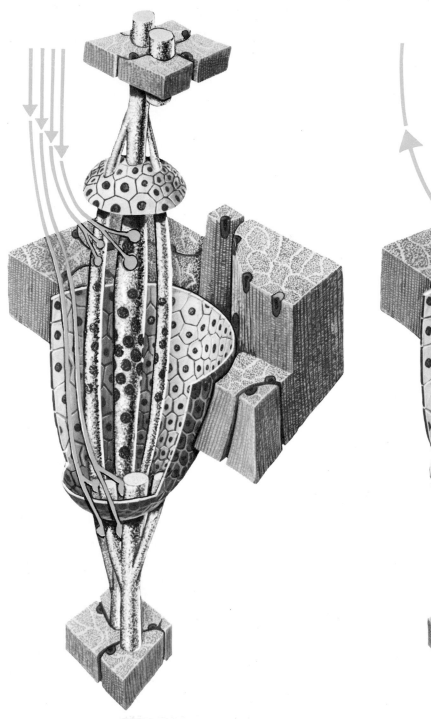

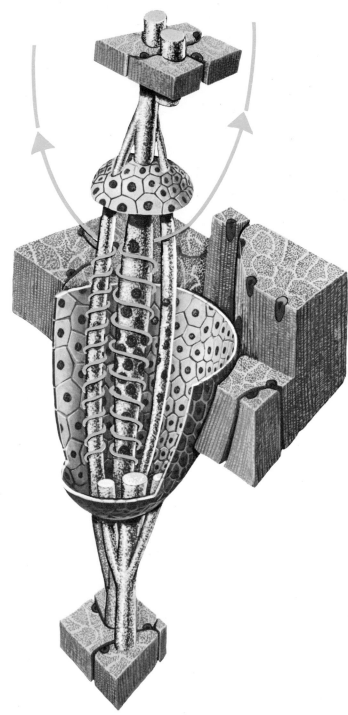

Fig. 163. Model of a typical muscle spindle (see Fig. 162). At the left is indicated the motor supply of the intrafusal fibers by endings of the γ-neurons.

Fig. 164. Primary sensory endings of the intrafusal fibers.

Even simple movements are deceptively complex in their underlying control mechanisms, since not only spinal and supraspinal processes determine the excitability state of the motoneuron, but also feed-back mechanisms from the motoneuron itself and from the sensory apparatus add information to the regulatory system. The many neuronal circuits serving an individual muscle are part of larger regulatory and feed-back networks serving a group of muscles. The striking feature is the multiplicity of pathways which converge on the motoneuron. Fig. 161 gives but a limited picture of this convergence for only part of the spinal inputs are shown, without an indication of the quantitative relationships and not taking into account the distribution of the synaptic inputs on the receptive surface of the motoneuron.

14.1.2 Sense organs of muscle and tendon

Figs. 162, 163, 164, 165. Two distinct sets of motoneurons innervate a striated muscle: The large α-neurons send messages to the extrafusal muscle fibers, whereas the small γ-neurons transmit action potentials to the intrafusal muscle fibers which are part of the muscle spindle.

This sensory apparatus – about 50 to 100 in each muscle – is a complex organ with afferent and efferent connections to the spinal cord. A typical spindle is made up of a number of intrafusal muscle fibers contained within a thick connective tissue sheath, expanded at the equator into a sac containing a lymphelike fluid. Generally a spindle consists of 6 intrafusal fibers, 2 large fibers with a thick equatorial part which is packed with nuclei (s1 fibers) and 4 small fibers (s2 intrafusal fibers) with a single chain of nuclei throughout the equatorial part. The intrafusal fibers are in mechanical parallel with the extrafusal fibers.

An extensive neuronal system transmits signals back and forth to the spinal cord. The sensory part of the system consists of primary and secondary fibers. The fibers of the primary neurons end in helical terminals that encircle the equatorial part of the s1-intrafusal fibers. Therefore, these endings are also known as annulospiral endings. The fibers of the secondary sensory neurons end in coils, rings and varicosities on the distal proximal poles of the intrafusal fibers. They are also called flower-spray endings. Both types of endings are so arranged that they can easily be mechanically distorted by stretch of the muscle.

The intrafusal fibers of the muscle spindle receive a motor supply from the spinal cord; the neurons end in endplates on both contractile poles of the intrafusal fibers. These endplates resemble the endplates on extrafusal fibers, with one exception: there is usually more than one endplate to an intrafusal fiber.

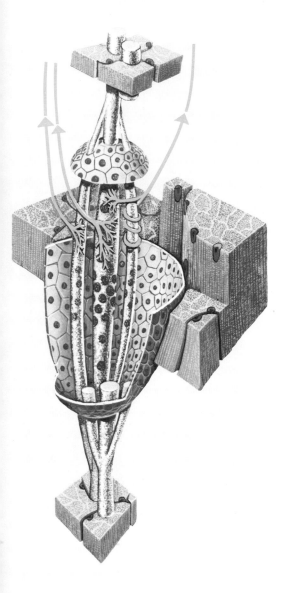

Fig. 165. Secondary sensory endings of the intrafusal fibers.

Thus the muscle spindle seems to be a highly organized sense organ by which muscle length can be said to be at the same time measured by the sensory system and controlled by the motor system. The sense organs of the muscle tell us of the moment to moment state of the muscle in respect to its tension and length, and there is also specific information on the relative length of the intrafusal and extrafusal muscle fibers.

The γ-system can be divided physiologically into a dynamic and a static part. The fibers belonging to the dynamic part of the system are able to increase the dynamic sensitivity of the primary sensory ending and do not usually modify the response of the secondary sensory ending. The neurons belonging to the static part of the system are able to increase the discharge of the primary sensory ending at constant length, but do not change the dynamic sensitivity of the ending. On the other hand, these fibers change greatly the discharge from the secondary sensory endings at constant length.

Fig. 166. The sense organ of the tendon has a relatively simple structure. The so-called Golgi-organ consists of numerous spray-like endings on the surface of a bundle of small tendon fascicles, the whole being enclosed in a delicate capsule. Tendon organs are in mechanical series with muscle fibers. This sense organ is not so fortunate as to have its own efferent nervous supply. However, this type of receptor will also be influenced by contraction of the muscle, and this will depend on the state of the muscle during contraction. The firing threshold of both types of sense organs differs considerably. In accordance with its structure the tendon organ is a stretch-sensitive unit; both active and passive contraction of the muscle causes the receptor to discharge.

The primary sensory endings rather than the tendon endings are the receptors for the myotatic or stretch reflex. The low threshold to muscle stretch of the primary ending, as opposed to the high threshold of the tendon organ, is a suggestive datum since the stretch reflex is elicited by exceedingly minute stretches.

Investigators and practising physicians concerned with the problems of patients with neurological deficits have become greatly interested in the function of the receptors in muscles and tendons. An important aspect is the observation that intramuscular injection of procain could abolish the exaggerated stretch reflexes of patients with hemiplegic spasticity. If a muscle is stretched in a hemiplegic patient, firing increases markedly in the antagonistic muscle. By injecting procain around the muscle the stretch reflex in the antagonistic muscle completely disappears, but the outburst of involuntary activity is as intense as before. This had led to the idea that the disordered function in spasticity is one of hyperactivity of the γ-neurons: the motor innervation of the muscle spindle.

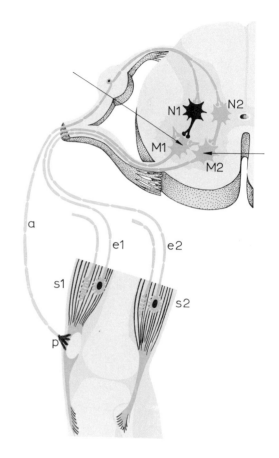

Fig. 166. Basic scheme of the neuronal circuit of a tendon organ (**p**). The afferent fiber (**a**) of the tendon organ makes synaptic contact via inhibitory interneurons (**N1**) and excitatory interneurons (**N2**) which synapse with motoneurons (**M1** and **M2**) respectively which innervate agonistic and antagonistic muscles (**s1** and **s2**).
e1 and **e2**, efferent fibers.

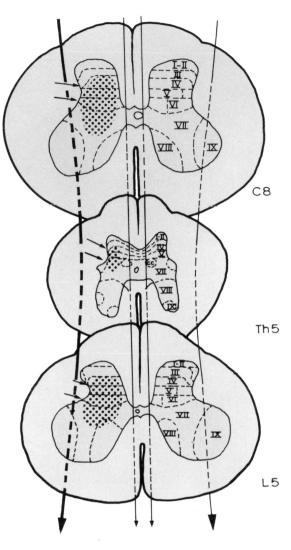

Fig. 167. Diagrammatic representation of the distribution of terminal fibers of the corticospinal tract from the primary sensory motor cortex (left side of figure). The Roman numerals in the right half of the grey matter refer to the laminae described by Rexed in the cat.

14.1.3 Supraspinal control system of the final common pathway

Fig. 167. The observations of Rexed that the grey matter of the spinal cord of the cat may be subdivided on a cytoarchitectonic basis into a number of laminae representing functionally different regions, have stimulated a more exact analysis of motor and sensory areas in the spinal cord. In the grey matter one can distinguish a primary sensory area (laminae I–IV) in which the fibers of the exteroceptive sense organs end, and a primary motor area (lamina IX) in which the efferent axons originate. Many other areas have an associative character, e.g. laminae V and VI which may be regarded as a reflex integration area, since here terminate the fibers of the proprioceptive sense organs and the lateral corticospinal tract.

It has become clear that the majority of fibers of the supraspinal pathways does not terminate directly on motoneurons, but that one or more interneurons are part of the system. In all major motor pathways spinal interneurons are intercalated, usually in the following way:

(a) in a pathway excitatory to extensor and inhibitory to flexor motoneurons, and

(b) in a pathway inhibitory to extensor and excitatory to flexor motoneurons.

These neurons are located within laminae V, VI and VII.

As far as the descending supraspinal pathways are concerned a lateral and a ventral system can be distinguished, located in the lateral and ventral funiculus respectively. The lateral system, made up of the lateral corticospinal, the rubrospinal and the medullo-reticulospinal tracts, give excitatory action on interneurons of spinal reflex paths. The endings of the lateral system are spatially closely related to the motoneurons which innervate the distal extremity musculature. These muscles are to a large extent concerned with phasic flexion movements.

The ventral system, made up mainly of the ponto-reticulospinal and vestibulospinal tracts, are spatially located to motoneurons innervating the proximal part of the extremity and the trunk muscles. These muscles are chiefly concerned with tonic extension movements. Recent microphysiological studies on animals have confirmed these morphological and macrophysiological investigations. Most of the fibers of the ventral system are found to convey impulses, primarily excitatory to extensor and inhibitory to flexor motoneurons, while the fibers of the lateral system chiefly exert the opposite effect on the spinal neurons. The ventral system thus contributes to the maintenance of postural tone and the lateral system exerts fascilatory influences on the flexor mechanisms and thus is instrumental in the performance of skilled voluntary movements.

14.1.4 The flow of information from sense organs to computing areas in the CNS

The cerebellum provides a great challenge to discern functional meaning in neuronal patterns, because there is such a beautiful geometrical arrangement of its unique neuronal constituents.

The cerebellum acts as a coordinating system for motor activities. It receives a continuous flow of signals a.o. from the spinal cord, the cerebral cortex and the vestibular nuclei. *Via* the spinal cord and brain stem it receives signals relayed from receptors in muscles, tendons, joints, the whole periphery of the body as well as from visual, auditory and vestibular end organs. This great volume of sensory input serves purely motor functions, chiefly regulatory in effect. The cerebellum is partly involved in the regulation of the stretch reflex and the background upon which phasic movements occur, particularly in relation to the motor control of the muscle spindles. This mechanism is part of a complex supraspinal feed-back system serving to regulate the length of muscle fibers upon integration of the multitude of signals of peripheral and central origin. There has been sufficient evidence from experimental and clinical data that the cerebellum acts as a position servomechanism.

Of particular importance is the way by which the continuous flow of signals from the receptors reaches the cerebellum. Since this latter part of the brain has no memory capacity of any size, the immediate information about length and tone of muscle fibers should provide the background activity necessary for unvoluntary movements. The cerebellum has in this respect a double function; as a monitor it watches every movement, and as computer it calculates all parameters for this movement.

Signals from the musculoskeletal apparatus reach the cerebellum by various pathways. Generally the dorsal spinocerebellar tract transmits information from muscle spindles to the ipsilateral side of the anterior lobe of the cerebellum. Only one tract fiber is engaged in transmitting signals from muscle and tendon receptors of a restricted group of muscles. This tract carries information of movement position of a whole limb. The ventral spinocerebellar tract relays signals from tendon organs of large groups of muscles. Also the olivocerebellar tract provides a major pathway by which information from muscle receptors reaches the cerebellum.

It is generally believed that the cerebellum functions as a type of computer that is particularly concerned with the smooth and effective control of movement. The cerebellum integrates and organizes the information flowing into it from the spinal cord, vestibular nuclei, reticular formation and cerebral cortex, and the consequent cerebellar output goes to major motor centers and so participates in the control of movement. It is therefore not surprising that a disturbance of the major flow of information from the spinal cord to the cerebellum leads to ataxias.

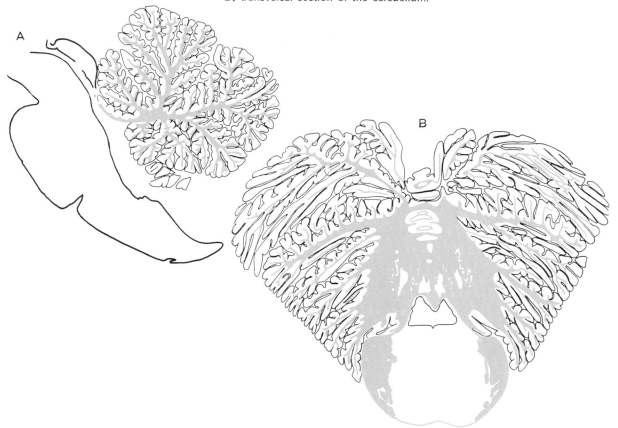

Fig. 168. Impulses conducted in the spinocerebellar tracts reach the cerebellar cortex which, due to folding, has a very large surface.
A, sagittal section of the cerebellum;
B, transversal section of the cerebellum.

14.2 The cerebellum

14.2.1 Cellular organization

Fig. 168. The cerebellum consists of many long parallel folia which are alike in structure. The inner part (green) of each folium is made up of myelinated fibers running to and from the cerebellar cortex.

Figs. 169, 170. The grey mantle of each folium consists of three layers (*cf.* Fig. 81, p. 92). The inner region or granular layer contains closely packed cellular elements: granule cells. It has been estimated that the packing density is more than 2 million granule cells per mm² in the monkey cerebellar cortex. In the human this figure ranges from 3 to 5 million cells per mm². The second region consists of a single layer of large nerve cells: the Purkinje neurons. The external portion of the grey mantle is known as the molecular or plexiform layer, for it contains relatively few nerve cells and it is a synaptic region, rich in dendritic ramifications and terminal axonal networks.

The mossy and climbing fibers are the afferents to the cerebellar cortex. The terminals of the mossy fibers are clasped by the claw-shaped dendrites of the granule cells. The climbing fibers run in a climbing-like pattern on the Purkinje cell's smooth branches, forming longitudinal axo-dendritic connections. These fibers also make connections with the cell bodies of Golgi cells.

The dendritic system of the *Purkinje neuron* – the central integrator of the cerebellum – arises from the summit of the pear-shaped cell body and spreads out in the molecular layer in a leaf-shaped formation with dimensions of 350 × 350 × 50 μ. Primary, secondary and tertiary branches with numerous spines form the basic structural substrate of the receiving pole of the Purkinje cell. An enormous number of spine-laden terminal branches sprout from the mentioned smooth branches.

The *stellate cells* (**g**) are also found in the molecular layer and their dendrites radiate in the transverse direction of the folium. The axons of the *basket cells* (**c**) cross transversely just above the Purkinje cell layer and give off ascending longitudinal and descending collaterals. The latter form complicated nests or baskets about the Purkinje cell bodies and terminate mostly on the Purkinje cells axonic cones. The basket cells exert their influence on a rectangular patch of Purkinje cells, about 20 cells in a transverse direction, and about 12 cells in a longitudinal direction.

The *Golgi cells* are located in the granular layer, usually near the Purkinje cells. Their dendrites ramify in the molecular layer and their axons break up immediately into dense plexuses permeating the granular layer and terminating as delicate nestlike endings. The presynaptic terminals synapse with the claw-shaped dendrites of the granule cells.

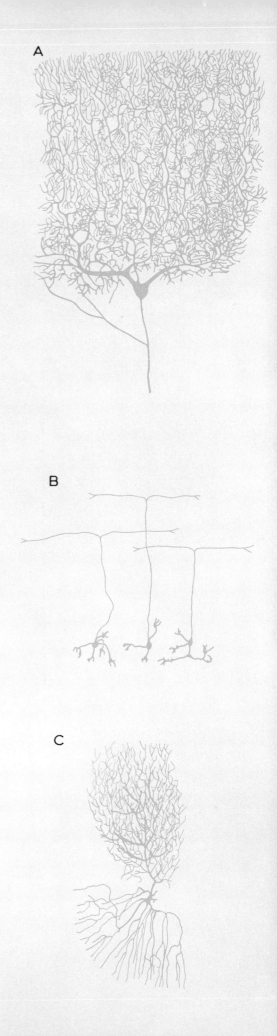

Fig. 169. Types of cerebellar neurons. **A**, Purkinje cell; **B**, granule cell; **C**, Golgi cell.

Each *granule cell* (**a**) has 3 to 6 slender dendrites that terminate in claw-like formations. The axon proceeds to the molecular layer where it bifurcates T-shaped. These bifurcating fibers, the parallel fibers, run longitudinally in the folium. The inferior thicker parallel fibers are about 3 mm in length and the superior thinner parallel fibers are about 1 mm in length.

14.2.2 The input channels

(a) *Mossy fibers*. The white matter of a folium contains the in- and output channels of the cerebellar cortex. The mossy fiber system (**d**) and the climbing fiber system (**h**) are two separate input-channels. The various types of neurons in the grey mantle take care of the processing of the information, while the axons of the Purkinje cell transmit the processed information to the other parts of the central nervous system. The mossy fibers are quantitatively the most important input channel and they bring information into the cerebellar cortex from four main sources: the vestibular system, the spinal cord, the reticular formation and the cerebral cortex.

The fibers from the *vestibular nuclei* convey information from receptors in the labyrinth. They inform the computing area of the cerebellum about acceleration of the head and its position in space. A number of separate pathways convey signals from the *spinal cord* to the cerebellar cortex. The fibers which make up these tracts are essentially those from second order neurons, *i.e.* neurons not directly connected to the receptors of the peripheral apparatus. Most of these pathways show a somatotopic pattern which means that fibers conveying information from adjacent regions of the body go to adjacent regions of the cerebellar cortex, resulting in a map of the body's periphery on the cerebellar surface. In the anterior lobe of the cerebellum the body is inverted: the representation of the hind limb is most anterior whereas that of the fore limb and head are more posterior. In the map on the paramedian lobules the body is oriented in a direction opposite to that in the anterior map.

Another mossy fiber system is made up of axons arising from cells in the basis pontis, which relay information from the cerebral cortex. In man, many fibers from the temporal and frontal regions of the cerebral cortex terminate on these nuclei in the pons. However, also fibers from the corticospinal and corticonuclear tracts give off collaterals to the pontine nuclei as they pass through. Through these collaterals, the cerebellar cortex is continuously informed about the influence that the cerebral cortex is exerting on the motor nuclei in the spinal cord and brain stem.

The projections from the *reticular formation* to the cerebellar cortex are rather diffuse and the entire cerebellar cortex receives fibers. These fibers come mainly from the lateral, the paramedian and the ponto-tegmental nuclei of the reticular formation.

In addition to these four major mossy fiber inputs there are several

Fig. 170. A, half folium of the cerebellar cortex with a.o. a Purkinje neuron, climbing fibers and granule cells.
a, granule cell; **b,** Purkinje cell; **d,** mossy fibers; **f,** Purkinje cell, side view; **h,** climbing fiber.

TABLE 6

MOSSY FIBER AND CLIMBING FIBER PATHWAYS IN CEREBELLAR CORTEX

	Excitatory			*Inhibitory*	
	Di-vergence number	*Con-vergence number*		*Di-vergence number*	*Con-vergence number*
Mossy fibers ↓ Granule cells	600	4	Mossy fibers ↓ Granule cells	600	4
Parallel fibers ↓ Purkinje cells	300	250 000	Parallel fibers ↓ Basket cells	~30	~20 000
Climbing fibers ↓ Purkinje cells	~10	1	Basket cell axons ↓ Purkinje cells	~50	20

other tracts of unknown function which also contribute to the mossy fiber system. It has been shown that auditory and visual stimulation have an influence on the excitability state of neurons in certain parts of the cerebellar cortex.

Climbing fiber system. Although there is still some confusion about the interpretation of degeneration studies, it is almost certain that the inferior olive is a major source of climbing fibers. The work of Brodal shows that there is a point-to-point mapping of the inferior olive on to the cerebellar surface, and that fibers from different parts of the brainstem and higher parts of the nervous system go on to different parts of the olive.

In order to delineate the significance of the two input channels, some quantitative data are of importance. As is shown in table 6, the mossy fiber channel is characterized by an enormous divergence, and it has both excitatory and inhibitory actions on Purkinje cells. In contrast, the climbing fiber channel is very restricted in its distribution. Each Purkinje neuron receives synapses from only one climbing fiber which exerts such a powerful excitatory action that the Purkinje cell responds by a brief repetitive discharge at high frequency.

Although it may seem remarkable that the Purkinje neurons receive two quite different inputs, it should be realized that these two channels convey information from approximately the same peripheral receptors. Moreover, the pathways from any particular zone of these receptors have an approximately concurrent distribution of climbing fibers and mossy fiber input to the cerebellar cortex.

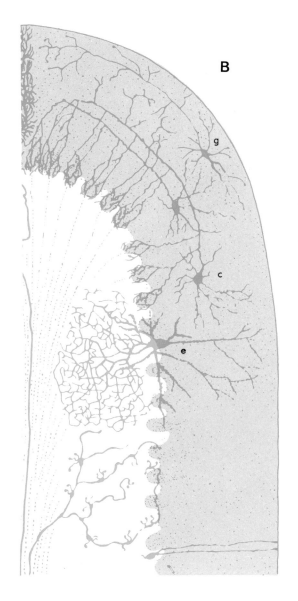

Fig. 170. B, half folium of cerebellar cortex with a.o. **c,** basket cell; **e,** Purkinje cell; **g,** stellate cell.

14.2.3 The output channels

Histological and electrophysiological investigations of the past decade have led to the surprising conclusion that the entire output of the cerebellar cortex is by way of the axons of the Purkinje cells and that this output is inhibitory. The terminations of the axons of the Purkinje cell release an inhibitory transmitter: gamma-aminobutyric acid (GABA). The transmitting part of these cells makes synaptic contacts with neurons located in the deep cerebellar nuclei and in the vestibular nuclei. The axons leaving the flocculus project exclusively to the vestibular nuclei, while all other areas of the cerebellar cortex project to both systems.

The connections between the Purkinje axons and the various nuclei are rather complex. Some of these relationships are somatotopically organized. This is the case with axons from the Purkinje cells in the vermis of the anterior lobe and of the pyramis which end in the lateral vestibular nucleus. It has been shown that fibers from the fore-limb and hind-limb regions of the anterior lobe of the cerebellum end in appropriate portions of the lateral vestibular nucleus.

Fig. 171. Pattern of output channels from the cerebellar cortex.
1, hemisphere; **2**, intermediate; **3**, vermis; **4**, dentate nucleus; **5**, nucleus interpositus; **6**, fastigial nucleus; **7**, nucleus thalami ventrolateralis; **8**, red nucleus; **9**, vestibular nuclei; **10**, reticular formation; **11**, motor cortex; **12**, motoneuron pool.

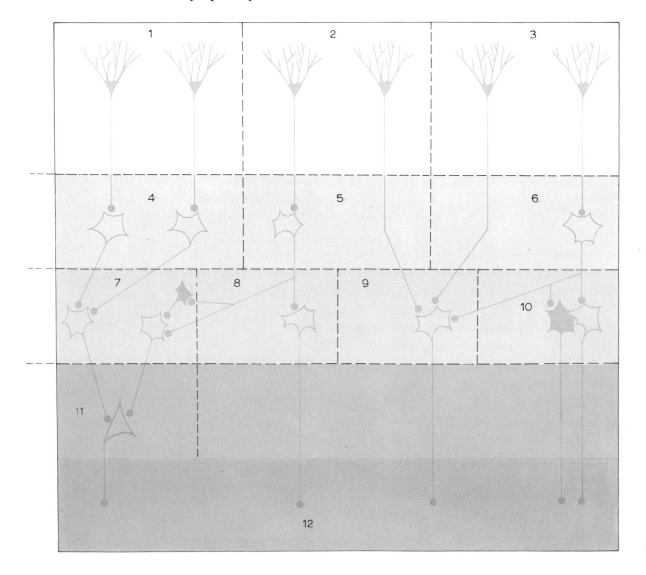

In addition to a direct route from the cerebellar cortex to the vestibular nucleus, there is also an indirect route. Axons from Purkinje cells go to a cerebellar nucleus from which a second set of neurons send their axons to the lateral vestibular nuclei.

Fig. 171. Scheme of the pattern of output channels from the cerebellar cortex through the deep cerebellar nuclei and the nuclei in the brain stem to the motor neurons. As can be seen from the scheme, the cerebellum does not affect the motor outflow directly, but does influence powerfully those cells which do. Fibers from the cerebellum make synaptic contacts with cells of origin of the vestibulospinal, the reticulospinal, and the rubrospinal tracts. Apparently, the action of the Purkinje neurons is to inhibit, or more exactly, to remove excitation from the neurons, giving rise to the descending and ascending fibers. The Purkinje neurons are inhibitory, the cells of the next stage are in general excitatory.

14.2.4 Computing properties of the cerebellar cortex

Speculation concerning the cerebellar function can be found in some of the earliest writings on the brain, since for more than a century physicians have recognized a group of clinical signs which are related to the control of motor activity as characteristic of cerebellar damage. An individual who suffers from damage of the cerebellum walks akwardly with feet well apart, and has difficulties in maintaining his balance.

With micro-electrode investigations in the past decades a vast amount of knowledge has been accumulated on the function of the cerebellar neurons. It is now generally believed that the cerebellum functions as a type of computer that is particularly concerned with the smooth and effective control of movement. It does not hold information for any length of time. There are no maintained information loops going around. It seems that the cerebellum only computes ongoing effects of movements. It is not programming, but purely servile and the initiative for control is elsewhere; it only modifies the timing or instructions of movements as the latter develops. The cerebellar neurons and networks do not have a memory function, but throughout life we learn how to use to the utmost the capabilities of this structure.

Figs. 172, 173, 174. Various neuronal elements and their specific task in the cerebellar circuitry.

(a) *Granule cell* and *parallel fiber*. The excitability state of the Purkinje cells is influenced by the granule cells in two various ways. The mossy fibers exert an excitatory effect upon the granule cells which discharge impulses along their axons–the parallel fibers–that make excitatory synaptic connections with Purkinje cells. The mossy fibers also exert an excitatory influence *via* the granule cells to basket cells which give a dense array of inhibitory synapses on the cell bodies of Purkinje neurons.

The parallel fibers, conducting action potentials with a speed of about 0.3 m/sec, make synaptic contacts with Purkinje, basket, stellate, and

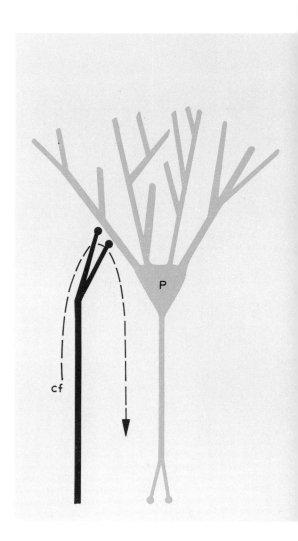

Fig. 172. Part of the cerebellar circuit. The broken line indicates the direction of the signals.
cf = climbing fiber; **P** = Purkinje cell.

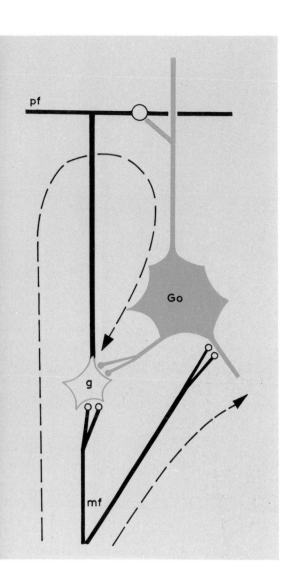

Fig. 173. Part of the cerebellar circuit. The broken line indicates the direction of the signals.

mf, mossy fiber; **g**, granule cell; **Go**, Golgi cell; **pf**, parallel fiber.

Golgi cells. The superficial fibers are thinner (ca. 0.1 μ) than the lower ones (about 1 μ). Since the superficial fibers have a lower conduction velocity, this difference in diameter may serve a temporal dispersion in impulses reaching the dendritic tree. The parallel fibers do not cross in passing along the folium and do retain their spatial relationship to each other.

(b) *Golgi cell*. The Golgi cell, some 150,000 in the human cerebellum, has dendrites in both the granular and molecular layer, the latter being contacted by parallel fibers. Collaterals of climbing fibers and recurrent collaterals of Purkinje cells make synaptic contacts with the cell body of Golgi cells. The Golgi cells participate in a recurrent inhibitory circuit of the granule cells.

(c) *Basket cell*. The cell bodies are located in the lower part of the molecular layer. The dendritic tree is oriented in the plane of the molecular layer as is that of the Purkinje cell. Only a small proportion of the parallel fibers makes synaptic contact with the dendritic tree of the basket cell. The axons of the basket cell form a dense plexus about the axon hillock and initial segment of the Purkinje cell axon. The activity of the basket cells inhibits the Purkinje cells.

(d) *Stellate cell*. The cell bodies are located in the outer part of the molecular layer. The axons of these small cells end on the smooth branches of the Purkinje dendrites, where they exert an inhibitory action.

(e) *Purkinje cell*. Each Purkinje neuron is bombarded by a large fraction of the 250,000 or so excitatory influences from parallel fibers and by a very powerful convergent inhibitory activity from about 20 basket cells. There is sufficient neurophysiological evidence to assume that the input by the mossy fiber system is sharply focussed by its negative feed-back pathway through Golgi cells. In this way, impulses will travel in parallel fibers in a beam for about 3 mm length. The basket cells will be excited by this beam and in turn will give lateral inhibition of extending Purkinje cells about 1 mm at either side of the folium.

The excitatory signals, transmitted by the mossy fiber system, are thus transported *via* the granule cells to inhibitory neurons which all contribute to the spatio-temporal organization of the output signal of the cerebellar cortex. The information in the output channel of the cerebellar cortex transmitted to the neurons of the deep cerebellar or vestibular nuclei is inhibitory in nature. These latter neurons, however, also receive excitatory inputs from collaterals of the climbing and mossy fibers. The Purkinje cell exerts an inhibitory influence upon the background excitation, so producing spatio-temporal forms in the pattern of firing of these neurons.

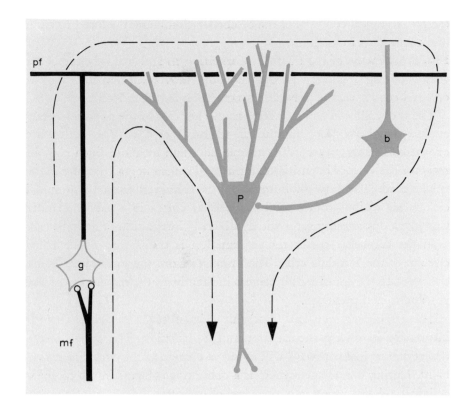

Fig. 174. Part of the cerebellar circuit. The broken line indicates the direction of the signals.
mf, mossy fiber; **g,** granule cell; **pf,** parallel fiber; **P,** Purkinje cell; **b,** basket cell.

The inhibitory action within the cerebellar cortex is the exclusive task of the Golgi, basket and stellate cells. Axon collaterals of the Purkinje cell also have a subsidiary task of exercising an inhibitory action within the cerebellar cortex.

The exclusive transformation of all input into inhibition with at most two synaptic relays gives the cerebellar cortex a dead-beat character in its response to input. It has been shown by Eccles and Llinás[117, 118] and coworkers that some 20 msec. after a given input there will be no further evoked discharges in the cortical neurons. By 100 msec. even the excitatory and inhibitory postsynaptic potentials will have faded and that area of the cerebellar cortex will have been cleared of all disturbance by the initial input. This region of the cerebellum will then be in an unbiased state for the computing of a new input. This has led to the statement that the cerebellum does not hold information for any length of time, but only computes ongoing effects of movement.

14.2.5 Dynamic cerebellar loops

We owe the bulk of the neurophysiological data about the operation of the cerebellum to Eccles and Llinás and coworkers. They have provided

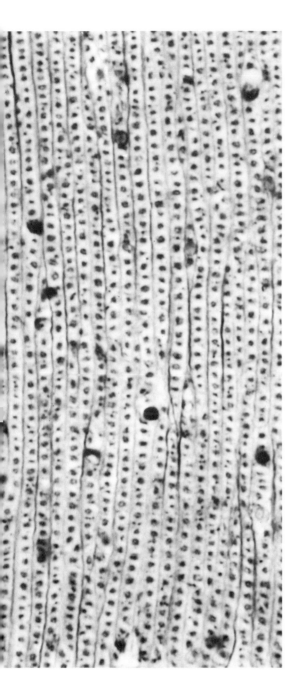

Fig. 175. Regular matrix formed by the parallel fibers and the dendritic branches of the Purkinje cell.

the physiological concepts of the cerebellar circuit and the interpretation of a more global function.

Fig. 176. Scheme of the flow of information to and from the cerebellar cortex during the carrying out of some movement initiated by the cerebral cortex, *via* the pyramidal tract. (Adapted from Eccles.)

The movement initiated in response to activity in the pyramidal tract evokes the discharge of impulses in various receptors. These latter are organized in subsets according to modality and location. Each class of receptor has various intensities of input, and some integrated center in the spinal cord. The flow of information is conveyed from these spinal centers *via* various routes to the cerebellar cortex in a patchy manner that gives opportunity for a widely differing integration of actions.

In the cerebellar cortex the information is transferred *via* neuronal circuits to the Purkinje cells. The impulses from the Purkinje cells are conveyed to the spinal motor centers indirectly *via* the reticulospinal and vestibulospinal pathways.

The cerebellar cortex is also organized in subsets and each of them is integrating its own particular inputs of information. The signals in the descending spinal pathways will induce a change in the evolving movement. During a movement there is a continuous change in the receptor activity and the input into the cerebellar cortex is also continuously revised and in turn gives corrective information *via* the descending spinal pathways. This is a perfect example of a dynamic loop control of an evolving movement by feed-back systems up to the cerebellar cortex. In this respect it is important to realize that in the resting state there is a background activity in all the pathways and neuronal aggregates of this dynamic system, and that the evolving movement merely decreases or increases the ongoing activity. The scheme only shows a part of the total system, *e.g.* there also exist reciprocal connections between the pyramidal tract and the Purkinje cells of the contralateral cerebellar hemisphere. In the cerebello-cerebral control loop the flow of information is also conveyed from the cerebellum *via* the thalamus to the motor areas of the cerebrum. The extensive connections with the vestibular system and reticular formation are not indicated.

In summary, it can be stated that there are three areas at which integration of a movement mechanism may occur: in the cerebral cortex with expression in the excitability state of the pyramidal neuron, in the cerebellar cortex with expression in the excitability state of the Purkinje cell, and in the spinal cord with expression in the motoneuron discharge.

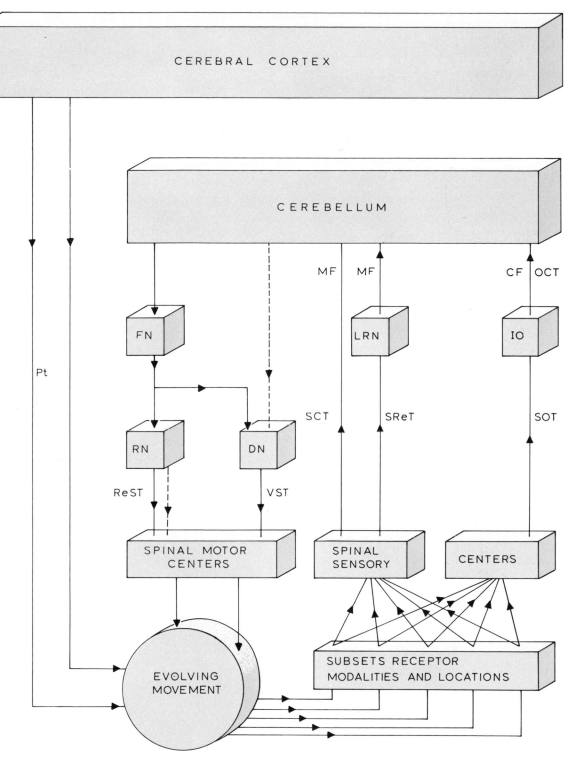

Fig. 176. Diagram showing in detail the pathways involved in the cerebellospinal and cerebrospinal circuits, the continuous and dotted lines showing respectively the excitatory and inhibitory neural pathways.

CF, climbing fibers; **DN,** Deiters' nucleus; **FN,** fastigial nucleus; **IO,** inferior olive; **LRN,** lateral reticular nucleus; **MF,** mossy fibers; **OCT,** olivocerebellar tract; **RN,** reticular nucleus; **ReST,** reticulospinal tract; **SCT,** spinocerebellar tracts; **SOT,** spino-olivary tract; **VST,** vestibulospinal tract; **Pt,** pyramidal tract.

14.3 The thalamus

Fig. 177. An old saying tells us that in the thalamus lie the keys to the secrets of the cerebral cortex. Classical histological investigations reveal conglomerations of nerve cells having a fairly homogeneous appearance and fiber pathways entering and leaving the thalamus. Fiber pathways include both thalamic projections to the cortex and cortical projections to the thalamus, the latter parallelling the thalamo-cortical system. The afferent and efferent relations of the thalamus clearly indicate a relay function for many, if not all, sensory systems. In agreement with the anatomical findings impulses, *e.g.* from cutaneous nerves, and afferent signals initiated by tactile and joint stimulation, produce potential changes in specific regions of the contralateral thalamus.

In the past decade many data have been compiled on postsynaptic inhibitory events in nuclear aggregates of the thalamus. Recently evidence has been obtained for a role of presynaptic inhibition in some specific relay activities. Andersen and coworkers[2] have performed a series of very elegant experiments which elucidate the significance of these inhibitory mechanisms. This short summary of the thalamic relay functions is primarily based on their data.

14.3.1 Thalamic interneuronal activity

Investigations with micro-electrodes have revealed that in addition to the thalamocortical relay cells (so-called TCR-neurons) there are in many regions of the thalamus interneurons (I) that are responsible for

Fig. 177. A, localization of the thalamus in the brain; **B**, scheme of the main nuclei of the thalamus.
1, right pulvinar; **2**, left pulvinar; **3**, medial geniculate body; **4**, lateral geniculate body; **5**, posterolateral ventral nucleus; **6**, anterior ventral nucleus.

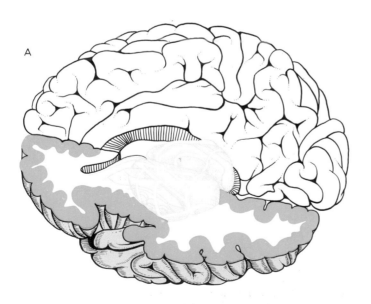

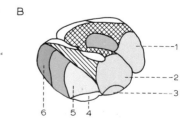

the production of inhibitory postsynaptic potentials. Apparently the thalamus does not act as a simple relay system, but the flow of information in the sensory pathway will be modulated on its way to the cerebral cortex.

Figs. 178, 179. Two types of interneurons (I) are intercalated in the relay pathway. Fig. 178 shows the pathway for postsynaptic inhibition: the axon collaterals of TCR-cells are seen to excite both TCR-cells and the postsynaptic inhibitory cells. In Fig. 179 branches of the afferent thalamic fibers (**a**) excite the presynaptic inhibitory interneurons which provide for axonal projection toward the TCR neurons to produce presynaptic inhibition at x of the thalamic afferents.

An important micro-physiological finding was the observation that many TCR-cells show a cyclic discharge pattern. Upon stimulation a short burst of action potentials is seen, followed by a large and long lasting hyperpolarization due to inhibitory postsynaptic activity.

These observations have significantly contributed to our understanding of the so-called spontaneous waves–the electroencephalogram–which can be recorded from the intact skull of man and animal.

Fig. 178. Neuronal pathway in the thalamus.
a, thalamic afferent; **TCR**, thalamocortical relay cell; **I**, interneuron, responsible for the production of inhibitory postsynaptic potentials.

Fig. 179. Thalamic pathway.
a, thalamic afferent; **TCR**, thalamocortical relay cell; **I1** and **I2**, interneurons responsible for the production of presynaptic inhibition at **x**.

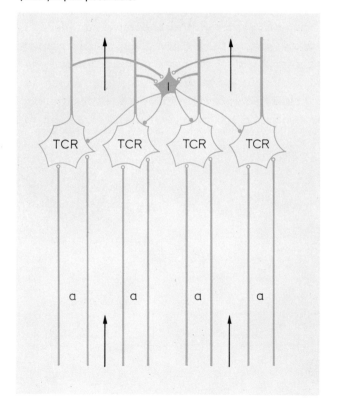

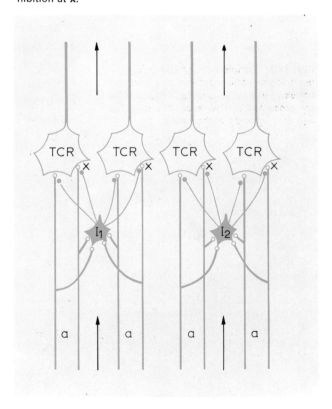

14.3.2 Interpretation of α-waves

There are some main problems concerning the interpretation of the alpha waves of the electroencephalogram. These are the basis for the remarkably constant rhythm of about 10/sec shown by the waves and the nature of the electromotive force generating the electroencephalographic waves themselves.

Figs. 180, 181. Ten per second spontaneous waves of undulating amplitude can only be recorded from the thalamus and the cortex. There is no doubt that the thalamic rhythmic activity is of essential importance for the cortical 10/sec activity. The experimental analysis of the alpha rhythm has been greatly facilitated by the presence of a similar activity in barbiturate anaesthetized animals. This activity takes the form of spindle-like formations of about 10/sec sinusoidal activity, lasting from 1-2 sec. These periods are called barbiturate spindles. Similar activity can be seen in drowsy humans and also in humans slightly anaesthetized with barbiturates. It is, therefore, probable that the animal spindle activity is homologous with the human alpha rhythm.

Since the cortical activity is abolished by removal of the thalamus or by cutting of the thalamocortical fibres, whereas the thalamic spindle activity remains unaltered after cortical removal, the thalamic rhythmic activity is apparently the prime mover, driving the cortical rhythm. This assumption is strengthened by the finding that local cooling depresses the amplitude but not the frequency of the spindle activity.

By simultaneous recording from various thalamic nuclei and different cortical areas, it has been possible to show that a given thalamic area is in fully synchrony with a small part of the cortex. This cortical region corresponds exactly to that point to which the thalamic region in question projects. Since rhythmic activity has been found in virtually all thalamic nuclei, the association and projection nuclei each seem to

Fig. 180. Spindle activity (**S**) in 2 of 3 recordings, obtained from the cerebral cortex of a conscious rabbit. The spindles are presented in the recordings **a** and **c** and they appear synchronously.

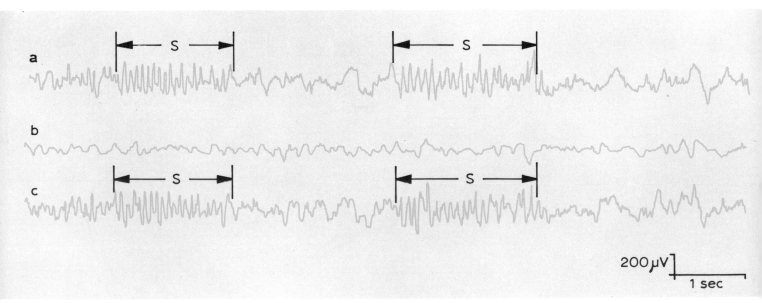

200 µV

1 sec

command one private area of the cortex. In contrast, the intralaminar and medial nuclei only seem to have direct effect at a thalamic level.

In the thalamic nuclear complex, no particular area preponderates over others in starting rhythmic activity. In other words, there is no obvious pacemaker as judged by multiple micro-electrode recordings. On the other hand, several thalamic areas have the capability of starting rhythmic activity by themselves. Although the midline and intralaminar nuclei have been proposed to act as a general pacemaker for human alpha activity as well, this theory can no longer be upheld in its original form. Complete removal by suction of the entire midline and intralaminar nuclei leaves the frontal cortical spindle activity completely unaltered. However, restricted lesions in the appropriate projection nucleus give a remarkable change in the spindle activity, exactly similar to that produced by ordinary deafferentiation. The main substrate of the bar-biturate spindle activity, therefore, seems to be the specific and not the unspecific thalamocortical system. Obviously, this theory does not deny the possibility that intralaminar and medial thalamic nuclei may modify the activity of other thalamic nuclei. In fact, many data seem to indicate that this happens during states of synchronization and desynchronization produced by midline thalamic stimulation.

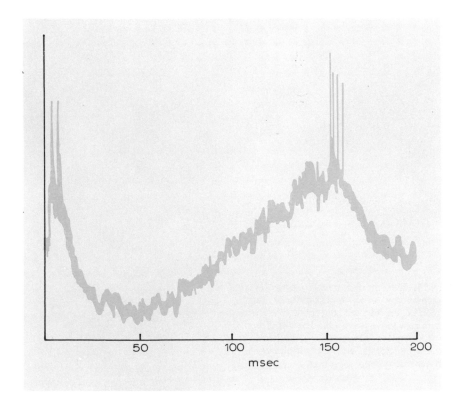

Fig. 181. Typical recording from a thalamic neuron showing a long inhibition. (after Andersen.)

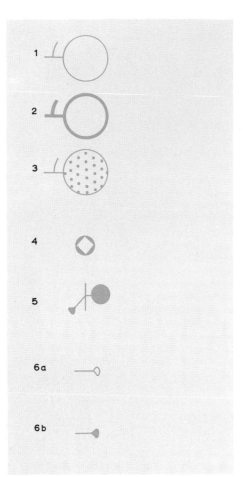

Fig. 182

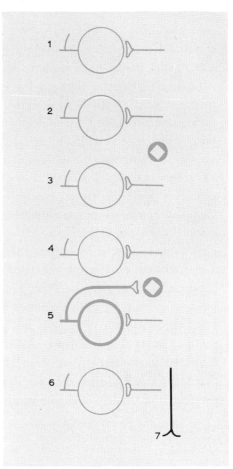

Fig. 183

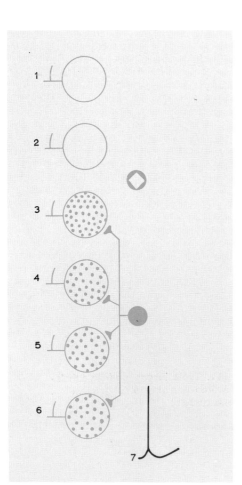

Fig. 184

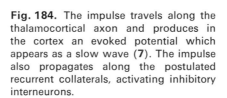

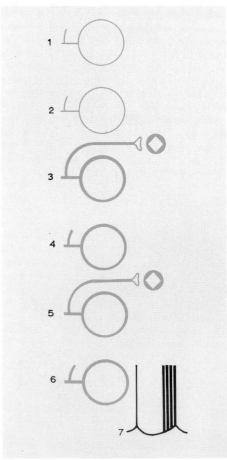

Fig. 185

Fig. 182. This and the following figures show a diagrammatic representation of the inhibitory phasing theory illustrating various stages during the development of the thalamic spindle. (After Andersen.) This figure gives an explanation of the various symbols: **1,** resting projection cell; **2,** discharging projection cell; **3,** inhibited projection cell; **4,** resting inhibitory interneuron; **5,** discharging inhibitory interneuron; **6a,** excitatory synapse; **6b,** inhibitory synapse.

Fig. 183. A thalamic spindle may start by a discharge of any neuron of a thalamic group, in this example neuron **5**. The resulting potential is indicated in **7**.

Fig. 184. The impulse travels along the thalamocortical axon and produces in the cortex an evoked potential which appears as a slow wave (**7**). The impulse also propagates along the postulated recurrent collaterals, activating inhibitory interneurons.

Fig. 185. Following the long lasting IPSP that is produced in a number of neighbouring cells by the inhibitory interneuron (cells **3** to **6** in Fig. **184**) these cells will be in a state of postinhibitory increased excitation.

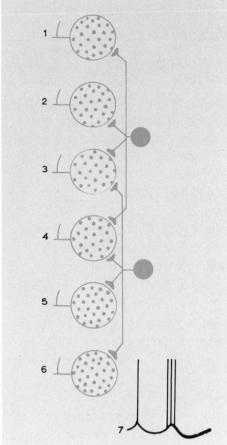

Fig. 186

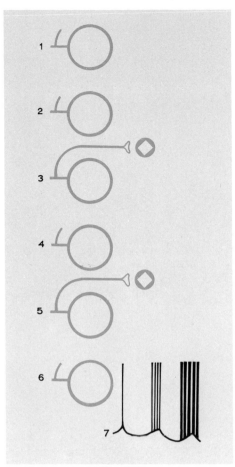

Fig. 187

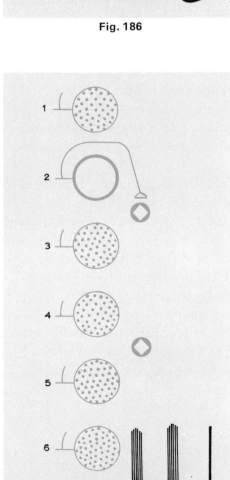

Fig. 188

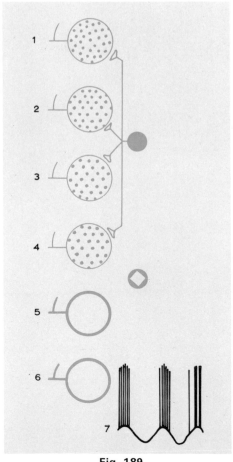

Fig. 189

Fig. 186. A large number of inhibitory neurons is activated in the second cycle, thereby expanding the number of thalamic projection cells that are inhibited.

Fig. 187. Subsequently, large IPSP's are produced in all 6 cells which again will be subject to a postinhibitory depolarization, and subsequent burst discharges.

Fig. 188. This figure shows a possible way by which the synchronous spindle activity may be disrupted. One of the neurons is firing prematurely, *i.e.* some time before the anticipated burst discharge of the major group of cells.

Fig. 189. The tendency to create more groups of neurons following their own rhythm will increase until a stage of low regularity is again attained.
(Figs. 182–189 according to Andersen; legends according to Andersen and Andersson: *Physiological Basis of the α-Rhythm*. Appleton–Century–Crofts, New York, 1969.)

14.3.3 Intrinsic mechanism of thalamic rhythmic activity

Figs. 182–189. A closer analysis of the rhythmic thalamic 10/sec activity has revealed the mechanism responsible for the rhythmic discharges. Through a comparison with the 10/sec rhythmic thalamic discharges which follow a single afferent volley through the medial lemniscus, it has been possible to unravel the mechanism behind the spontaneous 10/sec activity as well. After the initial excitation by a medial lemniscal volley, the thalamic ventro-basal cells undergo a large and prolonged inhibition. Since this inhibition can be mimicked by antidromic excitation of cells by stimulation of the white matter after cortical removal, the inhibition is of a recurrent inhibitory nature. Following this large and long-lasting (100 msec) postsynaptic recurrent inhibition, the cells undergo a stage of increased excitation. In fact, the cells very often show a phase of increased excitability as compared with the normal non-stimulated level. This increased excitability is signalled by a marked depolarization, often leading to a discharge of a series of spikes. Since the thalamic neurons are subject to a recurrent inhibition, a new inhibition will ensue. Thus, the process will repeat itself in a cyclic manner from 3 to 20 times.

Even without afferent stimulation, the cells undergo a series of cyclic excitability changes that apparently occur spontaneously. During such a series, the sequence of events is exactly similar to that produced by a single afferent volley. The process starts completely at random. A discharge of a given cell will produce inhibition in some surrounding neurons. When these neurons return from their hyperpolarization, some of them will be in a hyper-excitable state which will lead to the discharge of impulses as a post-inhibitory rebound phenomenon. The rebound discharge will lead to a new inhibition of the surrounding cells, this time of a greater number than the first time. In this way, the process will spread from a small to a larger number of cells through the wide distribution of the recurrent inhibition.

When the process is at its full stage, it will start to decay because of slight interference with the rhythm due to the uneven duration of the inhibition in various cells in the population. After some 5–30 cycles, the neurons are back to random firing.

Since the thalamic cells are coupled to various small cortical areas, the discharge of the thalamic cells will lead to a repeated 10/sec thalamo-cortical volley which in turn will create the corticographic waves. Thus, the rhythm seems to be dependent upon a peculiar property that the thalamic neurons have almost exclusively for themselves. It depends upon a widely distributed and strong recurrent inhibition that will lead to post-inhibitory rebound discharges.

14.4 The cerebral cortex

14.4.1 Introduction

A number of complex functions are attributed to the cerebral cortex, ranging from the faculties of mind to the command of motoneurons. Although a detailed investigation of both ultrastructure and function has provided a wealth of data we are still far from solving the sensation–perception mechanisms. The morphological and functional cartography of the cerebral cortex have been discussed in the anatomy section of this book. These data have provided a rough scheme of the organization of the cerebral cortex and have been a useful tool for clinicians to determine the localization of neurological disturbances.

By attributing such functions as the faculties of mind to this brain region we must first ask ourselves whether the cellular elements of the grey mantle of the forebrain are in any respect different from the neurons in other parts of the central nervous system. This statement holds for both the structural and functional characteristics of cortical neurons. The opinions about the structural organizations have ranged from a randomly connected aggregation of cells to an exquisitely ordered arrangement. In comparison with other cortical structures such as the cerebellar cortex and the hippocampus, we do not observe in the cerebral cortex the very regular arrangements of cell types and fiber bundles. There even exists a great variation in the detailed cellular and fiber arrangements from one cortical area to another. It seems unlikely that this variability has anything to do with the specific function of the different cortical regions.

Figs. 190, 191, 192, 193. The neurons in the cortex can be classified into pyramidal, stellate and fusiform cells. These three types, when the axons are taken into account, include both Golgi type I and Golgi type II cells. Only a small percentage of cells does not fall into one of these categories. Pyramidal cells make up about 60 to 70% and stellate cells about 20 to 25% of the cell population. A pyramidal cell is defined as a neuron possessing a conical perikaryon with in general one apical and many basal dendrites. The apical dendrite is directed towards the pial surface, usually at a right angle. The basal dendrites originate from the basal angles and from the surface of the perikaryon and extend horizontally or obliquely upward and downwards. The basal dendritic field usually extends in a half sphere in the center of which the perikaryon is localized. The ramifications of the apical dendrites extend roughly into a cone, the base of which is directed towards the pial surface. The dendritic surface is enlarged by small evaginations or spines which are also the places of synaptic contact. The dendrites of a stellate cell extend in all directions and the surface of the branches has a rather smooth appearance due to the absence of dendritic spines.

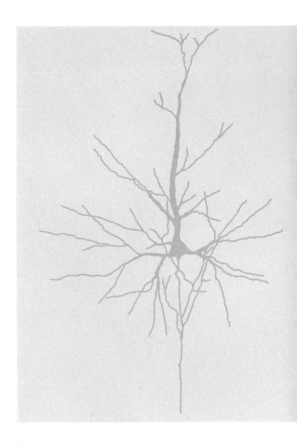

Fig. 190. Drawing of a typical pyramidal cell.

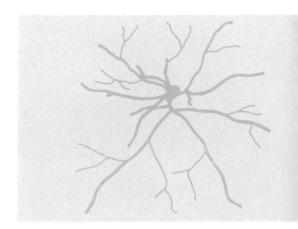

Fig. 191. Drawing of a typical stellate cell.

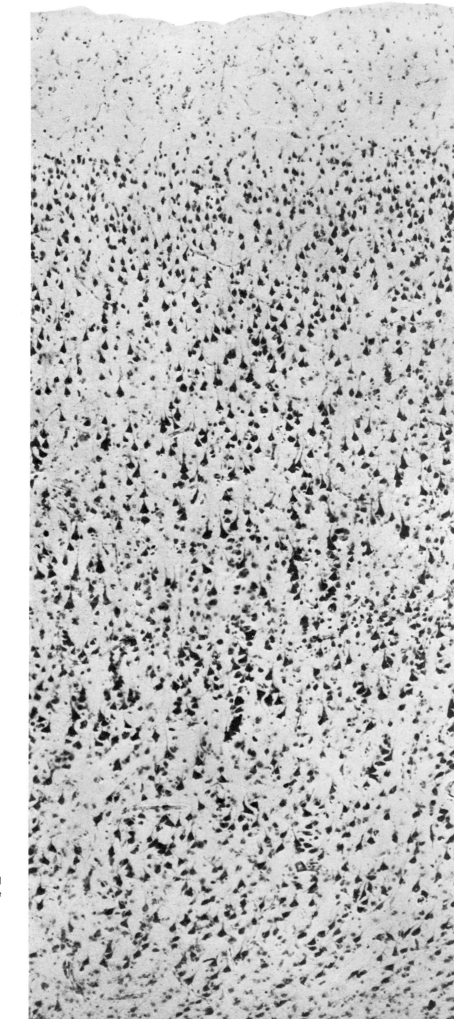

Fig. 192. Nissl staining of the cerebral cortex; **top,** pial surface; **bottom,** white matter.

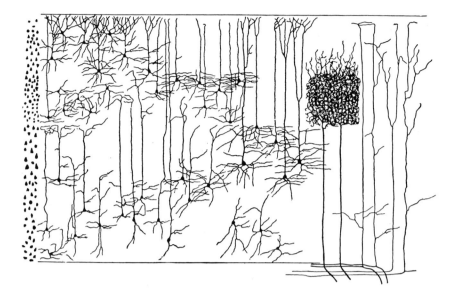

Fig. 193. Typical cortical neurons. (Scheme by Lorente de Nó.) *Cf.* Fig. 87, p. 99.

14.4.2 Patterns of neuronal organization

As has been shown for the large neurons which function as integrators in other brain areas (Purkinje cell and pyramidal cell in the hippocampus) the cortical pyramidal cells also show a remarkable organization as far as the receptive surface is concerned. With respect to pyramidal cells of the visual cortex the following structural pattern has been recognized.

(1) The specific sensory afferents synapse on the middle 2/3 of the apical shaft.

(2) The non-specific afferents contact the entire apical shaft.

(3) The commissural fibers project to oblique branches of the apical dendrites.

(4) The recurrent collaterals of the pyramidal cells synapse on the outer portion of the basilar dendrites and apical dendrites terminals.

Fig. 194. Another question to be asked is whether the circuitry of the neuronal elements is in any way different from the organization shown in other brain regions. In contrast to other regions in the central nervous system, *e.g.* the cerebellum, the circuits in the cerebral cortex are relatively simple. The figure shows the arrangements of pyramidal and stellate cells. The stellate cell may function as an inhibitory interneuron like the Renshaw cell in the spinal cord: an example of recurrent inhibition.

Fig. 195 shows another intracortical circuit in which inhibitory (S2) and excitatory (S1) stellate cells participate. The diagram shows the postulated synaptic connections of axon collaterals of pyramidal cells. The single inhibitory interneuron, together with its inhibitory synapses on the somata of the pyramidal cells are shown in green. The other two stellate cells and the pyramidal cells are assumed to be excitatory.

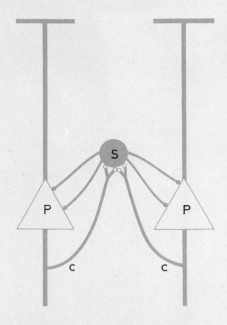

Fig. 194. Simple intracortical circuit. **P,** pyramidal cell; **c,** collateral of pyramidal cell; **S,** stellate cell.

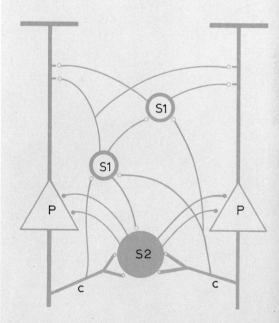

Fig. 195. Intracortical network of a more complex nature. **S1,** stellate cell producing excitatory synaptic action; **S2,** stellate cell producing inhibitory synaptic action.

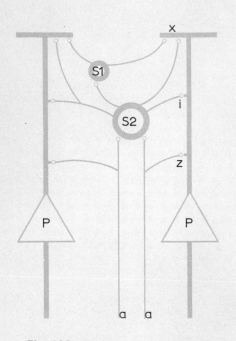

Fig. 196. Cortical circuit activated by thalamic afferents (a).
P, pyramidal cell; **S1** and **S2,** excitatory stellate cells; **x, j** and **z,** topographical distribution of the apical dendritic system of excitatory synaptic terminals.

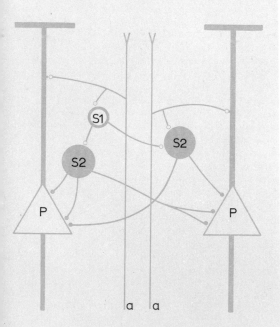

Fig. 197. Cortical network activated by thalamic afferents.
S1, excitatory interneuron; **S2,** inhibitory interneuron.

Figs. 196, 197. As suggested by experimental evidence, both the excitatory and inhibitory pathways can include interpolated excitatory interneurons. The pyramidal cells are exclusively excitatory, but the stellate cells may be either excitatory or inhibitory. The figures show the postulated connections of specific afferent fibers from the thalamus (**a**) to the cortical pyramidal cells. Excitatory terminals of the afferents may excite a portion of the apical dendrite of the pyramidal cell (**z**) either directly or *via* an excitatory interneuron (**S2**). Fig. 197 is an example of a cortical circuit with inhibitory and excitatory stellate cells, activated by thalamic afferents (**a**). The inhibitory path is through inhibitory cells that are activated either directly by the afferent fibers or by mediation of excitatory interneurons. The excitatory pathways to the pyramidal cells show various degrees of complexity.

14.4.3 Synaptic action of cortical neurons

Fig. 198. It has become clear from experimental evidence that the excitatory and inhibitory synaptic action resemble in the essential features the synapses in the spinal cord. As far as the electrical properties are concerned, cortical neurons resemble those at the lower levels of the central nervous system.

The membrane potentials are between −50 and −70 mV and the action potentials range from 60–100 mV. Numerous investigations reveal that the large pyramidal cells have many resemblances to spinal motor neurons. In general the excitatory and inhibitory postsynaptic potentials show the same essential features as the synaptic actions in the spinal cord and other brain areas.

14.4.4 Processing of sensory patterns

This account so far has dealt with the elementary components of brain action, of synapses, of neuronal circuits, and of simple patterns of neuronal interconnection, but so far no insight has been gained in the so-called 'higher functions' of the nervous system, *e.g.* the neuronal machinery, responsible for the perception of sensory patterns. The most successful efforts to shed some light on the perception mechanisms in the cerebral cortex have been made by the penetrating studies of Hubel, Wiesel and Mountcastle. The investigators have shown that neurons within vertical columns, extending from the pial surface to the subcortical white matter, have similar functions. Such functional columns of cortical grey matter appear to be universal in the visual, auditory and somato-sensory areas of many animals. Successive cells, excited by the same sensory stimulus, having the same peripheral field, can be recorded during an electrode penetration in a direction rectangular to the pial surface. The diameter of such functional columns is about 0.2 to 0.6 mm. Minute data have been collected on the analysis of electrical activities in neurons located in various stations of the visual pathway in cat and monkey in response to different incoming visual messages.

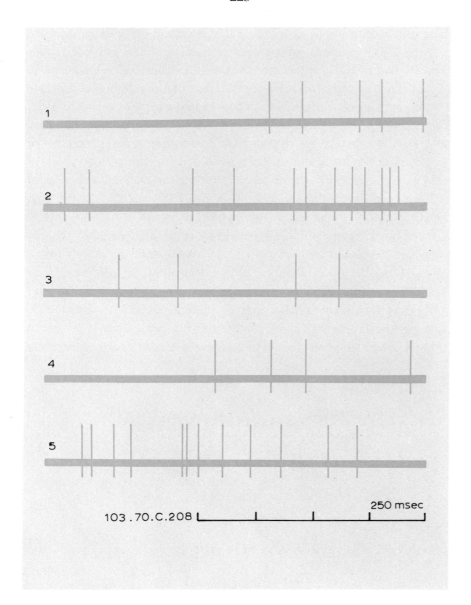

103.70.C.208

250 msec

Fig. 198. Firing pattern of a neuron in the cerebral cortex. The action potentials show the same characteristics as in other neuronal aggregates.

Fig. 199. The first analysis of visual patterns takes place in the retina where cellular elements are organized in receptive fields. These cells fire often at a fairly steady rate, even in the absence of stimulation, but the firing rate is increased or decreased by small illuminated circular regions in the retina. Upon the basis of these observations the retina can be divided into on- and off-receptive regions. The neurons in the next station, the lateral geniculate body, are organized in more or less the same manner.

The visual signals reach the primary visual area and they are mainly distributed to neurons located in the fourth cortical layer.

At least two types of nerve cells can be distinguished in this region. The so-called simple cells respond to light lines on a dark background and to straight line-boundaries between light and dark regions. Thus, these cells respond to lines and edges. The second category of cells are called complex neurons which also respond to lines and edges, but continue to fire as the stimulus moves over a substantial retinal area. It seems likely to assume from the reported data that the simple cells receive their input from a large number of neurons in the lateral geniculate body. Those on- and off-centers are arranged along straight lines. Complex cells, on the other hand, receive their input from a large number of simple cells. When the stimuli are transmitted from area 17 to areas 18 and 19 the complexity in the response of the individual neurons increases. So it has been shown that the neurons in area 18 receive their input from the complex cells of area 17. The cortical elements of area 18 are influenced by excitatory and inhibitory drives from the neurons in area 17. Therefore these elements are defined as hyper-complex cells of lower order. When the flow of information is transmitted from area 18 to area 19 the situation becomes even more complex. The cells in this region respond to two orthogonally directed stimuli, *i.e.* the receptor fields have an orientation 90° apart. Apparently the visual messages move through neuronal aggregates which show a hierarchical organization

Fig. 199. Concentric fields are characteristic of retinal ganglion cells and of geniculate cells. (after Hubel and Wiesel.) A, 'on'-center field. The oscilloscope recordings show strong firing (1) when a spot of light strikes the field center. If the spot hits an 'off'-area (2) the firing is suppressed until the light goes off. B, 'off'-center field. Responses of a cell of the 'off'-center type. a, light off; b, light on.

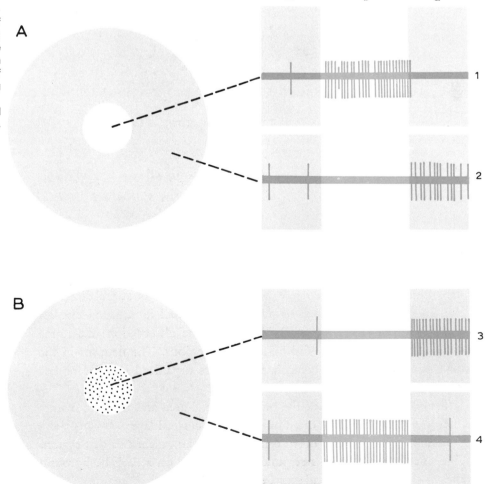

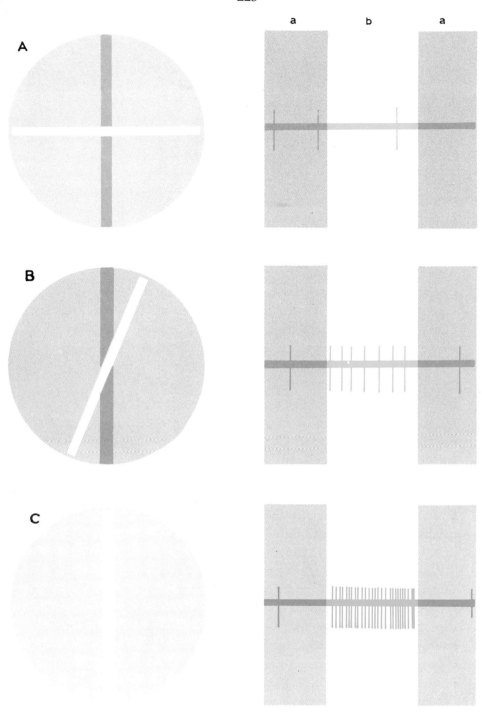

Fig. 200. The importance of orientation of simple cortical cells is indicated by various responses to a slit of light from a cell prefering a vertical orientation. The horizontal slit (**A**) shows no response. The vertical orientation (**C**) produces a maximal response. **a,** light off; **b,** light on

since the response patterns become more and more complex in moving step by step from area 17 to area 19. The association areas (18 and 19) apparently integrate sensation into more complex perceptions. The power of integration of neuronal circuits is still beyond all imagining. Hundreds of neurophysiologists are still searching for new insights in their efforts to understand the nervous system. Small pieces of an enormous jigsaw puzzle are at present being put together. However, we should realize that what we know at present are some elementary functional components, neurons linked by excitatory and inhibitory synapses into simple patterns which may have a specific functional meaning.

15. Integrative mechanisms: Sensory and motor systems

15.1 Introduction

The figures of this section illustrate in a schematic fashion certain of the more important primary pathways or connections, starting with receptor elements, which project into the central nervous system. With the motor system, these paths start at a cerebral cortical level to proceed *via* relays on motoneurons of the cord and brain stem to terminals on effector organs. The cellular areas or nuclei are indicated as boxes; the lines indicate the pathway projections to or from these nuclear zones. Note that synaptic connections are not always indicated in these figures. However, unless the structure is a ganglion, one or several synapses may usually be assumed to occur in the nuclear zones.

Fig. 201 deals with the transmission of pain-temperature (green lines) and light touch (black lines). The signals of these categories picked up from the body surface would be transmitted along nerve fibers having their cell bodies in the dorsal root ganglia (**DRG**) whose proximal rami (dorsal roots) terminate in the dorsal horn after extending for a short ascending and descending course. Cells in the dorsal horn activated by these signals may serve to initiate reflex responses at this or closely adjacent levels *via* interconnections in the intermediate grey (**IG**) substance. The neurons of the IG might then be expected to act on the ventral horn motoneurons (**VHC**) of the spinal cord.

A significant ascending projection arises from cells of the dorsal horn which crosses to the opposite side of the cord *via* the anterior white commissure to ascend in the anterolateral funiculus (**alf**). (These fibers used to be considered as ascending in the spinothalamic tract, but since so many of the fibers terminate at lower levels, this term is no longer appropriate for these units.) Connections may be seen to occur in the medial reticular formation (**MRF**), ventrolateral reticular formation (**VLRF**), central grey of the midbrain (**CG**), tectum (superior colliculus), the nucleus centralis (**CL**) and the ventroposterolateral nucleus of the thalamus (**VPL**). It is to be noted that pain and temperature ascend contralateral to the side of stimulus and that light touch appears to ascend bilaterally. Connections are made from the reticular formation and tectum to the motoneurons (**VHC**) *via* internucials in the **IG**, while

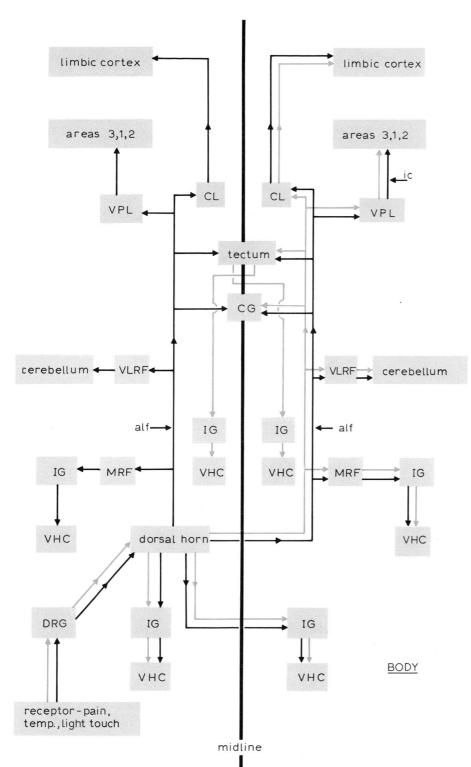

Fig. 201. Map of pain-temperature and light touch paths from the body.

the ventrolateral reticular formation (**VLRF**) projects to the cerebellar cortex. The afferent sensory signals finally are distributed to the cortex from the thalamic nuclei *via* fibers running in the internal capsule (**ic**). The paleothalamic nucleus (centralis lateralis—**CL**) projects to the limbic cortex (gyrus cinguli), while the neothalamic nucleus (**VPL**) projects to the neocortical region of the postcentral gyrus (**area 3, 1, 2**).

Visceral afferents subserving pain are directed towards the CNS from the internal organs *via* fibers which run in association with the autonomic system. The cell bodies of these afferents are also in the **DRG**. Comparable connections are made in the dorsal horn and the sensory information appears to ascend in the anterolateral funiculus toward higher levels with the same sort of intermediate connections being established before attaining the level of the thalamus. However, the input appears more diffuse. This could be because of the midline nature, particularly embryologically, of most of these organs so that they in effect have a bilateral innervation, or it could be because the afferent signals tend to enter the dorsal horn at a number of different levels.

Fig. 202. Signals of pain (**p**), temperature (**t**) and light touch (**lt. t**) from the face are mediated by components comparable to those found for the rest of the body. Thus, the input enters *via* peripheral nerves whose cell bodies are in a peripheral ganglion (**tr. g**). The proximal root enters the CNS at the level of the pons to terminate in two nuclei. Pain and temperature units (green lines) terminate in the spinal or inferior nucleus of the trigeminal nerve (**Sp. nu. V**) which descends as far caudally as the 4th cervical segment. Light touch (black lines) terminates in the main sensory nucleus of V (**m.s. V**) and in the rostral portion of the inferior nucleus. Secondary fibers arising from the inferior or spinal nucleus effect connections like those of the dorsal horn with the ventrolateral reticular formation (**VLRF**), dorsolateral reticular formation (**DLRF**) and medial reticular formation (**MRF**). As before, these reticular nuclei establish connections with the motoneurons (**VHC**) *via* the intermediate grey (**IG**) and cranial nerve nuclei and cerebellum. An important ascending fiber bundle, the ventral central trigeminal tract (**vctt**) crosses to the opposite side and passes rostrally toward the thalamus, establishing connections in the central grey (**CG**), tectum of the midbrain, nucleus centralis lateralis (**CL**) of the paleothalamus and finally the ventroposteromedial nucleus of the dorsal neothalamus (**VPM**). The cortical connections are again established *via* fibers to the postcentral gyrus (**areas 3, 1, 2**) and to the limbic cortex (**l.c.,** gyrus cinguli). Note again that light touch (black arrows) appears to have a bilateral pathway toward higher centers.

229

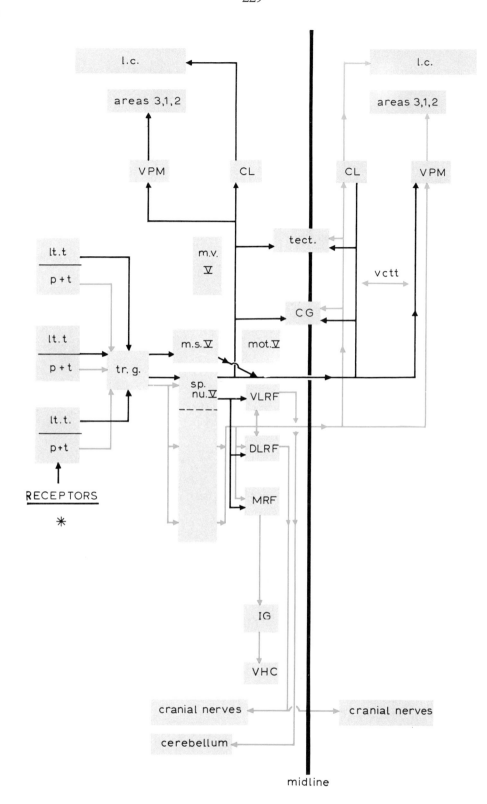

Fig. 202. Map of trigeminal pain, temperature and light touch pathways (face).

Figs. 203, 204 illustrate the routes and connections made for sensations coming in from the periphery which might be described as discriminative. These sensations have classically been listed as 2-point discrimination (the ability to discern whether or not one is being touched simultaneously by 2 sharp points close together or by one point), conscious proprioception (awareness of the position of one's body parts), vibratory sense (the appreciation of a buzzing when a vibrating tuning fork is applied to a bony prominence) and the ability to appreciate the form and texture of an object placed in one's hand.

As illustrated by Fig. 203, the receptor elements transmit impulses centrally to their cell bodies in the dorsal root ganglion (**DRG**). The central processes then pass through the dorsal root fibers (**dr**) into the spinal cord and ascend rostrally in the dorsal funiculus (**df**) to terminate on cells in the nuclei of gracilis and cuneatus at the junction of the lower medulla with the spinal cord. These processes are still part of the peripheral sensory neuron. Collateral connections are also made at the level of entry into the intermediate grey (**IG**) of the spinal cord which relays the signal to the ipsi and contralateral ventral horn motoneurons (**VHC**) for local reflex response. These cells, as the final common pathway elements, initiate the responses of the effector organs.

The two nuclear groups at the rostral end of the dorsal funiculus (gracilis and cuneatus) continue the rostral propagation of the afferent messages. These cells are called the central sensory neurons. Fibers arising from these cells cross and ascend as the medial lemniscus (**ml**) which terminates in the ventroposterolateral nucleus of the neothalamus (**VPL**). Cells in this nucleus relay the signals primarily to the sensory cortex of the post central gyrus (**areas 3, 1, 2**), the fibers passing through the posterior limb of the internal capsule (**ic**). Corticofugal fibers arising from the sensory cortex descend through the internal capsule to terminate on cells in the nuclei of gracilis and cuneatus. The precise role played by these cortical projections is uncertain, but it is considered that they may modulate the response of these cells to the ascending sensory input coming in from the periphery.

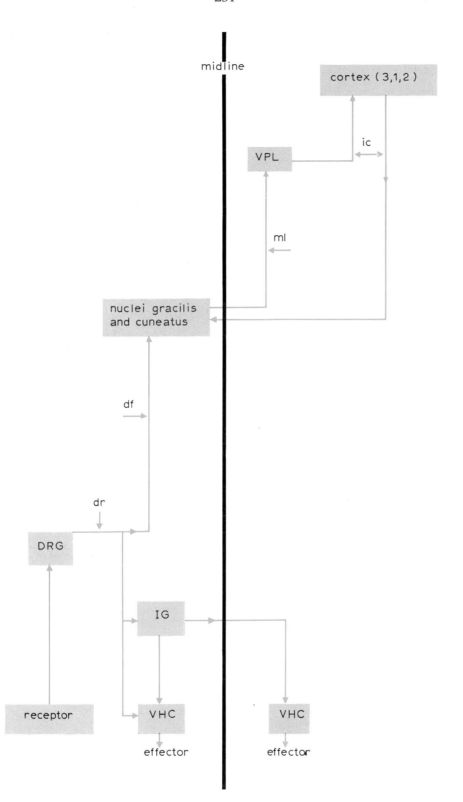

Fig. 203. Map of pathways for body discriminative sense.

In Fig. 204 the comparable system is schematically outlined for the face. The receptors for discriminative sense (**rec. dis.**) are indicated as having a triple nerve distribution to correspond to the 3 peripheral nerve trunks of the trigeminal nerve. Position sense (**pos. sen.**) which is another term for conscious proprioception is indicated as being present in only one of the 3 rami of the trigeminal nerves, the mandibular ramus. As with the body, the peripheral nerves transport the incoming signals toward the cell bodies in a trigeminal ganglion (**tr. g.**). Note that discriminative sense is carried by fibers which have their cell bodies in the trigeminal ganglion and that position sense is carried by fibers whose cell bodies are in the central nervous system itself: in the mesencephalic nucleus of the fifth nerve (**m. n. V**). There also appear to be some fibers which carry position sense from the extraocular muscles supplied by the IIIrd cranial nerve which also have their cell bodies in this nucleus.

Fibers carrying discriminative sensations terminate in the main sensory nucleus of the trigeminal nerve (**m. s. n. V**), which relays the information *via* fibers which seem to be mostly in what is called the dorsal central trigeminal tract (**dctt**) to the contralateral ventroposteromedial nucleus (**VPM**) of the neothalamus. The thalamic projection to the cortex is again *via* the posterior limb of the internal capsule (**ic**) to the primary sensory cortex (**areas 3, 1, 2**). As with somatic sensations from the body, a cortical projection is sent back to the main sensory nucleus.

The final series of interactions are concerned with those afferent projections which terminate in the mesencephalic nucleus. The efferent fibers of the cells in this nucleus appear to make contact with the cells in the motor nucleus of the Vth nerve (**m. n. V**) and with neurons in the dorsolateral reticular formation (**DLRF**). This nucleus is then in a position to distribute appropriate inputs to the nuclei of the motor cranial nerves (*i.e.* VII, X and XII) for associated reflex responses.

233

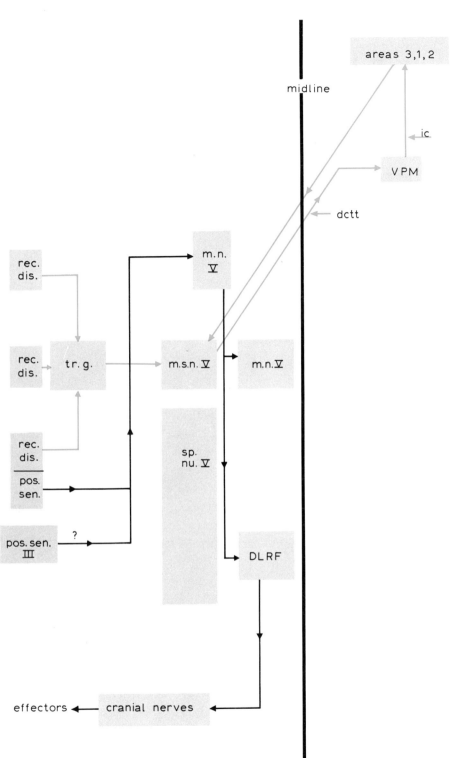

Fig. 204. Map of pathways for face discriminative sense.

15.2 The cerebellar system

Fig. 205. The connections within the central nervous system associated with the cerebellar system are considerably more complicated, inasmuch as the cerebellum functions in the areas of integration of motor activity. This function is based as much on sensory inputs from the periphery and cerebral cortex as it is on influencing the motor functions *via* the red nucleus (**RN**), midbrain reticular formation (**MBRF**) and the ventro-lateral (**VLN**) nucleus of the neothalamus.

Afferents mediating position sense (unconscious), pain (**p**) and temperature (**t**) originating from receptors at * transmit their signals toward the CNS *via* cells in the dorsal root ganglia (**DRG**), trigeminal ganglia (**trig. g.**) and the mesencephalic nucleus of the Vth nerve (**m. nu. V**). The signals referable to pain and temperature from the body are mediated *via* the anterolateral funiculus to the ventrolateral reticular formation (**VLRF**) of the medulla which relays the signals to the ipsilateral cerebellar cortex. Comparable information related to pain and temperature which arises from the face is relayed *via* cells in the inferior trigeminal nucleus to the ventrolateral reticular formation (**VLRF**), which, as before relays these signals to the cerebellum.

Position sense (unconscious) from the body is relayed rostrally in the spinal cord *via* the dorsal (and to a lesser extent by the ventral) spinal cerebellar tracts after a synapse in the nucleus dorsalis or on cells at the base of the dorsal horn. These fibers ascend and enter into the inferior cerebellar peduncle (**icp**) and again terminate in the cerebellar cortex. Most of this projection is ipsilateral although the ventral tract projects bilaterally. Comparable signals from the cervical areas ascend in the dorsal funiculus to synapse on cells of the external cuneate nucleus (**ext. cun.**) rather than in the nucleus dorsalis (**nu. dors.**). These cells also relay *via* the inferior cerebellar peduncle. Some 'unconscious' position sense arising from within the muscles of mastication is transmitted through nerve fibers in the mandibular ramus of the Vth nerve to their cell bodies in the mesencephalic nucleus of the Vth nerve (**m. nu. V.**). Though not yet clearly demonstrated on an anatomical basis, it is believed that there are some direct projections to the cerebellar cortex from this nucleus. All these fibers enter the cerebellar cortex as the mossy fiber system.

There is also a projection to the cerebellum from higher levels. Thus, there is the well established projection from the motor and premotor cortex (**areas 4, 6**) *via* the fibers of the internal capsule and cerebral peduncle (**cp**) to cells in the basal pons, where a synaptic connection occurs. These cells of the pons then project to the contralateral cerebellar cortex *via* the middle cerebellar peduncle (**mcp**). Another descending system has at least an established origin in the central grey of the midbrain (**CG**) plus unconfirmed origins from some area of cortex and perhaps other subcortical nuclear areas. The fibers in this system project ipsilaterally *via* the central tegmental fasciculus (**ctf**) to the inferior olive. The neurons of the inferior olive then relay the signal *via* internal arcuate fibers into the contralateral inferior cerebellar peduncle (**icp**) to the cerebellar cortex. These fibers enter the cerebellar cortex as the climbing fiber system.

The efferent projection of the cerebellum is achieved by the fibers which arise from the deep cerebellar nuclei (dentate, globosus, emboliform and fastigial). These fibers ascend as the superior cerebellar peduncle (**scp**) which projects into and decussates in the midbrain before terminating in part in the red nucleus (**RN**) and midbrain reticular formation (**mbrf**) of the opposite side. A few fibers may terminate in the reticular formation prior to decussation. Some fibers by-pass these nuclei and continue to ascend to the ventrolateral nucleus (**VLN**) and ventral anterior nucleus (**VAN**) of the neothalamus which relays the signal onto the motor and pre-motor cortices. Note that the red nucleus also serves to relay the information on to the **VLN**, but, in conjunction with the reticular formation provides for descending fiber systems which decussate (mainly) and form the rubrospinal and a part of the reticulospinal tracts. These descending elements terminate on internucial neurons of the intermediate grey (**IG**) and dorsolateral reticular formation (**DLRF**) which relay the cerebellar influence to the motoneurons in the brain stem and spinal cord.

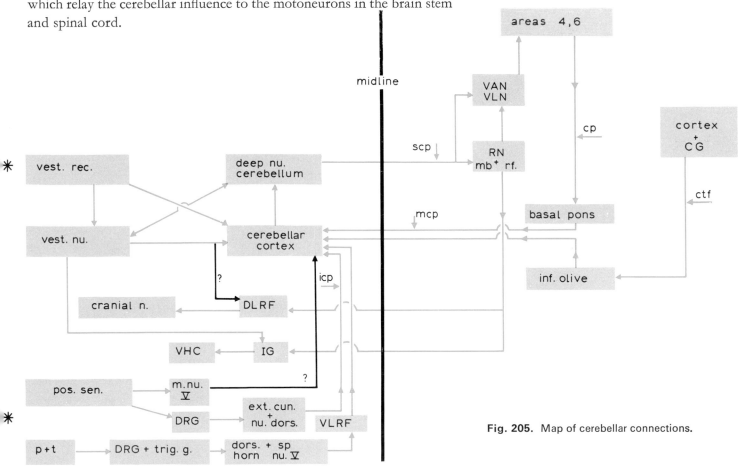

Fig. 205. Map of cerebellar connections.

15.2.1 Vestibulocerebellar connections

Fig. 206. The reflex adjustments which occur during equilibratory processes also necessitate the action of the cerebellum. In this instance the vestibular receptors appear to project directly to the cerebellar cortex in the region of the flocculus as well as by a relay through the vestibular nuclei in the pontine tegmentum and medulla. The deep cerebellar nucleus most concerned with these adjustments is the fastigial nucleus and most of its subsequent relay projections are back to the vestibular nuclei, though projections rostrally into the midbrain are claimed. Descending fiber tracts arising from the vestibular nuclei form the medial and lateral vestibulospinal tracts which act on the motoneurons *via* synapses on the cells of the intermediate grey matter (**IG**). Connections with the cranial nerve motor nuclei *via* the dorsolateral reticular formation (**DLRF**) have been claimed and seem likely. However, their existence has not yet been conclusively established.

The details of the vestibulocerebellar associations with other units are elaborated in Fig. 206. Here fibers arising from cells in the vestibular receptors (**vest. rec.**) are depicted as terminating in both the vestibular nuclei (**vest. nu.**) and the cerebellar flocculus (**flocc.**). The vestibular nuclear group is then observed to exert an influence on cranial nerve nuclei *via* fibers in the medial longitudinal fasciculus (**MLF**; which is often called the medial vestibulospinal tract in the spinal cord) and *via* the lateral vestibulospinal tract (**lat. vest. sp. tr.**) which descends primarily to spinal cord elements. Connections may also be made into the dorsolateral reticular formation (not shown) to influence the cranial nerve motor nuclei. However, the nuclei innervating the extra-ocular muscles (III, IV and VI) appear to receive fibers from all the vestibular nuclei *via* the **MLF**. Connections are illustrated in the flocculus, vestibular nuclei (**vest. nu.**), fastigial nucleus (**fast. nu.**) and the nodulus (**nod.**) which are inter-connected by what has often been termed the juxtarestiform body. These are associated with a fiber bundle (unicate fasciculus) arising from a fastigial nucleus which terminates in the contralateral vestibular area. The two units may logically be referred to as the fastigiobulbar tract. The fibers of the uncinate fasciculus have been demonstrated as having some terminations in the pontine reticular formation (**pont. RF**) as well as in the medial reticular formation (**MRF**) of the medulla. The latter may provide for additional reticulospinal components.

The rostral projections arising from the fastigial nucleus are not as well documented as the other connections. However, there is some evidence suggesting projections into the midbrain reticular formation (**MBRF**) and to the paleothalamic nuclei. This would include the centromedian nucleus (**cm**) and perhaps the parafascicular nucleus. Some terminals may also occur in the nucleus of the posterior commissure (**npco**) in the region of the rostral end of the cerebral aqueduct (**A**).

There are other connections of the vestibular system made *via* connections with various brain stem nuclei. One of these is related to the movements of the eye following acceleratory rotatory stimulation of the semicircular canals. As long as the stimuli applied to paired cristi in the semicircular canals (*i.e.* of the horizontal canals) is unequal, a condition known as 'nystagmus' occurs. This appears to the observer as rapid to-and-fro movements of the eyes, the movement to one side being quicker than the other. The 'quick component' is to the side on which the stimulus to the crista is maximal. While these eye movements can be easily produced in normal persons by spinning them in a chair with the head held at an appropriate angle, this is not always correctly undertaken. Therefore techniques whereby warm or cold fluids are flushed through the ears have been divised. The temperature of the fluid will alter the temperature of the endolymph of the semicircular canals, causing convection currents to be set up which will cause the crista (receptor) of a particular semicircular canal to be maximally or minimally stimulated as compared with the equivalent crista of the opposite side. This inequality of stimulus to the two cristi induced by caloric stimuli will then also produce a nystagmus.

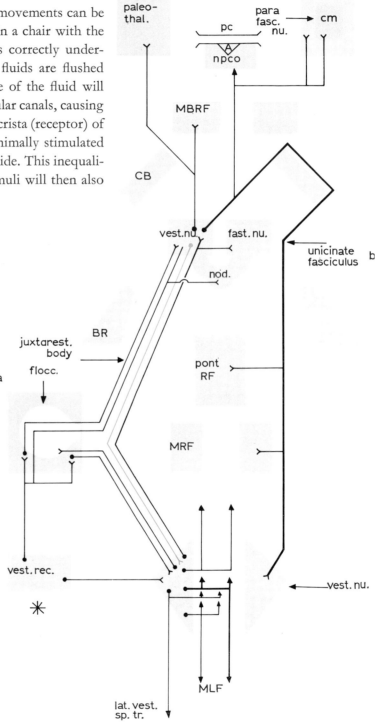

Fig. 206. Vestibular cerebellothalamic associations via fastigiobulbar tracts **a** and **b**; **CB**, brachium conjunctivum or superior cerebellar peduncle; **BR**, restiform body of inferior cerebellar peduncle.

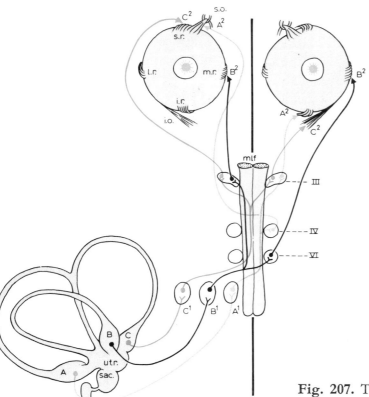

Fig. 207. Vestibular canals as related to pairs of extra-ocular muscles. (based on Szentagothai.)

Fig. 207. This principal of caloric induction of convection currents in the endolymph to produce unequal stimulation of the semicircular canals receptors was utilized to relate specific semicircular canals to the response of specific pairs of extraocular muscles. The semicircular canals have been coded such that the anterior canal is **C,** the horizontal canal is **B** and the posterior canal **A.** These canals are then connected by nerve fibers to unspecified nuclear groups in the vestibular nuclear complex in the lateral floor of the fourth ventricle, labeled A^1, B^1 and C^1, to correspond to the similarly coded semicircular canals. Fiber projections from the vestibular nuclear zones ascend in the medial longitudinal fasciculus (**mlf**) to reach the nuclei for the extra-ocular muscles: III-oculomotor, IV-trochlear and VI-abducens. Connections are then made to the extra-ocular muscles which are grouped in pairs and coded A^2, B^2 and C^2 to match the proper semicircular canals. Thus, caloric stimulation of the crista of the horizontal canal (**B**) induces impulses relayed by vestibular nuclear group B^1 to the abducens and oculomotor nuclei *via* the **mlf.** The cranial nerve nuclei then in this instance projects to the medial rectus muscle (**m.r.**) and the lateral rectus muscle (**l.r.**).

Comparable connections to pairs of extra-ocular muscles following stimulation of the anterior or posterior semicircular canal cristi lead to responses of other pairs of extra-ocular muscles, which are the inferior rectus (**i.r.**), superior rectus (**s.r.**), superior oblique (**s.o.**), and inferior oblique (**i.o.**) muscles. The caloric method for stimulating the cristi of the semicircular canals has often proven a useful procedure in the physical diagnosis of patients suspected of having a disorder of the vestibular system.

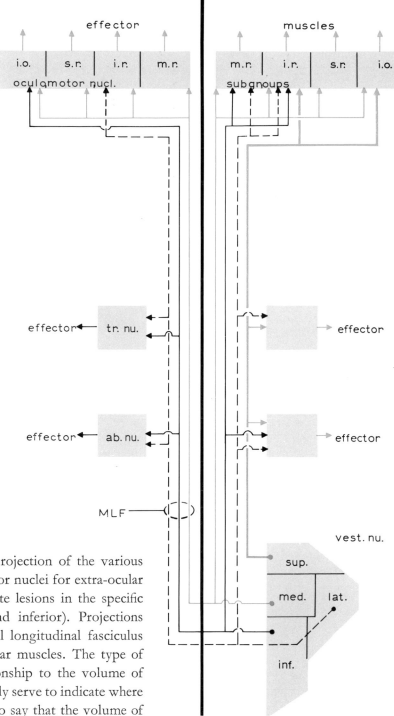

Fig. 208. Vestibular connections with eye muscles. (based on McMasters *et al.*, 1966.)

Fig. 208. A more detailed analysis of the projection of the various components of the vestibular nuclei to the motor nuclei for extra-ocular muscles was based on the placement of discrete lesions in the specific vestibular nuclei (superior, medial, lateral and inferior). Projections arising from these nuclei ascend *via* the medial longitudinal fasciculus to terminate in all of the nuclei for extra-ocular muscles. The type of line denoting these connections has no relationship to the volume of fibers ascending from each nucleus. The lines only serve to indicate where vestibular projections are terminating. Suffice to say that the volume of projection varied considerably from one vestibular nucleus to another. Thus, it is apparent that connections are made in the abducens (**ab. nu.**), trochlear (**tr. nu.**) and oculomotor nuclei. In the case of the latter, terminals were reported in the nuclear subgroups supplying the inferior obliques (**i.o.**), superior rectus (**s.r.**), inferior rectus (**i.r.**) and medial rectus (**m.r.**) muscles.

15.3 The auditory system

Fig. 209. Auditory projections may also be outlined in a similar schematic plan. The receptor cells in the cochlear (indicated by *) project their signals to the dorsal and ventral cochlear nuclei (**co. nu.**). Two types of relays arise from the cochlear nuclei, both of which pass through the trapezoid body (**trb**) in the caudal pontine tegmentum and ascend to higher levels *via* the lateral lemniscus (**l.l.**). Thus, one group of fibers provides an input into the superior olive (**s.ol.**) and reticular formation (**RF**). Fibers arising from cells in the superior olive ascend in the lateral lemniscus to terminate in the medial geniculate body (**MG**) which in turn relays the signal to the auditory cortex of the transverse temporal gyrus (areas 41, 42). This ascending bundle provides for collaterals to the nucleus of the lateral lemniscus (**n.l.l.**) which is reciprocally connected with the comparable nucleus of the other side. The ascending fibers of the lateral lemniscus may also make a small contribution to the superior colliculus (**SC**). Note that the nucleus of the lateral lemniscus sends out fibers *via* the lateral lemniscus which terminate in the inferior colliculus (**IC**). These fibers in turn, project to the superior colliculus and to the medial geniculate body. The inferior colliculi are also reciprocally interconnected *via* commissural fibers.

The other pathway taken to higher levels from the cochlear nuclei has terminals entering the reticular formation, the nucleus of the lateral lemniscus (**n.l.l.**) and finally the inferior colliculus (**IC**).

A series of descending connections which are associated with the auditory system may also be mapped. These arise from the cortex of the parietal or temporal lobe and descend through the internal capsule to terminate in the medial geniculate body (**MG**). A continuing relay passes *via* the inferior colliculus to the superior olive nucleus and there are also direct geniculo-olivary fibers. Some of the cells of the superior olive (**s. ol.**) then appear to project back through the contralateral cochlear nuclei (without a synapse) and cochlear nerve to the receptor cells of the organ of Corti in the cochlea.

A final sequence of connections may be visualized to follow the occurrence of a sharp sound. This signal is relayed toward the inferior colliculus which transmits this stimuli to the superior colliculus. The reflex adjustment (eye, head and body turning to this stimuli) is then mediated to a large extent by impulses descending over the tectospinal tract (**tec. sp. tr.**) which arises as a decussating fiber bundle from the superior colliculus.

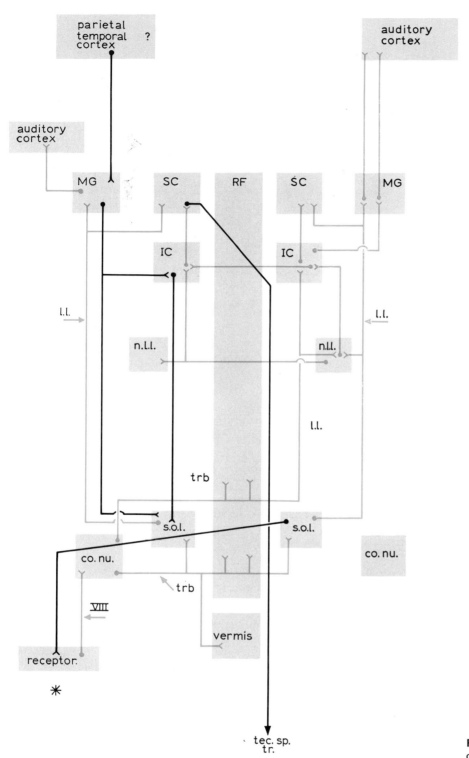

Fig. 209. Auditory projections. (based on Ades, 1959.)

Fig. 210. Transmission of visual information in the eye. **18,** retinal pigment.

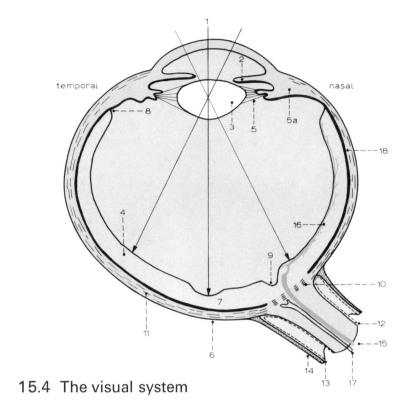

15.4 The visual system

Fig. 210. The receptors transmitting visual information are of course in the eye. Rays of light arising from the object which is 'seen' pass through the cornea at the anterior pole (**1**) of the eye; through the pupillary opening formed by the iris (**2**); through the lens (**3**) and finally a relatively dense medium behind the lens known as the vitreous humour before reaching the receptor cells of the retina (**4**). In the process of passing through these various refractive media, the image projected onto the retina is reversed, left for right and top for bottom. Thus, light rays arising from an object to the left of the eye (left visual field) stimulate receptors on the right side of the retina. The lens is held in place just behind the iris by the ciliary zonule (**5,** zonular fibers) which appears to rise from the epithelium of the ciliary body (**5a**) as straight homogenous filaments forming a ligamentous structure. The entire ciliary body is actually a circular structure encircling the lens. The origin of the muscle fibers within the ciliary body is in the region of the base of the iris. Contraction of the smooth muscle fibers within the ciliary body shifts the ciliary body toward the anterior pole of the eye. It serves to decrease the diameter of the ciliary body and the suspending ligament of the lens. This has the effect of decreasing the tension applied by the ciliary zonule to the margin of the lens. In this way the elastic lens expands in an anteroposterior direction. The process wherein the lens changes its shape is known as accommodation and it is necessary to provide for focussing of the light rays on the retina when the object examined is closer to the eye than 20 feet.

The region of the posterior pole (**6**) of the eye is characterized by having a shallow pit in the retina-the fovea centralis (**7**) which is the region of the greatest visual acuity. The receptor elements found here are all cone cells (color receptors in bright light). The region of the 'ora serrata' at the anterior margin of the retina (**8**) is the region of least visual acuity. The light receptors in this area are all rod cells (most effective when light is of low intensity and are considered to be 'black and white' receptors). Moving anteriorly from the fovea to the ora serrata, the proportion of the cones slowly decreases and that of the rods slowly increases.

The optic disc (**9**), which is medial to the fovea centralis on the nasal side of the eye is the region where the fibers arising from the retinal receptor system will converge to form the optic nerve. The nerve fibers are unmyelinated up to this point. As they pass through openings (**10**, lamina cribrosa) in the wall of the sclera (**11**), the fibers will become myelinated. The large nerve trunk which arises from the eyeball at this point is the optic nerve. Since the eye is embryologically derived as an outgrowth from the diencephalon, it is really an extension of the brain. The optic nerve can then be considered as being comparable to one of the tracts which run through the central nervous system. Further, as an extension of the brain, the optic nerve is encased by the same meningeal layers as the rest of the brain. Thus, there is a layer of pia (**12**) adhering to the nerve which reflects back at the eyeball and becomes continuous with the arachnoid membrane (**13**). Covering both is a layer of dura mater (**14**) which fuses to the sclera (**11**). Note that the central artery (**15**) in the optic nerve distributes in the retina only to the innermost surface (**16**, retinal vessels). Thus, cells along the outermost margin of the retina receive no direct blood supply. Drainage is *via* the central vein (**17**).

Fig. 211. The cellular components of the retina are illustrated schematically. The outer capsule of the eyeball is formed by the sclera which continues to curve around rostrally forming the cornea at the anterior pole (Fig. 210, **1**). The deeper layers of the sclera (**1**) are characterized by the presence of many pigmented cells and two layers of blood vessels (**2, 3,** choroid layer). Deep to the choroid is the pigmented layer of the retina (**4**). These cells have processes which can extend up around the excitable terminals of the receptor cells (**5**), shielding them from light of too great an intensity. The neural part of the retina is adjacent to the pigmented layer. It contains essentially 3 layers of cells: layer **5**, rod (**r**) and cone (**c**) cells, layer **7** of *bipolar cells* (**bp**) and finally layer **8** of larger *ganglion cells* (**g**) whose axonal processes form the optic nerve. The receptor cells are of two types, cones with plump peripheral receptor processes and rods with very thin receptor processes projecting toward the pigmented layer.

Fig. 211. Cellular components of the retina.
2, large blood vessels; **3,** capillary layer; **9,** capillary plexus.

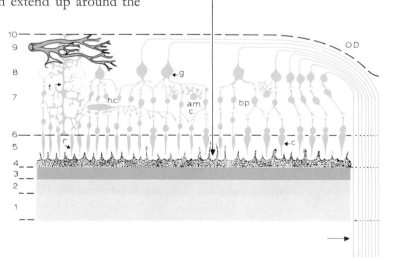

In the diagram, the right side of the figure would be in the region of the fovea centralis and the left side near the ora serrata. Note on the right that each cone cell (**c**) synapses with a bipolar cell (**bp**) and that each bipolar cell synapses with a ganglion cell (**g**). As one moves toward the left this one-to-one synaptic relationship changes so that one bipolar cell may synapse with several rods (and or cones) and each ganglion cell will also synapse with several bipolar cells. Thus, visual acuity tends to be sharper when associated with cells which possess a one-to-one synaptic relationship, as on the right side and to be less sharp where there is convergence of cell elements on the left of the figure.

The capillary vessels (**9**) are essentially restricted to the retinal layer containing the large ganglion cells and to a lesser extent the terminal processes of the bipolar cells. The rods and cones appear to have no direct blood supply. However, their nourishment is considered to be mediated through the *Müller fibers* (**f**). These cells appear to be modified astroglial elements which, like the comparable astroglia in the rest of the brain, establish a close contact with the capillaries and with the various neuronal elements. Thus, they may be considered as providing a pathway for transport of dissolved gases and nutrients to the neurons. These Müller fibers also provide processes which form an external limiting membrane (**6**) and an internal limiting membrane (**10**). The processes arising from the ganglion cells are diagrammed as forming a thin layer of fibers along the inner surface of the retina which converge in the region of the optic disc (**OD**).

There are additional types of cells to be considered in the retina. The first is the *amacrine cell* (**am. c.**). These elements are located in the inner aspect of the bipolar cell zone. They lack axons but have one or more processes which are in contact with bodies of the ganglion cells. Despite the lack of a fiber with anatomical characteristics of an axon, there is reason to believe that these cells do have a role in transmitting the visual signals (based on comparative studies of lower forms). The second type to consider is the *horizontal cell* (**h.c.**). These are of different size and are found in the outer part of the bipolar zone. The dendrites are in contact with the processes of groups of cone cells. The axon runs horizontally for some distance and has terminals on both rods and cones. In addition to these two cells, which seem to represent associative cells, there are bipolar cells which project in a centrifugal rather than in a retinofugal manner. The dendrites of these cells are in contact with the dendrites and cell bodies of the ganglion cells and possibly the axons of the centripetal (retinofugal) bipolar cells. The axons of these cells arborize and terminate on the rods and cones.

15.4.1 Visual system pathway

Fig. 212. The pattern of distribution of visual signals from the object seen by the subject (visual fields as seen by the left eye) through the visual pathway is illustrated. The visual field is depicted as being divided into quarters for the sake of simplicity. As the light rays which arise from this object are transmitted through the lens to impinge upon the retina, the image is inverted and switched right for left. This may be noted by following the projection of each visual field component to the appropriate retinal field as indicated by the symbols. Thus, a signal arising from the upper (**up**) left temporal visual field is received by cells in the lower right retinal field (**low**, right nasal quadrant). The subsequent projection from the retina is such that fibers on the nasal side of the retina cross through the optic chiasma (**o.c.**) to the contralateral geniculate body (**l.g.**) while the fibers arising from the temporal side of the retina remain uncrossed and terminate on cells in the ipsilateral geniculate body. The fibers which reach the geniculate bodies do so by passing through the optic tracts (**o.t.**). One should also note that fibers arising from the lower part of the retina terminate in the more lateral part of the lateral geniculate body. Finally, the optic radiation fibers reach the visual cortex. Those arising from the lateral part of the lateral geniculate body sweep down over the inferior horn of the lateral ventricle in the temporal lobe and then curve caudally, passing under the posterior horn of the lateral ventricle to reach the inferior aspect of the visual cortex bordering the calcarine fissure. The fibers leaving the medial part of the geniculate body follow a slightly more direct course to arrive at the primary visual cortex (also known as area 17) in the medial aspect of the occipital lobe.

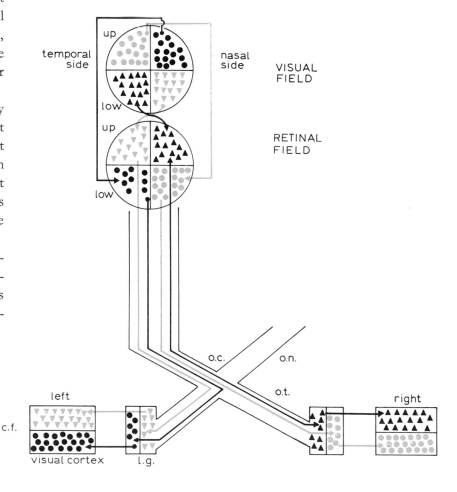

These fibers swing out laterally passing just rostral or in front of the antrum of the lateral ventricle. They then turn and run caudally, passing over the posterior horn of the ventricle to terminate in the cortex along the upper margin of the calcarine fissure (**c. f.**).

These projections represent only the primary projection to the visual cortex. Subsequent connections made from area 17 to the adjacent visual cortical area 18 and from 18 to 19, both of which are in the occipital lobe, represent other less clearly understood connections which seem significant in interpreting the signals relayed by the visual system.

The fiber pathway arising from the geniculate body with its wide distribution throughout the temporal, parietal and occipital lobes represents the optic radiations (geniculocalcarine tract).

Fig. 212. Pattern of distribution of visual signals from object seen by subject through the visual pathway. Visual fields as seen by the left eye.

15.4.2 Visual reflex response

Fig. 213. There are two highly important reflex responses which occur in relation to the visual system. These are the 'light' and 'accommodation' reflexes.

The 'light' reflex refers to the pupillary constriction which occurs when a bright light is directed into the eye. This acts effectively to reduce the amount of light which impinges upon the retina. As the test for determining the adequacy of pupillary response to light is usually performed, a bright light is directed toward the cornea which then impinges on the retina in the region of the posterior pole of the eye, as illustrated for the left eye. Such signals are transmitted from both nasal and temporal retinal halves and pass through both the decussated and undecussated fibers of the optic nerve (**o.n.**).

The pathway which such an impulse would follow in order to elicit pupillary constriction is as follows. The signal would pass along the optic nerve (**o.n.**) and optic tract (**o.t.**) to terminate primarily in the pretectal area (**prt**) just rostral to the superior colliculus (**SC**). The course of these fibers between the region of the lateral geniculate body and the pretectal area is by way of a fiber bundle known as the brachium of the superior colliculus (**bsc**). None of the fibers involved in transmitting the signals for the light reflex terminate in the lateral geniculate body (**LGB**). Some authors believe that there may be a relay for some of these fibers *via* the pregeniculate body (**p.g.b.**) as shown in the figure. However, this has not been clearly shown by anatomical techniques.

Connections are effected through the pretectal area (**prt**) to the nucleus of Edinger Westphal (**EW**) directly and *via* fibers which pass through the posterior commissure (**p.c.**) to attain the opposite side. The presence of the fibers passing through the posterior commissure is said to insure that a concensual light reflex response (constriction of the non stimulated pupil) will also occur. Preganglionic fibers arise from this autonomic nucleus of the midbrain and pass out through the oculomotor nerve to terminate in the ciliary ganglion (**c.g.**). This ganglion appears to possess two populations of cells. The minority group is concerned with the constriction of the pupil (**p.cn.**) and the majority with the process of accommodation. Postganglionic fibers pass out from the ganglion to the pupillary constrictor muscle of the iris (**2**).

While the shining of a bright light into the eye clearly causes pupillary constriction on what appears to be an active basis, the converse: pupillary dilatation in response to light of low intensity is less clearly an active reflex. The absence of a light stimulus to the retina does set up an active reflex response leading to pupillary dilation. The signals may be relayed by cells in either the pregeniculate body (**p.g.b.**) or the pretectal area (**prt**). In this instance the relay would appear to be into some region of the midbrain reticular formation (**R.F.**) which would in turn relay the signals to the preganglionic sympathetic neurons (**p.g.s.**) in the intermediolateral cell column of the spinal cord from the first to the fourth thoracic segment (T1-4). These sympathetic neurons would then transmit the signals rostrally *via* the sympathetic trunk to terminate on postganglionic cells of the superior cervical ganglion (**s.c.g.**). The postganglionic cells could then induce active pupillary dilation through their connections on the dilator muscle. However, pupillary dilation may simply result passively, in part at least, from the lack of stimulation to produce constriction.

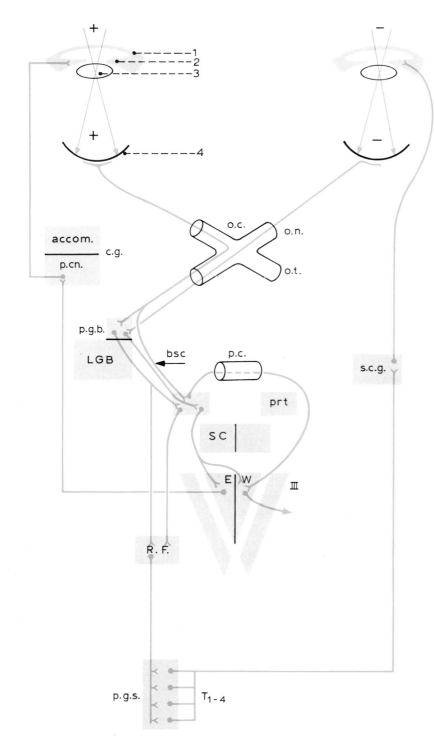

Fig. 213. Pupillary light reflexes. +, positive and — negative stimulus. **1**, cornea; **2**, iris; **3**, lens; **4**, retina.

Fig. 214. In the response of the eye to accommodation, the impulses are not generally restricted to a single region of the retina as illustrated, but are delivered to a larger area, presumably in the area of the fovea centralis under normal conditions. In this instance the stimulus which sets up the response is presumed to be the failure to focus a clear image on the retinal surface which may be interpreted by the visual cortex. Here again the signal is relayed over the optic nerve (**o.n.**) and tract (**o.t.**). Observe that fibers from the nasal retinal surface (medial) cross through the optic chiasma (**o.c.**) and that fibers from the temporal retinal (lateral) surface do not. In this reflex path, the first termination made is on cells of the lateral geniculate body (**LGB**) which relays the signal to the primary visual cortex (area **17**) of the medial occipital lobe *via* fibers which pass through the geniculocalcarine tract. Cells in the primary visual cortex (**17**) project to the secondary visual cortex (area **18**) which then relays the signal that some form of accommodation is required back to the pretectal area (**prt.**) *via* the internal sagittal stratum (**int. sag.**). This thin band of fibers is just medial to the external stratum and laterally adjacent to fibers (from the corpus callosum) forming parts of the wall of the inferior and posterior horn of the lateral ventricle. Cells of the pretectum then establish connections with the nucleus of Edinger-Westphal (**EW**) whose efferent projections of preganglionic fibers pass within the oculomotor nerve (**III**) to reach the ciliary ganglion (**c.g.**).

In this instance the synapses are made on both components of the ciliary ganglion population. Some fibers terminate on cells which innervate the ciliary body, inducing its muscle to contract. This releases the tension on the suspensory ligament of the lens, permitting it to increase in its anteroposterior axis. This alters the focal length of the lens to bring the image into focus on the retina. Other connections are made into that part of the ciliary ganglion which induces a pupillary constriction (**p.cn.**). This serves to increase the depth of focus.

A third part of the accommodation reflex is convergence of the eye in near vision so that both eyes are looking at the same visual field. At one time midbrain centers of convergence were postulated. However, there is no proof for the existence of such centers and it is believed that convergence is mediated *via* cortical connections. Of several possibilities, two are diagrammed which may both actually be in operation. One is *via* connections in the pulvinar of the thalamus from area **18**. The pulvinar in turn projects to the association centers in the temporal-parietal-occipital lobe. These in turn may be envisaged as projecting to the midbrain reticular formation (**MBRF**), superior colliculus (**SC**) and the dorsolateral reticular formation (**DLRF**). *Via* these interconnections with the **DRLF** signals may be projected to the cells innervating the medial rectus muscle (**m.r.m.**) of the oculomotor nerve (**III**) and to the abducens nucleus to inhibit the innervation of the lateral rectus muscle of the eye.

Another potential link could be *via* the striatum to the ventrolateral nucleus of the thalamus (**VLN**) and from there to areas **4** and **6** (motor and premotor cortex). These cortical areas could then act on the cranial nerve nuclei through the **DRLF**. In this latter instance connections *via* the pons to the cerebellum and red nucleus introduce the coordinative role of the cerebellum into the circuit.

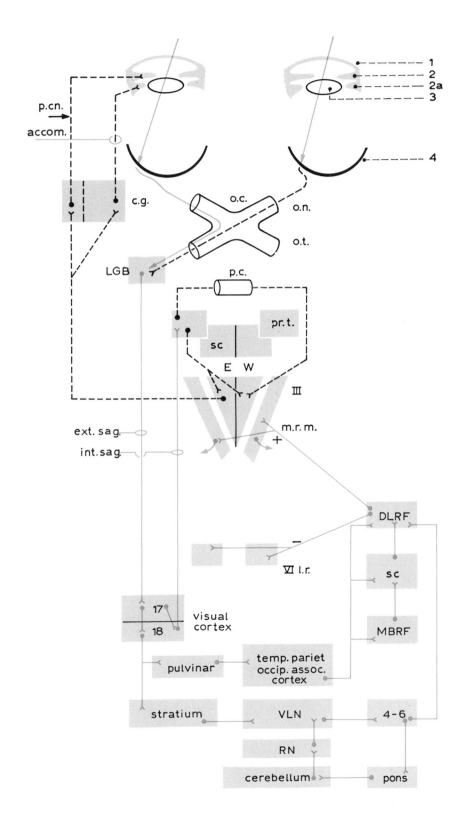

Fig. 214. Accommodation reflex pathways.
1, cornea; **2**, iris; **2a**, ciliary body; **3**, lens; **4**, retina.

15.5 The motor systems

Fig. 215. For many years it has been customary to consider the motor system of man as having two distinctly different parts, the 'pyramidal' and 'extrapyramidal' systems. This concept was based in part on clinical observations by neurologists who observed that lesions involving any part of the fiber projection system arising from the cerebral cortex (which went through the pyramids of the medulla) were associated with certain characteristic symptoms. These were paralysis or paresis of extremities, spasticity, increased deep tendon reflex responses, loss of superficial reflexes and the presence of certain abnormal reflexes such as dorsiflexion of the big toe with fanning of the other toes (Babinsky sign). Thus, the fibers passing into the lateral corticospinal tract which eventually synapse in relation to spinal motoneurons (directly or *via* internuncials) were considered the final projection of the pyramidal system. However, it was very quickly observed that lesions could occur in other parts of the brain, which also produced disturbances in motor function. Since a pyramidal system had been defined which excluded these other areas, the various structures which were associated with these disturbances were lumped together as the 'extrapyramidal system'. The subcortical nuclei which were considered to be primarily related to this system were the caudate nucleus, putamen, globus pallidus, subthalamic nucleus and the substantia nigra. However, various investigations revealed that there were also important cortical associations with these nuclei. Further, the connections of the vestibular and cerebellar system could then be considered a part of this system, since they also influenced motor function.

Two basic types of disorders are associated with disease of these 'non pyramidal' structures. First there are disturbances in which there are various types of abnormal movements (dyskinesia) and secondly there are disturbances in tone. The tremors found in the dyskinesias are rhythmical with a relatively regular frequency. When the tremor is associated with disease of the substantia nigra, it is the 'tremor at rest' seen in Parkinsonism. When the tremor is associated with cerebellar disease, it is manifest only during the period of muscle activity and therefore has been called an 'intention tremor'.

The clinical entities which became associated with this 'other' motor system are as follows:

(a) *Parkinsonism* in which there is tremor at rest, paucity of movement, rigidity, a masking of facial expression and a loss of the associated movements which occur during locomotor pregression;

(b) *athetosis* which is characterized by the presence of slow writhing wormlike movements;

(c) *chorea* in which there are brisk purposeless movements most evident in the distal parts of the extremities and face; and

(d) *ballismus* in which there are violent flinging movements involving primarily the proximal appendicular muscle groups.

To classify briefly the most frequent site of pathology with the major 'extrapyramidal' disorders:

Parkinsonism — substantia nigra

Athetosis — lesions in the striatum and cerebral cortex

Chorea — widespread lesions in cortex and striatum (in the hereditary form, it is referred to as Huntington's Chorea)

Ballismus — subthalamic nucleus

Despite the above localizations, there is a considerable degree of variability in the lesion site. Anatomically, the globus pallidus appears to possess a rather central point in these problems inasmuch as the various pathways arising from subcortical components of the 'extrapyramidal system' converge on it or utilize it as their efferent pathway to other subcortical regions.

This so-called 'extrapyramidal system', considered as a separate motor system for so many years, is not actually separate from the pyramidal system at all. It is phylogenetically older and has within itself components which are extremely primitive. Initially, in lower animal forms such as fish, the sensorimotor system was comprised of the globus pallidus and the primitive thalamic nuclei. As organisms became more complex, both the sensory and the motor systems also evolved by addition of newer nuclei to pre-existing ones culminating finally in the systems found in primates. At this point, it should be clear that we do not really have two motor systems, but a series of additions of neural components to pre-existing units. Each acquisition made for a more sophisticated and responsive motor system. Thus, in retrospect one can say that the terms 'pyramidal' and 'extrapyramidal' refer more to various symptoms which may be observed in patients when there is disease in various regions of the motor system. While these classifications can not be clearly related to discrete anatomical systems, they are convenient on a clinical basis, almost as a kind of shorthand defining certain types of clinical problems.

The anatomical connections of the various subcortical nuclei of the 'extrapyramidal' system will not be specifically diagrammed. However, if one considers that the vestibular and cerebellar systems are a part of the overall system, the diagrams relating to them can be turned to (Figs. 205, 206 and 208). Further, other figures in which cortical-striatum-thalamic-cortical associations are indicated will include some of the connections of this system.

To turn now to what is referred to as the 'pyramidal system' (Fig. **215**), it should be noted that it arises from the cerebral cortex from areas **4, 6, 8, 5,** and **7.** Only area **4** constitutes the primary motor cortex, while the other cortical areas are regions which also project *via* the striatum into the so-called 'extrapyramidal' system. Inasmuch as area **4** also has projections to the striatum, it is clear at the outset that even the cortical components of the 'pyramidal' system project to subcortical nuclei which are part of the 'extrapyramidal' system.

The primary cortical connections (heavy line) project into the cerebral white matter to pass through the genu and posterior limb of the internal capsule (**ic**). The fibers then pass through the pes pedunculi (**pp**) of the mesencephalon, the basis pontis and merge along the under surface of the medulla as the pyramids. At this point about 85% of the fibers pass through the pyramidal decussation to enter the lateral corticospinal tract (**lcspt**) of the spinal cord. These fibers descend through the lateral funiculus and terminate on cells in the ventral horn. This is probably done *via* an internucial cell relay in the intermediate grey (**IG**) in most instances. However, it is known that there may be direct synapses on the ventral horn motoneurons (**VHC**) as well.

As this descending bundle of fibers passes through the mesencephalon, pons and medulla, some fibers terminate in the dorsolateral reticular formation (**DLRF**) which serves a.o. to relay the signal to the cranial nerve nuclei. Again there may be some direct cortical connections being made on the motoneurons.

Note that just prior to the site of decussation some of the fibers (about 15%) continue to proceed along the ipsilateral side of the brain stem. These pass into the spinal cord as the fibers of the anterior corticospinal tract (**acspt**). Some of the undecussated fibers will actually enter the ipsilateral lateral tract. A few connections may be made from this fiber bundle to the DRLF and hence to cranial nerve nuclei while most fibers proceed to the intermediate grey (**IG**) and thus to the ventral horn motoneurons. Many of the fibers in this undecussated tract may eventually cross over near the region at which they terminate, passing through the anterior white commissure of the spinal cord. Note further, that the nuclear groups of cells which innervate muscles of the trunk and the upper 1/3 of the face receive fibers from both cerebral hemispheres, while the nuclear regions which serve to innervate the extremities and the lower 2/3 of the face are innervated only from the contralateral cortex.

Cortical connections are also made to the cerebellum. Thus, corticopontine (**cp**) fibers arising from the motor cortex as well as from a wider cortical distribution in the temporal–parietal–occipital cortex provide for fibers which, after passing through the pes pedunculi, terminate in the basis pontis. From here the signals are relayed through the opposite middle cerebellar peduncle (**mcp**) to reach the cerebellar cortex. The Purkinje cells of the cerebellar cortex then act through the deep nuclei of the cerebellum, the red nucleus (**RN**) and the midbrain reticular formation (**mbrf**) to relay a modified signal to the ventrolateral and ventral anterior nuclei of the thalamus. Note that this signal may reach the thalmus directly without a relay. These two components of the neothalamus complete the circuit by projections back to the motor and premotor cortex. Another rather indirect pathway also exists. This consists of a projection from the motor cortex to the ipsilateral red nucleus and reticular formation, which then relay the signal into the spinal cord *via* the rubrospinal and reticulospinal tracts, eventually activating motoneurons.

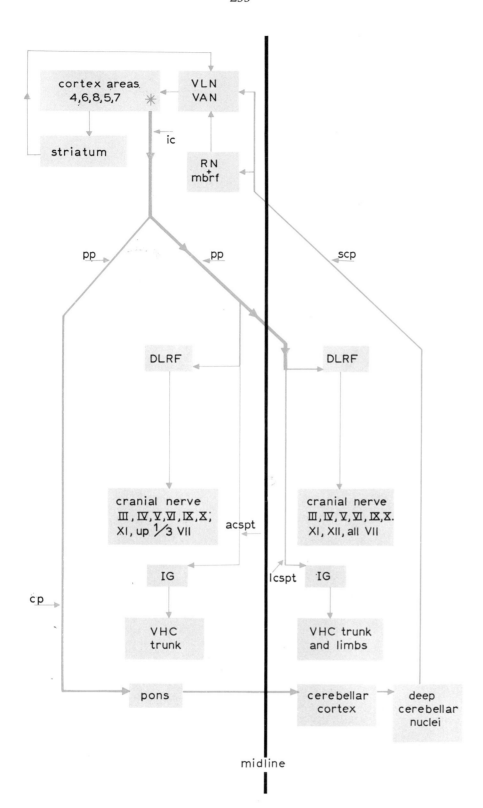

Fig. 215. Map of neomotor (pyramidal or direct) pathways.

References

1 ADRIAN, E. D. and BRONK, D. W. (1929) The discharge of impulses in motor nerve fibers. Part II. The frequency of discharge in reflex and voluntary contractions. *J. Physiol. (Lond.)*, *67*, 119–151.

2 ANDERSEN, P., ECCLES, J. C. and SEARS, T. A. (1964) The ventrobasal complex of the thalamus: types of cells, their responses and their functional organization. *J. Physiol. (Lond.)*, *174*, 370–399.

3 ARAKI, T., ITO, M. and OSCARSSON, O. (1961) Anion permeability of the synaptic and non-synaptic motoneurone membrane. *J. Physiol., (Lond.)*, *159*, 410–435.

4 ARAKI, T. and TERZUOLO, C. A. (1962) Membrane currents in spinal motoneurons associated with the action potential and synaptic activity. *J. Neurophysiol.*, *25*, 772–789.

5 BERGER, H. (1929) Über das Elektroenkephalogramm des Menschen. *Arch. Psychiat.*, *87*, 527.

6 BIRKS, R., HUXLEY, H. E. and KATZ, B. (1960) The fine structure of the neuromuscular junction of the frog. *J. Physiol.*, *150*, 134–144.

7 BLANKENSHIP, J. E. (1968) Action of tetrodotoxin on spinal motoneurons of the cat. *J. Neurophysiol.*, *31*, 186–194.

8 BLANKENSHIP, J. E. and KUNO, M. (1968) Analysis of spontaneous subthreshold activity in spinal motoneurons of the cat. *J. Neurophysiol.*, *31*, 195–209.

9 BODIAN, D. (1963) The generalized vertebrate neuron. *Science*, *137*, 323–326.

10 BRAZIER, M. A. B. (1959) The historical development of neurophysiology. *Handbook of Physiology.* Section I: Neurophysiology, Vol. I. J. Field, H. W. Magoun and V. E. Hall, Editors. Washington, American Physiological Society (pp. 1–58).

11 BRAZIER, M. A. B. (1960) *The electrical activity of the nervous system.* New York, MacMillan.

12 BRAZIER, M. A. B. (1961) *A history of the electrical activity of the brain.* London, Pitman.

13 BRAZIER, M. A. B. (1961) Editor, *Computer techniques in EEG analysis.* Electroenceph. clin. Neurophysiol., Suppl. 20. Amsterdam–New York, Elsevier.

14 BRAZIER, M. A. B. (1962) The analysis of brain waves. *Scientific American*, *206*, 142–153.

15 BROCK, L. G., COOMBS, J. S. and ECCLES, J. C. (1953) Intracellular recording from antidromically activated motoneurones. *J. Physiol. (Lond.)*, *122*, 429–461.

16 BROOKS, C. McC., ECCLES, J. C. and MALCOLM, J. (1948) Synaptic potentials of inhibited motoneurones. *J. Physiol. (Lond.)*, *11*, 417–430.

17 BULLOCK, J. H. and HORRIDGE, G. A. (1965) *Structure and Function in the Nervous System of Invertebrates.* Freeman and Co., San Francisco–London.

18 CALDWELL, P. G., HODGKIN, A. L., KEYNES, R. D. and SHAW, T. I. (1960) The effects of injecting "energy-rich" phosphate compounds on the active transport of ions in the giant axons of *Loligo*. *J. Physiol., (Lond.)*, *152*, 561–590.

19 CARLSSON, A. (1966) Pharmacological depletion of catecholamine stores. *Pharmac. Rev.*, *18*, 541–549.

20 CATON, R. (1875) The electric currents of the brain. *Brit. Med. J.*, *2*, 278.

21 CATON, R. (1887) Researches on electrical phenomena of cerebral grey matter. *Trans. 9th Int. Med. Congress*, *3*, 246.

22 COOMBS, J. S., CURTIS, D. R. and ECCLES, J. C. (1957) The interpretation of spike potentials of motoneurones. *J. Physiol. (Lond.)*, *139*, 198–231.

23 COOMBS, J. S., ECCLES, J. C. and FATT, P. (1955) The electrical properties of the motoneurone membrane. *J. Physiol. (Lond.)*, *130*, 291–325.

24 COOMBS, J. S., ECCLES, J. C. and FATT, P. (1955) Excitatory synaptic action in motoneurones. *J. Physiol. (Lond.)*, *130*, 374–395.

25 CURTIS, D. R. and ECCLES, J. C. (1959) The time courses of excitatory and inhibitory synaptic actions. *J. Physiol. (Lond.)*, *145*, 529–546.

26 CURTIS, D. R. and RYALL, R. W. (1966) The synaptic excitation of Renshaw cells. *Exp. Brain. Res.*, *2*, 81–96.

27 DALE, H. H. (1914) The action of certain esters and ethers of choline and their relation to muscarine. *J. Pharmacol. exp. Therap.*, *6*, 147–190.

28 DALE, H. H. (1935) Pharmacology and nerve endings. *Proc. roy. Soc. Med.*, *28*, 319–332.

29 DALE, H. H. (1937) Transmission of nervous effects by acetylcholine. *Harvey Lectures*, *32*, 229–245.

30 DALE, H. H. (1938) Acetylcholine as a chemical transmitter substance of the effects of nerve impulses. The William Henry Welch Lectures 1937. *J. Mt. Sinai Hosp.*, *4*, 401–429.

31 DE ROBERTIS, E. D. P. and BENNETT, H. S. (1954) Submicroscopic vesicular component in the synapse. *Fed. Proc.*, *13*, 35.

32 DE ROBERTIS, E. D. P. and BENNETT, H. S. (1955) Some features of the submicroscopic morphology of synapses in frog and earthworm. *J. biophys. biochem. Cytol.*, *1*, 47–58.

33 ECCLES, J. C. (1953) *The neurophysiological basis of mind. The principle of neurophysiology.* Oxford, Clarendon Press.

34 ECCLES, J. C. (1957) *The physiology of nerve cells.* Baltimore, The Johns Hopkins Press.

35 ECCLES, J. C. (1959) Neuron physiology-introduction. *Handbook of Physiology.* Section I: Neurophysiology, Vol. I. J. Field, H. W. Magoun and V. E. Hall, Editors, Washington, American Physiological Society (pp. 59–74).

36 ECCLES, J. C. (1961) The nature of central inhibition. *Proc. roy. Soc. B*, *153*, 445–476.

37 ECCLES, J. C. (1961) The mechanisms of synaptic transmission. *Ergebn. Physiol.*, *51*, 299–430.

38 ECCLES, J. C. (1963) Presynaptic and postsynaptic inhibitory actions in the spinal cord. Brain Mechanisms. *Progress in Brain Research*, *Vol. I.* G. Moruzzi, A. Fessard and H. H. Jasper, Editors. Amsterdam–New York, Elsevier (pp. 1–22).

39 ECCLES, J. C. (1964) *The physiology of synapses.* Berlin, Springer.

40 ECCLES, J. C. (1964) The excitatory responses of spinal neurones. Physiology of spinal neurons. *Progress in Brain Research, Vol. 12.* J. C. Eccles and J. P. Schadé, Editors. Amsterdam–New York, Elsevier (pp. 1–34).

41 ECCLES, J. C. (1964) Presynaptic inhibition in the spinal cord. Physiology of spinal neurons. *Progress in Brain Research, Vol. 12.* J. C. Eccles and J. P. Schadé, Editors. Amsterdam–New York, Elsevier (pp. 65–91).

42 ECCLES, J. C., ECCLES, R. M. and FATT, P. (1956) Pharmacological investigations on a central synapse operated by acetylcholine. *J. Physiol. (Lond.)*, *131*, 154–169.

43 ECCLES, J. C., ECCLES, R. M., IGGO, A. and LUNDBERG, A. (1961) Electrophysiological investigations on Renshaw cells. *J. Physiol. (Lond.)*, *159*, 461–478.

44 ECCLES, J. C., FATT, P. and KOKETSU, K. (1954) Cholinergic and inhibitory synapses in a pathway from motor-axon collaterals to motoneurons. *J. Physiol. (Lond.)*, *216*, 524–562.

45 ECCLES, J. C., ITO, M. and SZENTÁGOTHAI, J. (1967): *The Cerebellum as a Neuronal Machine.* Springer-Verlag. Berlin–Heidelberg-N.Y.

46 ECCLES, J. C., LLINÁS, R. and SASAKI, K. (1966a) The excitatory synaptic actions of climbing fibres on the Purkinje cells of the cerebellum. *J. Physiol. (Lond.)*, *182*, 268–296.

47 ECCLES, J. C., LLINÁS, R. and SASAKI, K. (1966b) The action of antidromic impulses on the cerebellar Purkinje cells. *J. Physiol. (Lond.)*, *182*, 316–345.

48 ECCLES, J. C., LLINÁS, R. and SASAKI, K. (1966c) The inhibitory interneurones within the cerebellar cortex. *Exp. Brain. Res.*, *1*, 1–16.

49 ECCLES, J. C., LLINÁS, R. and SASAKI, K. (1966d) Parallel fibre stimulation and responses induced thereby in the Purkinje cells of the cerebellum. *Exp. Brain Res.*, *1*, 17–39.

50 ECCLES, J. C., LLINÁS, R. and SASAKI, K. (1966e) The mossy fibre-granule cell relay of the cerebellum and its inhibitory control by Golgi cells. *Exp. Brain Res.*, *1*, 82–101.

51 ECCLES, J. C., LLINÁS, R. and SASAKI, K. (1966f) Intracellularly recorded responses of the cerebellar Purkinje cells. *Exp. Brain Res.*, *1*, 161–183.

52 ECCLES, J. C. and RALL, W. (1951) Repetitive monosynaptic activation of motoneurones. *Proc. roy. Soc. B*, *138*, 475–498.

53 ECCLES, J. C. and SCHADÉ, J. P (1964) Editors. Organization of the spinal record. *Progress in Brain Research, Vol. 11.* Amsterdam–New York, Elsevier.

54 ECCLES, J. C. and SCHADÉ, J. P. (1964) Editors. Physiology of spinal neurons. *Progress in Brain Research, Vol. 12.* Amsterdam–New York, Elsevier.

55 ECCLES, J. C., SCHMIDT, R. F. and WILLIS, W. D. (1962) Presynaptic inhibition of the spinal monosynaptic reflex pathway. *J. Physiol. (Lond.)*, *161*, 282–297.

56 ECCLES, J. C., SCHMIDT, R. F. and WILLIS, W. D. (1963) Pharmacological studies on presynaptic inhibition. *J. Physiol. (Lond.)*, *168*, 500–530.

57 FATT, P. (1950) The electromotive action of acetylcholine at the motor end-plate. *J. Physiol. (Lond.)*, *111*, 408–422.

58 FATT, P. (1954) Biophysics of junctional transmission. *Physiol. Rev.*, *34*, 674–710.

59 FATT, P. (1957) Electric potentials occurring around a neurone during its antidromic activation. *J. Neurophysiol.*, *20*, 27–60.

60 FATT, P. (1957) Sequence of events in synaptic activation of a motoneurone. *J. Neurophysiol.*, *20*, 61–80.

61 FATT, P. (1959) Skeletal neuromuscular transmission. *Handbook of Physiology.* Section I: Neurophysiology, Vol. I, J. Field, H. W. Magoun and V. E. Hall, Editors. Washington, American Physiological Society (pp. 199–213).

62 FESSARD, A. (1959) Brain potentials and rhythms-introduction. *Handbook of Physiology*. Section I: Neurophysiology, Vol. I. J. Field, H. W. Magoun and V. E. Hall, Editors. Washington, American Physiological Society (pp. 255–259).

63 FRANK, G. B. and INOUE, F. (1966) Large miniature end-plate potentials in partial denervated skeletal muscle. *Nature (Lond.)*, 212, 596–598.

64 FRANK, K. and FUORTES, M. G. F. (1957) Presynaptic and postsynaptic inhibition of monosynaptic reflexes. *Fed. Proc.*, 16, 39–40.

65 FRANK, K. (1959) Basic mechanisms of synaptic transmission in the central nervous system. *I.R.E. Trans. Med. Electronics*, ME-6, 85–88.

66 FUORTES, M. G. F., FRANK, K. and BECKER, M. C. (1957) Steps in the production of motoneurone spikes. *J. gen. Physiol.*, 40, 735–752.

67 FURSHPAN, E. J. (1959) Neuromuscular transmission in invertebrates. *Handbook of Physiology*. Section I: Neurophysiology, Vol. I. J. Field, H. W. Magoun and V. E. Hall, Editors. Washington, American Physiological Society. (pp. 239–254).

68 GRANIT, R. (1955) *Receptors and sensory perception*. New Haven, Yale University Press.

69 GRANIT, R., KERNELL, D. and SHORTESS, G. K. (1963) Quantitative aspects of repetitive firing of mammalian motoneurones, as caused by injected currents. *J. Physiol. (Lond.)*, 168, 911–931.

70 GRAY, E. G. (1959) Axo-somatic and axodendritic synapses of the cerebral cortex, an electron microscope study. *J. Anat. (Lond.)*, 93, 420–433.

71 GRAY, E. G. (1961) Ultra-structure of synapses of the cerebral cortex and of certain specialisations of neuroglial membranes. *Electron microscopy in anatomy*. I. Boyd, Editor. London, Edward Arnold (pp. 54–73).

72 GRAY, E. G. (1962) A morphological basis for presynaptic inhibition. *Nature*, 193, 82–83.

73 GRAY, E. G. (1963) Electron microscopy of presynaptic organelles of the spinal cord. *J. Anat. (Lond.)*, 97, 101–106.

74 GRAY, J. A. B. (1947) A single sensory-ending preparation. *J. Physiol. (Lond.)*, 106, 34P.

75 GRAY, J. A. B. (1959) Initiation of impulses at receptors. *Handbook of Physiology*. Section I: Neurophysiology, Vol. I. J. Field, H. W. Magoun and V. E. Hall, Editors. Washington, American Physiological Society (pp. 123–145).

76 GRAY, J. A. B. (1962) Coding in systems of primary receptor neurons. Symposia of the Society for Experimental Biology, XVI. *Biological Receptor Mechanisms*. J. W. L. Beament, Editor. Cambridge, Cambridge University Press (pp. 345–354).

77 GRAY, J. A. B. and MALCOLM, J. L. (1950) The initiation of nerve impulses by mesenteric Pacinian corpuscles. *Proc. roy. Soc.*, 137, 96–114.

78 GRAY, J. A. B. and SATO, M. (1953) Properties of the receptor potential in Pacinian corpuscles. *J. Physiol. (Lond.)*, 122, 610–636.

79 GRAY, J. A. B. and SATO, M. (1955) The movement of sodium and other ions in Pacinian corpuscles. *J. Physiol. (Lond.)*, 129, 594–607.

80 GRUNDFEST, H. (1959) Synaptic and ephatic transmission. *Handbook of Physiology*. Section I: Neurophysiology, Vol. I. J. Field, H. W. Magoun and V. E. Hall, Editors. Washington, American Physiological Society (pp. 147–197).

81 HAAPANEN, L., KOLMODIN, G. M. and SKOGLUND, G. R. (1958) Membrane and action potentials of spinal interneurones in the cat. *Acta physiol. scand.*, 43, 315–348.

82 HARRIS, J. B. and LEACH, G. D. H. (1968) The effect of temperature on end-plate depolarization of the rat diaphragm produced by suxamethonium and acetylcholine. *J. Pharm. Pharmac.*, 20, 194–198.

83 HODGKIN, A. L. (1937) Evidence for electrical transmission in nerve. Part I. *J. Physiol. (Lond.)*, 90, 183–210.

84 HODGKIN, A. L. (1937) Evidence for electrical transmission in nerve. Part II. *J. Physiol. (Lond.)*, 90, 211–232.

85 HODGKIN, A. L. (1951) The ionic basis of electrical activity in nerve and muscle. *Biol. Rev.*, 26, 339–409.

86 HODGKIN, A. L. (1958) Ionic movements and electrical activity in giant nerve fibers. *Proc. roy. Soc. B*, 148, 1–37.

87 HODGKIN, A. L. (1964) *The Conduction of the Nervous Impulse*. Liverpool, Liverpool Univ. Press.

88 HODGKIN, A. L. and HUXLEY, A. F. (1952) Currents carried by sodium and potassium ions through the membrane of the giant axon of *Loligo*. *J. Physiol. (Lond.)*, 116, 449–472.

89 HODGKIN, A. L. and HUXLEY, A. F. (1952) The components of membrane conductance in the giant axon of *Loligo*. *J. Physiol. (Lond.)*, 116, 473–496.

90 HODGKIN, A. L. and HUXLEY, A. F. (1952) The dual effect of membrane potential on sodium conductance in the giant axon of *Loligo*. *J. Physiol. (Lond.)*, 116, 497–506.

91 HODGKIN, A. L. and HUXLEY, A. F. (1952) A quantitative description of membrane current and its application to conduction and excitation in nerve. *J. Physiol. (Lond.)*, 117, 500–544.

92 HODGKIN, A. L. and KATZ, B. (1949) The effect of sodium ions on the electrical activity of the giant axon of the squid. *J. Physiol. (Lond.)*, 108, 37–77.

93 HODGKIN, A. L. and KEYNES, R. D. (1952) Methods of investigating sodium transport in *Sepia* axons (T). *J. Physiol. (Lond.)*, 117, 54P.

94 HODGKIN, A. L. and KEYNES, R. D. (1953) The mobility and diffusion coefficient of potassium in giant axons from *Sepia*. *J. Physiol. (Lond.)*, 119, 513–522.

95 HODGKIN, A. L. and KEYNES, R. D. (1955) Active transport of cations in giant axons from *Sepia* and *Loligo*. *J. Physiol. (Lond.)*, 128, 28–60.

96 HUBBARD, J. I., LLINAS, R. and QUASTAL, D. M. J. (1969) Electrophysiological analysis of synaptic transmission. Arnold, London.

97 HUNT, C. C. and KUNO, M. (1959) Properties of spinal interneurones. *J. Physiol. (Lond.)*, 147, 346–363.

98 INMAN, D. R. (1962) The electrophysiology of single mammalian mechanoreceptors. Symposia of the Society for Experimental Biology XVI. *Biological Receptor Mechanisms*. J. W. L. Beament, Editor. Cambridge, Cambridge University Press (pp. 317–344).

99 ITO, M. and YOSHIDA, M. (1964) The cerebellar-evoked monosynaptic inhibition of Deiters' neurones. *Experientia*, 20, 515–516.

100 ITO, M. and YOSHIDA, M. (1966) The origin of cerebellar-induced inhibition of Deiters' neurones. I. Monosynaptic initiation of the inhibitory postsynaptic potentials. *Exp. Brain Res.*, 2, 330–349.

101 KATSUKI, Y. (1960) Editor. *Electrical activity of single cells*. Tokyo. Igaku Shoin Ltd.

102 KATZ, B. (1950) Action potentials from a sensory nerve ending. *J. Physiol. (Lond.)*, 111, 248–260.

103 KATX, B. (1950) Depolarization of sensory terminals and the initiation of impulses in the muscle spindles. *J. Physiol. (Lond.)*, 111, 261–282.

104 KATZ, B. (1966) *Nerve, Muscle and Synapse*. New York, McGraw Hill.

105 KATZ, B. (1962) The transmission of impulses from nerve to muscle, and the subcellular unit of synaptic action. *Proc. roy. Soc. B*, 155, 455–479.

106 KATZ, B. and MILEDI, R. (1965a) Propagation of electric activity in motor nerve terminals. *Proc. roy. Soc. B*, 161, 453–483.

107 KATZ, B. and MILEDI, R. (1965b) The measurement of synaptic delay and time course of acetylcholine release at the neuromuscular junction. *Proc. roy. Soc. B*, 161, 483–495.

108 KATZ, B. and MILEDI, R. (1965c) The effect of calcium on acetylcholine release from motor nerve endings. *Proc. roy. Soc. B*, 161, 496–503.

109 KATZ, B. and MILEDI, R. (1965d) The effect of temperature on the synaptic delay at the neuromuscular junction. *J. Physiol. (Lond.)*, 181, 656–670.

110 KATZ, B. and MILEDI, R. (1965e) Release of acetylcholine from a nerve terminal by electric pulses of variable strength and duration. *Nature Lond.*, 207, 1097–1098.

111 KATZ, B. and MILEDI, R. (1967c) The release of acetylcholine from nerve endings by graded electric pulses. *Proc. roy. Soc. B*, 167, 23–28.

112 KATZ, B. and MILEDI, R. (1967d) The timing of calcium action during neuromuscular transmission. *J. Physiol. (Lond.)*, 189, 535–544.

113 KATZ, B. and MILEDI, R. (1967e) Ionic requirements of synaptic transmitter release. *Nature (Lond.,)* 215, 651.

114 KUFFLER, S. W. (1947) Physiology of neuro-muscular junctions: electrical aspects. *Fed. Proc.*, 7, 437–446.

115 KUFFLER, S. W. (1949) Transmitter mechanism at the nerve-muscle junction. *Arch. Sci. physiol.*, 3, 585–601.

116 LILEY, A. W. (1956) An investigation of spontaneous activity at the neuromuscular junction of the rat. *J. Physiol. (Lond.)*, 132, 650–666.

117 LLINÁS, R. and TERZUOLO, C. A. (1964) Mechanisms of supraspinal actions upon spinal cord activities. Reticular inhibitory mechanism on alpha-extensor motoneurons. *J. Neurophysiol.*, 27, 579–591.

118 LLINÁS, R. and TERZUOLO, C. A. (1965) Mechanisms of supraspinal actions upon spinal cord activities. Reticular inhibitory mechanisms upon flexor motoneurones. *J. Neurophysiol.*, 28, 413–422.

119 LOEWENSTEIN, W. R. (1956) Excitation and changes in adaptation by stretch of mechanoreceptors. *J. Physiol. (Lond.)*, 133, 588–602.

120 LOEWENSTEIN, W. R. (1959) The generation of electrical activity in nerve ending. *Ann. N.Y. Acad. Sci.*, 81, 367–387.

121 MACINTOSH, F. C. (1959) Formation storage and release of acetylcholine at nerve endings. *Canad. J. Biochem.*, 37, 343–356.

122 MACINTOSH, F. C. (1961) Effect of HC-3 on acetylcholine turnover. *Fed. Proc.*, 20, 562–568.

123 MACINTOSH, F. C., BIRKS, R. I. and SASTRY, P. B. (1956); Pharmacological inhibition of acetylcholine synthesis. *Nature*, 178, 1181.

124 MAEKAWA, K. and PURPURA, D. P. (1967) Properties of spontaneous and evoked synaptic activities of thalamic ventrobasal neurones. *J. Neurophysiol.*, 30, 360–381.

125 MAGOUN, H. W. (1962) *The waking brain*. Springfield, Thomas.

126 MARTIN, A. R. (1955) A further study of the statistical composition of the end-plate potential. *J. Physiol. (Lond.)*, *130*, 114–122.

127 MARTIN, A. R. (1966) Quantal nature of synaptic transmission. *Physiol. Rev.*, *46*, 51–66.

128 MARTIN, A. R. and PILAR, G. (1963) Transmission through the ciliary ganglion of the chick. *J. Physiol. (Lond.)*, *168*, 464–475.

129 PRESTON, J. B. and WHITLOCK, D. G. (1961) Intracellular potentials recorded from motoneurons following precentral gyrus stimulation in primate. *J. Neurophysiol.*, *24*, 91–100.

130 PURPURA, D. P. (1967) Comparative physiology of dendrites. In *The Neurosciences: A Study Program*. G. C. Quarton, T. Melnechuk, and F. O. Schmitt, Editors. pp. 372–393. New York, Rockefeller Univ. Press.

131 PURPURA, D. P. and SHOFER, R. J. (1963) Intracellular recording from thalamic neurons during reticulocortical activation. *J. Neurophysiol.*, *26*, 494–505.

132 RALL, W. (1967) Distinguishing theoretical synaptic potentials computed. for different soma-dendritic distributions of synaptic input. *J. Neurophysiol.*, *30*, 1138–1168.

133 RENSHAW, B. (1941) Influence of discharge of motoneurons upon excitation of neighbouring motoneurons. *J. Neurophysiol.*, *4*, 167–183.

134 ROSE, J. E. and MOUNTCASTLE, V. B. (1959) Touch and kinesthesis. *Handbook of Physiology*. Section I: Neurophysiology, Vol. I. J. Field, H. W. Magoun and V. E. Hall, Editors. Washington, American Physiological Society (pp. 387–429).

135 RUCH, T. C., PATTON, H. D., WOODBURY, J. W. and TOWE, A. L. (1962) Editors. *Neurophysiology*. Philadelphia, Saunders.

136 SCHMIDT, R. F. (1964) The pharmacology of presynaptic inhibition. Physiology of spinal neurons. *Progress in Brain Research, Vol. 12*. J. C. Eccles and J. P. Schadé, Editors. Amsterdam–New York, Elsevier (pp. 119–134).

137 SHERRINGTON, C. S. (1925) Remarks on some aspects of reflex inhibition. *Proc. roy. Soc. B*, *97*, 519–545.

138 SHERRINGTON, C. S. (1932) *Inhibition as a co-ordinative factor*. Nobel Lecture 1932. Stockholm. P. A. Norstedt.

139 STAMPFLI, R. (1959) Is the resting potential of Ranvier nodes a potassium potential. *Ann. N.Y. Acad. Sci.*, *81*, 265–284.

140 TAKEUCHI, A. and TAKEUCHI, N. (1960) On the permeability of the endplate membrane during the action of transmitter. *J. Physiol. (Lond.)*, *154*, 52–67.

141 TASAKI, I. (1953) *Nervous transmission*. Springfield, Thomas.

142 TASAKI, I. (1959) Conduction of the nerve impulse. *Handbook of Physiology*. Section I: Neurophysiology, Vol. 1. J. Field, H. W. Magoun and V. E. Hall, Editors. Washington, American Physiological Society (pp. 75–121).

143 TERZUOLO, C. A. and ARAKI, T. (1961) An analysis of intra versus extracellular potential changes associated with activity of single spinal motoneurons. *Ann. N.Y. Acad. Sci.*, *94*, 547–558.

144 TERZUOLO, C. A., LLINÁS, R. and GREEN, K. T. (1965) Mechanisms of supraspinal actions upon spinal cord activities. Distribution of synaptic inputs in cat's alpha motoneurons. *Archs. ital. Biol.*, *103*, 635–651.

145 WALTER, W. G. (1959) Intrinsic rhythms of the brain. *Handbook of Physiology*. Section I: Neurophysiology, Vol. I. J. Field, H. W. Magoun and V. E. Hall, Editors. Washington, American Physiological Society (pp. 279–298).

146 WHITTAKER, V. P. (1965) The application of subcellular fractionation techniques to the study of brain function. *Prog. Biophys. molec. Biol.*, *15*, 39–96.

147 WHITTAKER, V. P. (1966) Some properties of synaptic membranes isolated from the central nervous system. *Ann. N.Y. Acad. Sci.*, *137*, 982–998.

148 WOODBURY, J. W. (1962) The cell membrane: ionic and potential gradients and active transport. *Neurophysiology*. T. C. Ruch, H. D. Patton, J. W. Woodbury and A. L. Towe, Editors. Philadelphia, Saunders (pp. 2–30).

149 WOODBURY, J. W. and PATTON, H. D. (1962) Action potential; cable and excitable properties of the cell membrane. *Neurophysiology*. T. C. Ruch, H. D. Patton, J. W. Woodbury and A. L. Towe, Editors. Philadelphia, Saunders (pp. 32–65).

150 WOODBURY, J. W. and RUCH, T. C. (1962) Muscle. *Neurophysiology*. T. C. Ruch, H. D. Patton, J. W. Woodbury and A. L. Towe, Editors. Philadelphia, Saunders (pp. 97–127).

Annotated Bibliography

The following annotated bibliography includes some 100 titels of recent books, reviews and conference proceedings, dealing with the anatomy, physiology and chemistry of the central and peripheral nervous system, and with the role of brain in behavior. They have been chosen with a view to providing a guide line to the most advanced knowledge in the basic neurological sciences and will be especially useful to advanced students, physicians, and those engaged in research.

ADRIAN, E. D. (1932) The Mechanism of Nervous Action. University of Pennsylvania Press, Philadelphia.
An excellent small book, illustrating the ideas and results of one of the founders of modern physiology. It gives a lucid account of many basic ideas in neurophysiology before 1930.

ADRIAN, E. D., BREMER, F. and JASPER, H. H. (Editors) (1954) Brain Mechanisms and Consciousness. A symposium. Thomas, Springfield, Ill.
A select group of distinguished research workers in the brain sciences discusses the relationships of brain mechanisms and consciousness. Excellent reviews are given on the structure and function of the reticular formation and its relation to sleep mechanisms and the action of anesthetics. All those interested in the neurological basis for conscious mental processes and behavior should read this volume. A good account is given of the discussions of the various subjects by such prominent scientists as Jasper, Penfield, Adrian, Magoun, Moruzzi, and others.

AKERT, K., BALLY, C. and SCHADÉ, J. P. (Editors) (1965) Sleep Mechanisms. Progress in Brain Research, vol. 18. Elsevier, Amsterdam, London, New York.
This volume provides an overall account of the structural and functional aspects of the many mechanisms involved in sleep. A survey is given of the following fields: micro-electrical and molecular aspects, clinical studies, and therapeutic aspects.

AKERT, A. and WASER, P. G. (Editors) (1969) Mechanisms of Synaptic Transmission. Progress in Brain Resaerch, vol. 31. Elsevier, Amsterdam, London, New York.
Since processing and storage of information depends upon the structure, biochemistry and electrophysiology of contacts between nerve cells, synaptic mechanisms are among the principle areas of interest in modern brain research. Concise reviews by leading scientists on recent developments as well as laboratory reports of selected topics by a group of prominent scientists are collected in this volume.

ANDERSEN, P. and JANSEN, J. K. S. (Editors) (1969) Excitatory Synaptic Mechanisms. Universitetsforlaget, Oslo-Boston.
The mechanisms involved in transmission of impulses across excitatory synapses form a crucial part of our knowledge about the function of the nervous system. This book contains the lectures and discussions by an international group of neurobiologists. It presents a critical and comprehensive review of the present state (up to 1969) of knowledge concerning excitatory synaptic mechanisms. A presentation of original research is given in the field of ultrastructural and molecular aspects, integration at a neuronal level, the action of neuronal circuits, etc.

ARIËNS KAPPERS, C. H., HUBER, G. C. and CROSBY, E. C. (1936) The Comparative Anatomy of the Nervous System of Vertebrates, including Man. MacMillan, New York.
A monumental work from two famous schools of comparative neurology. Still a standard work in the field. The book has recently been reprinted by Haffner. Every student interested in this field should have this volume on his desk.

BAN, T. A. (1969) Psychopharmacology. Livingstone, Edinburgh.
The author comprehensively reviews current theory and progress in psychopharmacology. The first part is devoted to the general principles of psychopharmacology and pharmacological research, the second part to a systematic description of the different groups of psychotrophic drugs, and the third part to principles and practice of psychopharmacological treatment. It is a very useful introduction for all those interested in this rapidly expanding branch of pharmacology.

BARGMANN, W. and SCHARRER, B. (Editors) (1970) Aspects of Neuroendocrinology. Springer, Berlin.
The collection of articles presented in this volume provides a good source of information on the most recent data and concepts concerning neurosecretory phenomena and their role in neuroendocrine integration. Several topics are comprehensively treated: neurosecretion in invertebrates, adrenergic neurons as sources of neurohormones, the release of neurosecretory substances, and the control of adenohypophysical influences.

BASS, A. D. (Editor) (1959) Evolution of Nervous Control: from Primitive Organisms to Man. Amer. Assoc. Advancement Science, Washington.
A direction in current neuroanatomical research of the functional systems has been an orientation along phylogenetic lines. It is for this reason that the book, devoted to the evolution of nervous control is of interest attempting to understand the functional state in primate brains.

BEACH, F. A., HEBB, D. O., MORGAN, C. T. and NISSEN, H. W. (Editors) (1960) The Neurophysiology of Lashley. McGrawHill, New York.
This book represents a good selection of the papers of the great neurophysiologist. It gives in chronological order a view of a lifetime of research and study in the relationship of brain and behavior. One can read the growth and maturation of this concept in neurophysiology.

BERNHARD, C. G. and SCHADÉ, J. P. (Editors) (1967) Development Neurology. Progress in Brain Research, vol. 26. Elsevier, Amsterdam, London, New York.
This volume contains research reports about two interdisciplinary projects in developmental neurology: A Swedish group reports on the prenatal development of function and structure of the cortex of sheep, and a group from the Netherlands reports on developmental patterns in the central nervous system of birds.

BOGOCH, S. (Editor) (1969) The Future of the Brain Sciences. Plenum, New York.
Discussions are given of the methods of investigation and the application of new techniques of many aspects of research, both from a physical and chemical point of view.

BRADY, R. O. and TOWER, D. B. (1960) The Neurochemistry of Nucleotides and Amino Acids. John Wiley, New York, London.
Those having considerable knowledge of biochemistry will benefit from the presentations of detailed topics in this collection of papers which emphasizes the dynamic and metabolic aspects of amino acids and nucleotides. Contains also a survey of protein metabolism in the brain.

BRAZIER, M. A. B. (Editor) (1958, 1959, 1960) The Central Nervous System and Behavior. Vol. I, II, III. Josiah Macy Jr. Foundation, New York.

These volumes, like many of the Macy publications, are difficult to read, but contain much valuable information on the relationship of neurophysiology and behavior. The excellent editorship of Mary Brazier of the Brain Research Institute in California is noticeable everywhere. The books represent outstanding lectures on the much needed inter-disciplinary cooperation in the fields of neurophysiology and behavior. The 1st volume contains Magoun's pictorial presentation of the evolution of human brain, an intro-duction to the history of recent physiology, reversible decortication, orienting reflexes and affection. The 2nd volume contains interesting articles by Mac-Lean on the limbic system, by Grastyan on the hippocampus, and by Bureš on the relation between EEG studies and the formation of conditioned reflexes. The 3rd volume con-tains discussions on the latest results of neurophysiological investigations in the Sovjet Union.

BRAZIER, M. A. B. (1961) A History of the Electrical Activity of the Brain. MacMillan, New York.
This booklet is a wonderful history of neurophysiology and electroencephalography. Biographical sketches are given of the early workers Caton, Beck, Sechenov, Hans Berger, and others. A nice collection of illustrations ac-companies the chapters. The biographies are used as a framework for a chronological discussion of the discoveries and techniques in basic and applied neurophysiology. Everybody will find it a great pleasure to read these inter-esting stories.

BRAZIER, M. A. B. (Editor) (1961, 1964) Brain and Behavior. Vol. I, II. Amer. Inst. of Biol. Soc., Washington, D.C.
These two volumes are a continuation of the Macy Con-ferences series on the central nervous system and behavior. The 1st volume gives again much needed access to neuro-physiological research data from Eastern Europe. The lectures deal mainly with the somato-sensory, auditory and visual system. Weddell summarizes his classical views on the receptor endings subserving human cutaneous sen-sation. Szentagothai discusses very instructive problems of neural activity based on experiments with individual eye muscles. Purpura gives a lucid account on the experimental analysis of the relation between electrophysiological patterns and the histological structure of the cerebral cortex during postnatal development. Anokhin and Smirnov discuss in length the research projects of two Russian laboratories. The projects deal mainly with the non-specific arousal system (Anokhin), and comparative neurobiological aspects of the visual system (Smirnov). Also Creutzfeldt deals with the visual system. He discusses the various patterns of unit activity in the visual system. Teuber gives a concluding and summarizing chapter. The 2nd volume discusses exclusively alimentary reflexes and behavior. It contains interesting lectures and discussions on the inter-relations between central regulation, body temperature and food- and water intake, the significance of interoceptive signals in the food behavior, the influence of digestive receptors on conditional and unconditional reflexes.

BRAZIER, M. A. B. (Editor) (1964) Brain Function–Cortical Excitability and Steady Potentials; Relations of Basic Research to Space Biology. University of California Press, Berkeley.
A series of lectures by distinguished neurophysiologists, dealing with the factors and mechanisms, maintaining and controlling the excitability of the brain. Specific reference is paid to the physiological role of steady and slow potentials in the central nervous system. The book is recommended for experienced neurobiologists who are interested in slow potential changes in relation to learning, wakefulness, sleep and seizures.

BRODAL, A. (1969) Neurological Anatomy in Relation to Clinical Medicine. The Clarendon Press, Oxford.
The neuroanatomy is presented along classical lines. While many interesting details are included in this text it is not a book easily understood by neophytes in the field of neuro-anatomy. For a neuroanatomy text it is rich in illustrative material which is of considerable importance for pre-liminary studies, it will serve as an excellent guide for the application of the principles of neuroanatomy to the problems of clinical neurology.

BUREŠ, J., PETRÁŇ, M. and ZACHAR, J. (1960) Electro-physiological Methods in Biological Research. Transl. by P. HAHN. Publishing House of the Czechoslovak Academy of Sciences, Prague.
This practical laboratory book for the advanced student in neurophysiology discusses almost any of the standard electrophysiological procedures. A detailed description is given of the elementary electronic principles and the use, servicing and troubleshooting of all basic neurophysio-logical instruments. The book concludes stereotaxic at-lasses of rabbit, rat and cat. It can be recommended to teachers in neurophysiology and to advanced students alike.

BURNS, B. D. (1968) The Uncertain Nervous System. Arnold, London.
In this interesting volume analyses are given between the nervous system and computers. The author begins by discussing the physical nature of analogous machines, proceeds to the physiology of the nervous system, enters the psychology of memory and learning, and ends with an interesting discussion of some philosophical implications. A major contribution lies in the discussion of how the analogy of brains and computers can be valuable to neurophysiologists in the interpretation of their research findings.

CAJAL, R. RAMON Y. (1909–1911) Histologie du Système Nerveux de l'Homme et des Vertébrés. Tome I, II. Malorie, Paris.
The contributions made by Cajal to the histologic anatomy of the nervous system were certainly underestimated in his days. In recent years it has become apparent that many of his initial observations were much more exact than those of many workers who followed him. This is particularly true in relation with the limbic system. This two-volume series summarizing much of his work is a true classic in neuro-anatomy.

CAJAL, R. RAMON Y. (1960) Studies on Vertebrate Neuro-genesis. Transl. by LLOYD GUTH. Thomas, Springfield, Ill.
A translation of a series of papers by the renowned histolo-gist Ramon y Cajal. This volume is devoted to neuronal histogenesis. Important studies and observations of the histogenesis in the spinal cord, cerebellum, cerebral cortex, retina and peripheral nervous systems are reproduced. The development of many of the specialized cell types is discussed. Almost all observations are still valid and important for neuroanatomists, neurophysiologists and clinicians alike.

COLE, S. (1969) Membranes, Ions and Impulses. University of California Press, Berkeley.
An analytical account is presented of the advance from cell membranes to nerve impulses during the past fifty years. Dr Cole, often called the "father of biophysics" gives an intriguing biography of the work in an entire field of research, and also provides an extensive lesson in the methods of scientific reasoning.

CROSBY, E. C., HUMPHREY, T. and LAUER, E. W. (1962) Correlative Anatomy of the Nervous System. MacMillan, New York.
This text appears to be based to a certain extent on the

lectures given by Crosby in her courses on neuroanatomy during the past years. There are many excellent illustrations and interesting presentations. The contributions of Crosby and Humphrey in neuroanatomy have been extensive throughout the past years. Unfortunately these contributions have not been included in the text.

DAVIDSON, A. N. and DOBBING, J. (Editors) (1968) Applied Neurochemistry. Blackwell, Oxford.

This book covers not only many basic neurochemical techniques and research results, but also anatomical aspects, biochemistry, growth factors and mental disorders related to amines and amino acids. The reader will also find a lucid account of the biochemical basis for memory. Efforts are made to apply the results of animal work to the human subject. This makes the book even more readable.

DE ROBERTIS, E. D. P. and CARREA, R. (Editors) (1965) Biology of Neuroglia. Progress in Brain Research, vol. 15. Elsevier, Amsterdam, London, New York.

This book attempts to coordinate the increasing volume of data yielded by new cytochemical and ultrastructural techniques, physiological methods for the study of the movement of ions and water between the different compartments of the brain, micro-physiological techniques for recording potentials at the glial membranes, and biochemical studies of isolated glial cells in different physiological conditions.

DE WIED, D. and WEIJNEN, J. A. W. N. (Editors) (1970) Pituitary, Adrenal and the Brain. Progress in Brain Research, vol. 32. Elsevier, Amsterdam, London, New York.

The concepts and theories of various disciplines can be applied to identify sites and modes of action of physiological and pharmacological agents within the nervous system. This book surveys many important aspects in the field of neuroendocrinology. Special emphasis is placed on the influence of the nervous system on pituitary adrenal activity and on the action of the pituitary adrenal axis of the nervous system.

DUNCAN, C. J. (1967) Evolution and Molecular Properties of Excitable Cells. Pergamon Press, Oxford.

The author presents a hypothesis, together with supporting evidence, for the way in which the excitation of nerve cells is achieved. Details of the suggested transducer mechanism of sense organisms and postsynaptic membranes of axonal conduction and the mechanism of transmitter release are presented.

ECCLES, J. C. (1953) The Neurophysiological Basis of Mind. The Principles of Neurophysiology. Clarendon Press, Oxford.

(1957) The Physiology of Nerve Cells. Johns Hopkins Press, Baltimore.

(1964) The Physiology of Synapses. Springer, Berlin.

These three books show clearly the remarkable development of microphysiology of neurons in spinal cord and brain. The famous neurophysiologist Sir John Eccles describes the extensive research by the Canberra group on intra- and extracellular recordings of spinal neurons. This method of research has revealed all the general principles of synaptic action and has demonstrated a remarkable uniformity of essential mechanisms of synaptic action in a wide variety of synapses. The subject of these books is the research for which Eccles was awarded the Nobel Prize for medicine and physiology in 1963.

ECCLES, J. C. and SCHADÉ, J. P. (Editors) (1964) Physiology of Spinal Neurons. Progress in Brain Research, vol. 12. Elsevier, Amsterdam, London, New York.

In the past decade much of the remarkable progress in our understanding of the function of the nervous system has been the result of studies on single nerve fibres and cells,

using micro-techniques. All fundamental modes of operation of the nervous system appear to be present at the spinal level, with the result that the physiology of the spinal neurons has been the focus of considerable attention.

This volume of reviews presents a complete account of the Nobel price winner's work of the Canberra laboratories, as well as that of the leading research laboratories in various countries.

ECCLES, J. C. and SCHADÉ, JP.(. Editors) (1964) Organization of the Spinal Cord. Progress in Brain Research, vol. 11. Elsevier, Amsterdam, London, New York.

The book presents a series of lectures on the current state of knowledge in the anatomy of the spinal cord, and on the part played by neuroanatomy in the neurological sciences, providing the basis for the design of neurophysiological experiments and the interpretations of results. The influence of neurophysiological studies such as the discovery of Renshaw cells and γ-motoneurons are extensively discussed.

ECCLES, J. C., ITÔ, M. and SZENTÁGOTHAI, J. (1967) The Cerebellum as a Neuronal Machine. Springer, Berlin.

The book is a publication of extraordinary importance and should surely be read by anybody interested in the fundamental physiology of movement, even though in itself it contains very little direct clinical information in this area. It will form the background against which all experimental data on movement coordination will have to be judged. Having this material available in book form is a major contribution to our understanding of the physiology of motor coordination.

ELLIOT, K. A. C., PAGE, I. H. and QUASTEL, J. M. (Editors) (1968) Neurochemistry, Thomas, Springfield, Ill., 2nd ed.

This book of over 1000 pages presents in detail a wide range of aspects of neurochemistry, ranging from descriptions of chemical constituents of brain and nerve to comparative, developmental and pathological aspects. While a wealth of facts is presented, complexity is never allowed to obscure clarity, and thus both the elementary and advanced student will find this book very useful.

EULER, C. VON, SKOGLUND, S. and SÖDERBERG, U. (Editors) (1968) Structure and Function of Inhibition Neuronal Mechanisms. Pergamon, Oxford, 1968.

This multi-author volume contains research reports of intensive studies of the last years on the ultrastructure, physiology, pharmacology and neurochemistry of the inhibitory processes in the nervous system. An integrated picture is given of present knowledge and current views (up to 1966) of one of the fundamental problems of the nervous system.

Contained in this volume are the proceedings of an international symposium which consists of more than fifty papers.

FESSARD, A., GERARD, R. W. and KONORSKI, J. (Editors) (1961) Brain Mechanisms and Learning. A Symposium. Thomas, Springfield, Ill.

A sequel to the book on brain mechanisms and consciousness. It gives very valuable surveys on learning, memory and behavior patterns. In an interdisciplinary way such problems are discussed as the fixation of experiences, early learning periods in birds, fundamentals of conditioned connections and reflexes, neurophysiological bases of behavior and the relation of various brain areas to learning and conditioning. The volume offers a very informative blend of interdisciplinary approaches to the problem of learning.

FIELD, J., MAGOUN, H. W. and HALL, V. E. (Editors) (1960) Handbook of Physiology. Neurophysiology, Vol. I, II, III. Williams and Wilkins, Baltimore, Md.

The section Neurophysiology of this handbook provides a

comprehensive survey of the experimental findings and the concepts of neurophysiology. An attempt has been made to present everything known about neurophysiology. The several dozens of authors with different backgrounds approach this goal with a different degree of success. Many prominent neurophysiologists of many nations have contributed to this monumental work. Every advanced student in neurophysiology will find many chapters of interest.

Volume I is concerned with the historical development of neurophysiology, neuron physiology, brain potentials and rhythms, sensory mechanisms and vision.

Volume II contains many surveys on motor mechanisms and central regulatory mechanisms.

Volume III contains reviews on the neurophysiological basis of the higher functions of the nervous system, central nervous system circulation, fluids and barriers, neuronal metabolism and function, and a final chapter by R. W. GERARD on neurophysiology: an integration.

FOLCH-PI., J. (Editor) (1961) Chemical Pathology of the Nervous System. Pergamon Press, London, New York.
For advanced students interested in the biochemical aspects of neuropathology this book offers a wide but very specialized choice of material. The following topics are discussed:

the chemistry of metabolic disorders;
the chemical pathology of copper;
the chemistry of demyelination;
the chemical pathology of fluids and electrolytes;
the neurochemistry of convulsive states and allied disorders;
the biochemistry of muscle diseases.

FOX, C. A. and SNIDER, R. S. (Editors)(1967) The Cerebellum. Progress in Brain Research, vol. 25. Elsevier, Amsterdam, London, New York.
A detailed structure of the cerebellum, its fibre connections, the organization of the components within these connections and their physiological significance are intensively discussed in this book. The comparative anatomy and phylogenetic development of the cerebellum, the structure and fibre connections of the mature cerebellum, the functional localization within its anatomy, and the organization of projections to the spinal cord and to the cerebellar cortex are extensively discussed.

GARLAND, H. (Editor) (1961) Review of Scientific Aspects on Neurology. Williams and Wilkins, Baltimore, Md.
A series of post-graduate lectures covering many aspects of the neurological sciences. The contributions include: the problem of the origin of the pyramidal tract, the applied physiology of sleep and the pharmacology of the reticular activating system. Many other chapters deal with clinical observations. The book gives a good survey of recent scientific foundations and the trends of thought of present-day neurology.

GAZE, R. M. (1970) The Formation of Nerve Connections. Academic Press, London.
This book sets out to examine the mechanisms involved in the formation of nerve connections during neural development and regeneration. Neural connectivity is essential for an understanding of the working of the nervous system. A description is given of neuromuscular connections, cutaneous sensory innervation, retinotectal projections and certain intracentral connections within the visual system.

GELLHORN, E. and LOOFBORROW, G. M. (1963) Emotions and Emotional Disorders. Harper and Row, New York.
This 500-page study, a result of a great number of years' research discusses in detail the physiological mechanisms underlying emotional reactions. Related fields also are discussed in the second part of the book, e.g. sensory deprivation and experimental neurosis. The references give about 1000 publications, most after 1950. Advisable as well as an introduction as for the advanced student.

GEORGE, F. H. (1961) The Brain as a Computer. Pergamon Press, London, New York.
In this book an attempt is made to outline the principles of cybernetics and to relate them to what we know of behavior. Both the points of view of experimental physiology and of neurophysiology are taken into account. The book can very well serve as a general introduction to the theory of computers and their relation to behavior and the nervous system.

GLASER, G. H. (Editor (1963) EEG and Behavior. Basic Books, New York.
This work represents an interdisciplinary endeavor of scientists who have been using the EEG as an indicator of brain functions. The emphasis is focussed on the EEG. The book is based upon the "Conference on Electroencephalographic Correlates of Behavior" at Yale University in 1961. There are studies in the general rubrics sensory system and learning, neuropharmacological aspects, epilepsy and behavior disorders. The wide scope of articles gives a good general view of the field and some detailed information.

GRANIT, R. (1970) The Basis of Motor Control. Academic Press, London.
This book begins with a presentation of the basic physiological facts pertaining to the triad of muscles, their sense organs, and motoneurons. It gives a lucid account of the knowledge of the commands to alpha and gamma motoneurons from specific structures such as the respiratory centres, motor cortex and the brain stem. The author who received a Nobel price for this type of stimulating investigations discusses the integration of the activity of muscles, motoneurons and their control systems.

HARLOW, H. F. and WOOLSEY, C. N. (Editors) (1958) Biological and Biochemical Basis of Behavior. University of Wisconsin Press, Madison.
This volume of nearly 500 pages is a well balanced collection of articles on interdisciplinary behavior research. Some of the studies are of more general nature and are excellent as an introduction, others report experimental data of high quality. Especially important is that biochemical data are discussed.

HEBB, D. O. (1949) Organization of Behavior. Wiley and Sons, New York, London.
This is a classic introduction and presents the first integrated neurophysiological theory of behavior. It is based upon the physiology of the nervous system and although time made some revisions necessary it is a stimulating work. The concepts of "cell assemblies" and "phase sequence" are developed in this study. Attention is paid to emotions and motivational aspects of behavior. Much research has been stimulated by this book, which makes it indispensable for the neurophysiologist.

HOUSE, E. L. and PANSKY, B. (1960) A Functional Approach to Neuroanatomy. McGraw Hill, New York.
This text represents a relatively simple approach to the study of neuroanatomy, which is ideally suited for undergraduate courses and various adjuncts to the medical profession such as nursing, physical therapy and so on. The figures prepared by Pansky are almost all of original composition and are very useful in a three-dimensional manner. Some attempts have also been made to relate the anatomy to clinical problems.

ISAACSON, R. L. (Editor) (1964) Basic Readings in Neuropsychology. Harper and Row, New York.
This book represents a number of articles which can be

regarded as milestones in psycho-physiological research. Groups of papers deal with the neural basis of sensory processes, the neural correlates of behavior (Papez' original paper published in 1937), with lesions of the forebrain and the effects of amygdalectomy on emotional behavior. Moruzzi and Magoun's original paper on the physiology of the reticular formation is also represented. Furthermore original contributions on the following subjects are represented:

the role of the hypothalamus in motivated behavior;
the discovery of pleasure centers;
processes underlying the formation of "temporary connections".

The book ends with a lucid account by SPERRY on the neurology of the mind–brain problem.

JANSEN, J. and BRODAL, A. (Editors) (1954) Aspects of Cerebellar Anatomy, Johan Grundt Tanum Forlag, Oslo. While a considerable literature devoted to the cerebellum has been written since the publication of this book, the information pertaining to the cerebellum at the time of publication is most illustrative. In this respect the book should serve as a good survey and introduction to the anatomy and connections of the cerebellum up to 1954.

KONORSKI, J. (1968) Integrative Activity of the Brain. University of Chicago Press, London. The purpose of this book is to show that the principles which Sherrington proposed for the basis of function in the spinal cord are compatible with the principles worked out by Pavlov on the development of the concept of the conditioned reflex. The book presents in early sequence the whole structure of the Pavlovian animal physiology.

KRIEG, W. J. S. (1953) Functional Neuroanatomy. 2nd ed. Blakiston–McGraw, New York, N.Y. This book, which is somewhat out of date from a functional standpoint, is organized almost completely along longitudinal functional systems. The greatest asset of this book is the excellent series of three-dimensional illustrations which are very useful for gaining an impression of the relative positions of nuclear and fibre tract structures.

KRIEG, W. J. S. (1957) Brain Mechanisms in Diachrome. Brain Books, Evanston, Ill. This book contains a description of some aspects of the structural organization and the functional patterns of the nervous system. Interesting chapters are the ones on cortical analysis and synthesis, cortical control and stereotyped motor mechanisms. A set of 12 figures in color, printed on transparent plastic material, gives a good schematic three-dimensional impression of nuclei and fiber tracts of the brain. The book is illustrated by excellent phantom illustrations.

KRIEG, W. J. S. (1961) A Polychrome Atlas of the Brain Stem. Brain Books, Evanston, Ill. This atlas is based on the standard sketches of Pal–Weigert preparations, presented in earlier books by Krieg, wherein an attempt has been made to indicate the location of cells as seen in the Nissl preparation in parallel with sections in which the various tract systems are presented in different colors.

KRONEBERG, G. and SCHÜMANN, H. J. (Editors) (1970) New Aspects of Storage and Release Mechanisms of Catecholamines. Springer, Berlin. The papers contained in this volume were presented at an International Symposium attended by the leading authorities in this research field. Sessions were devoted to the origin and axonal transport of adrenergic nerve granules, the mechanism of transmitter release with special reference to the problem of exocytosis, chemical sympathectomy, and the effects of drugs and hormones on the uptake and release mechanisms of catecholamines.

LABORIT, H. (1969) Aspects Métaboliques et Pharmacologiques. Masson, Paris. This textbook covers the field of basic physiology, cerebral metabolism and neuropharmacology. A major part of the book deals with the significant relationship of chemical changes to electrical activity in the brain. The book is a significant contribution to the whole field of neurobiology since it aims to relate metabolism to function and its electrophysiological substrate.

LAJTA, A. and FORD, D. H. (Editors) (1968) Brain Barrier Systems. Progress in Brain Research, vol. 29. Elsevier, Amsterdam, London, New York. The permeability patterns of the brain are unique for this organ. The presence of the blood–brain barrier is one of the characteristics in which the nervous system is differing from the rest of the organism. Numerous structural, biochemical, electrophysiological and pathological aspects of this intriguing mechanisms are discussed.

LEIBOVIC, K. N. (Editor) (1970) Information Processing in the Nervous System. Springer, Berlin. This symposium volume presents a series of papers with the objective of correlating neuronal "machinery" with psychophysiological phenomena. The "theoretical" and "experimental" contributions are thus an attempt to reflect the biological unity, which is often dismembered conceptually into anatomy, physiology and psychology.

LOEWENSTEIN, W. R. (Editor) (1970) Principles of Receptor Physiology. Springer, Berlin. Receptor biology is a new field onto which many disciplines have begun to converge. It has become a meeting ground for the physiologist, the psychologist, the biochemist and the biophysicist. The present volume is a collection of related topics written by a group of outstanding scientists.

LIVANOV, M. N. and ROSINOV, V. S. (Editors) (1968) Mathematical Analysis of the Electrical Activity of the Brain. Oxford University Press, London. Mathematical methods, with the possibility of numerical quantification are the major advances in EEG analysis. All the papers in the book make use of various types of computer analysis, not only special purpose computers, but also general purpose digital machines. This collection of papers gives a useful insight into the methods of EEG analysis in the Soviet Union.

McILWAIN, H. (1962) Chemical Exploration of the Brain. A Study of Cerebral Excitability and Ion Movement. Elsevier, Amsterdam, London, New York. This is an up to date account of the behavior of cerebral tissue in excitation under various conditions, with emphasis on the attempt to relate function with electrical events, ionic movements and metabolic responses. In addition, much attention is given to membranes, their structure and constituents, and relations of these factors to ion movements. This little book does invaluable duty in explaining biochemistry to electrophysiologists and electrophysiology to biochemists.

McLENNAN, H. (1968) Synaptic Transmission. 2nd ed. Saunders, Philadelphia, London. This volume discusses the general principles of synaptic action. It gives an extensive and well documented account of the neurochemistry and neuropharmacology of synaptic action.

MILLER, G. A., GALANTER, E. and PRIBRAM, K. (1960) Plans and the Structure of Behavior. Holt and Company, New York. This is a theoretical study in which various aspects of behavior are discussed from the viewpoint of "test-operate-test-exit mechanisms", a concept that the writers develop in this study, and that is based upon simple feedback mechanisms. They discuss motor skills, speaking, habit formation and remembering in some detail. This is a useful book as it takes modern neurological views into account and bases the discussion of behavior upon these views. Some neurological data are discussed.

NAUTA, W. J. H. and EBBESSON, S. O. E. (Editors) (1970) Contemporary Research Methods in Neuroanatomy. Springer, Berlin.

This is a modern contemporary treatise on neuroanatomical methodology. Each chapter contains a historical sketch, a detailed description of the methods, abilities and limitations of the technique, and causes of misinterpretation.

PEELE, T. L. (1961) The Neuroanatomical Basis for Clinical Neurology. 2nd ed. McGrawHill, New York.

This is a large, well illustrated text which many students find difficult to use. This may be due to the introductory chapters which perhaps assume too much knowledge on the part of the students. However, this deficiency is greatly offset by the last two thirds of the book, particularly by those chapters pertaining to the cerebral cortex and motor systems which are very well done. Despite the difficulty which many students have in handling this text, it is frequently the book to which many students turn for references in later years. In this respect it is probably of more value than many of the less detailed textbooks on neuroanatomy.

PENFIELD, W. and ROBERTS, L. (1959) Speech and Brain-Mechanisms. Princeton University Press, New Yersey.

This book is the result of a 10-years study of the neurological mechanisms of speech. A very considerable account of the anatomy of the areas concerned with speech and a review of the pertinent literature are given. A survey is given on the recent physiological conclusions derived from electrical stimulation of the cerebral cortex. The final chapter deals with the learning of languages. The study will appeal to neurologists, physicists and anatomists.

POLYAK, S. (Editor) (1957) The Vertebrate Visual System. University of Chicago Press, Chicago.

This monumental work containing more than 10000 references deals with everything known about the neuroanatomy of the visual system. The chapter of the historical survey of the growth of man's understanding is wonderful reading. Obviously a fine reference book.

PURPURA, D. P. and SCHADÉ, J. P. (Editors) (1964) Growth and Maturation of the Brain. Progress in Brain Research, vol. 4. Elsevier, Amsterdam, London, New York.

Two factors have contributed to the renaissance of interest in the developing nervous system in the past decade: (1) The application of new operational methods in neurocytology, neurochemistry and neurophysiology to studies of the immature brain, and (2) the growing recognition of the value of ontogenesis as the analytical tool in neurobiological research.

Topics of special interest in this volume include: investigations of brain mitochondria, patterns of cell development, electronmicroscopy studies of the immature brain, and comparative ontogenesis of structure and function relations.

ROSENBLITH, W. A. (Editor) (1961) Sensory Communication. M.I.T. Press, Cambridge, Mass.

Problems of sensory communications are discussed by the life-scientists, physicists, and communication and computer engineers. The biophysics and physiology of sense organs and the transmission of information is discussed at a high level by an outstanding group of scientists. An excellent book for research workers interested in sensory physiology.

ROSS ADEY, W. and TOKIZANE, T. (Editors) (1967) Structure and Function of the Limbic System. Progress in Brain Research, vol. 27. Elsevier, Amsterdam, London, New York.

This book brings together much new work on the correlates of limbic electrical and metabolic functions with behavioural processes, including many new data on the interrelations of the limbic system with cortical and subcortical structures and processes of attention and learning.

RUCH, T. C., PATTON, H. D., WOODBURY, J. W. and TOWE, A. L. (1961) Neurophysiology, Saunders, Philadelphia, London.

This book contains the neurophysiological chapters of the well-known textbook on "Medical Physiology and Biophysics" by Ruch and Fulton. The book is an ideal course for post-graduate training of neurologists and psychiatrists. Of specific importance are the chapters on the biophysics of the cell membrane (Section I, by WOODBURY) and the biophysics of nerve and muscle (Section II, by WOODBURY, PATTON and RUCH). Anatomical data are introduced in the chapters on motor and sensory functions. It makes them particularly useful for medical students.

SCHADÉ, J. P. and SMITH, J. (Editors) (1970) Computers and Brains. Progress in Brain Research, vol. 33. Elsevier, Amsterdam, London, New York.

The brain possesses both properties of digital and analogue computers. This book is aimed to stimulate a cross fertilization between the computer sciences and the brain sciences.

SHOLL, D. A. (1956) The Organization of the Cerebral Cortex. Wiley and Sons, New York, London.

In his short life Sholl made a great number of contributions to the quantitative analysis of the cerebral cortex. His studies are based on Golgi–Cox staining of neurons. The plates of his histological sections are the best ever produced. Every student interested in the quantitative analysis of cortical neurons should read this excellent booklet.

SCHMITT, F. O. (Editor) (1962) Macromolecular Specificity and Biological Memory. M.I.T. Press, Cambridge, Mass.

This monograph contains 25 lectures in a new discipline, called "molecular neurology". It stresses the importance of a biophysical and biochemical approach to the studies of mental processes. Biological memory in general, and long term memory and learning in particular, are discussed in relation to a chemical writing of experiences in macromolecular coding. Interesting reading for all those interested in molecular bases of function and behavior of the nervous system.

TASAKI, I. (1967) Nerve Excitation: A Macromolecular Approach. Thomas, Springfield.

The process of nerve excitation is explained in accordance with the physicochemical principles. The experimental data which form the basis of this book were derived predominantly from studies on the giant axon of the squid. The axon membrane is seen as a macromolecular structure with its cation exchange properties underlying the process of excitation in which the transition occurs between two stable states. A most interesting monograph for those interested in the physicochemical concepts of nerve action.

TOWER, D. B., LUSE, S. A. and GRUNDFEST, H. (1962) Porperties of Membranes and Diseases of the Nervous System. Springer, New York.

This book contains three major essays on the neurobiology of membranes. Particularly interesting for the advanced student in neurophysiology and biochemistry. TOWER outlines the theoretical aspects of the transport of large particles through membranes. A clear distinction is made between passive transport and carrier transport across neuronal membranes.

LUSE discusses the electron microscopy of the morphogenesis of myelin. Her data give further support to the view that oligodendroglia are the principal cells involved in myelin formation.

GRUNDFEST gives a lucid account of the distribution of ions inside and outside of cells, the resting potential and the ionic diffusion altering this potential.

A number of interesting discussions makes the book even more valuable.

TRUEX, R. C. and CARPENTER, M. (1969) Strong and Elwyn's Human Neuroanatomy. Williams and Wilkins, Baltimore, Md.

The latest editions of Strong and Elwyn's classical textbook on neuroanatomy have been largely rewritten. The major revisions, however, appear to be mainly in the areas of particular interest to the new authors TRUEX and CARPENTER. This has unfortunately resulted in a lack of changes in the ideas concerning the blood-brain barrier and other less directly anatomical concepts. In the process of revision many of the excellent illustrations from METTLERS "Neuroanatomy" have been included. The style of writing is clear and the book should be easily read and comprehended by most students.

VON BONIN, G. (1950) Essay on the Cerebral Cortex. Thomas, Springfield.

This essay presents a classification of the architecture of the cerebral cortex which differs somewhat from the older descriptions of the early architectonicists who may at times have been perhaps somewhat too enthusiastic in subdividing the cortex. Von Bonin's contribution in a sense, therefore, represents a simplification which is probably more in line with the actual facts.

VON MÖLLENDORFF, W. and BARGMANN, W. (Editors) (1928–1964) Handbuch der Mikroskopischen Anatomie des Menschen. Band IV. Nervensystem. Springer, Berlin, Göttingen, Heidelberg.

Handbook of Human Microscopic Anatomy. Part IV. The Nervous System. Springer, Berlin, Göttingen, Heidelberg.

A monumental work on the anatomy of the nervous system. Each volume of this famous handbook gives a complete covering of the subject, particularly important for those interested in the historical development of concepts. Although some volumes are already out of date the thousands of reference constitute a most valuable compilation of the older literature.

1. Teil. Nervengewebe. Das peripherische Nervensystem. Das Zentralnervensystem. Bearbeitet von M. BIELSCHOWSKI, S. T. BOK, R. GREVING, A. JAKOB, G. MINGAZZINI, PH. STÖHR, JR., G. VOGT und O. VOGT (1928).

2. Teil. Plexus und Meningen. Saccus vasculosus. Bearbeitet von G. SCHALTENBRAND und E. DORN (1955).

3. Teil. Sensibele Ganglien. Von J.-H. SCHARF (1958).

4. Teil. Das Neuron. Die Nervenzelle. Die Nervenfaser. Bearbeitet von W. HILD, K. A. REISER und H.-J. LEHMANN (1959).

5. Teil. Mikroskopische Anatomie des vegetativen Nervensystems. Bearbeitet von PH. STÖHR, JR. (1957).

6. Teil. Glia. Bearbeitet von K. NIESSING.

7. Teil. Der Hypothalamus. Bearbeitet von R. DIEPEN (1962).

8. Teil. Das Kleinhirn. Bearbeitet von J. JANSEN und A. BRODAL (1958).

9. Teil. Allocortex. Bearbeitet von H. STEPHAN.

10. Teil. Subcorticale Ganglien und Fasersysteme des Grosshirns. Bearbeitet von R. HASSLER.

11. Teil. Das Rückenmark. Bearbeitet von K. FLEISCHHAUER.

12. Teil. Das Subcommissuralorgan. Bearbeitet von A. OKSCHE.

VON NEUMANN, J. (1958) The Computer and the Brain. Yale University Press, New Haven.

A small booklet by one of the greatest mathematicians of this century. He gives a clear personal account of the analogies of computer machines and the living human brain. In a final chapter he concludes that the brain operates in part digitally, in part analogically, but uses a peculiar statistical language. A worthy introduction in the difficult field of communication sciences. His thoughts have had a great impact on many young scientists.

WAELSCH, H. (Editor) (1955) Biochemistry of the Developing Nervous System. Academic Press, New York, London.

These reports from the First International Neurochemical Symposium discuss, from the developmental point of view, morphological and functional ontogeny, chemical composition and dynamic metabolism, enzymatic differentiation in relation to function, cellular chemistry and the effects of intrinsic and extrinsic factors in development. While the facts are detailed, the treatment of so many aspects of development in one book allows the reader to synthesize his own theories on a broad basis.

WIENER, N. (1961) Cybernetics or Control and Communication in the Animal and the Machine. 2nd ed. M.I.T. Press, Cambridge, Mass.

A famous introduction in the rapidly growing field of the communication sciences. Specifically interesting for students in basic neurology are the chapters on computing machines and the nervous system; cybernetics and psychopathology; on learning and self-reproducing machines, and on brain waves and self-organizing systems.

WIENER, N. and SCHADÉ, J. P. (Editors) (1965) Cybernetics of the Nervous System. Progress in Brain Research, vol. 17. Elsevier, Amsterdam, London, New York.

In this volume special attention is paid to the application of cybernetics to neurological problems such as inhibitory mechanisms, adaptation, information processing and thinking, sensory mechanisms, pattern recognition, human perception and reaction, mathematical methods of verbal learning, and probability statistical models of brain organization.

WINDLE, W. F. (Editor) (1958) Biology of Neuroglia. Thomas, Springfield, Ill.

In recent years the thoughts of neuroanatomists concerning the role of neuroglial cells in the nervous system have become directed towards roles which are other than structural. It is in this area of thinking that the interesting concept of neuroglial units as functional components in conjunction with the nerve cells has developed. Therefore this book on the biology of neuroglia, while certainly far from conclusive, provides a step forward in our evaluation of the importance of the glial cells as physiological and biological contributors to the overall function of nerve cells.

ZOTTERMAN, Y. (Editor) (1963) Olfaction and Taste. Pergamon, London, New York.

Some 30 papers by eminent authorities on sensory mechanisms related to olfaction and taste. There are stimulating chapters on the generation and transmission of signals in the olfactory system, electrophysiology of human taste nerves, chemical coding in taste, and a number of comparative studies. Students in neurophysiology and zoology will learn many things from the printed lectures and discussion.

Index

The index has been compiled on the basis of the illustrations; the first number refers to the relevant illustration and is followed by the appropriate page number in parentheses.